AF647493

Anatomy of the Head and Neck

For Dental and Medical Students

Anatomy of the Head and Neck
For Dental and Medical Students

A. HALIM

M.B.B.S., M.S. (Anat.), F.I.M.S.A.
Formerly Professor and Head, Department of Anatomy,
King George's Medical College,
Lucknow (India)
W.H.O. Fellow in Medical Education (U.K.)
Fellow International Medical Sciences Academy,
Ex-Member Academic Council King George's Medical University
and King George's Dental University

Ane Books Pvt. Ltd.

New Delhi ♦ Chennai ♦ Mumbai
Bangalore ♦ Kolkata ♦ Thiruvananthapuram ♦ Lucknow

Anatomy of Head and Neck—For Dental and Medical Students

A. Halim

© Author

Second edition 2009

First edition 1989
First reprint 1992

Published by

Ane Books Pvt. Ltd.
4821, Parwana Bhawan, 1st Floor, 24 Ansari Road,
Darya Ganj, **New Delhi** - 110 002, India
Tel.: +91(011) 23276843-44, Fax: +91(011) 23276863
e-mail: kapoor@anebooks.com, Website: www.anebooks.com

Branches

- Avantika Niwas, 1st Floor, 19 Doraiswamy Road, T. Nagar,
Chennai - 600 017, Tel.: +91(044) 28141554, 28141209
e-mail: anebooks_tn@airtelmail.in
- G-012, Ground Floor, Jui Nagar Railway Station Building, Jui Nagar (East),
Navi Mumbai - 400 706, Tel.: +91(022) 27720842, 27720851
e-mail: anebooksmum@mtnl.net.in
- 38/1, 1st Floor, Model House, First Street, Opp. Shamanna Park,
Basavannagudi, **Bangalore** - 560 004, Tel.: +91(080) 41681432
e-mail: anebang@airtelmail.in
- Flat No. 16A, 220 Vivekananda Road, Maniktalla,
Kolkata - 700 006, Tel.: +91(033) 23547119
e-mail: anekol@vsnl.net
- # 6, TC 25/2710, Kohinoor Flats, Lukes Lane, Ambujavilasam Road,
Thiruvananthapuram - 01, Kerala, Tel.: +91(0471) 4068777, 4068333
e-mail: anebookstvm@airtelmail.in

Representative Office

- C-26, Sector-A, Mahanagar, **Lucknow** - 226 006
Mobile - +91 93352 29971

Disclaimer: Please be informed that the author and the publisher have put in their best efforts in producing this book. Every care has been taken to ensure the accuracy of the contents. However, we make no warranties for the same and therefore shall not be responsible or liable for any loss or any commercial damages accruing thereof. Neither the publisher nor the author is engaged in providing services of any professional nature and shall therefore not be responsible for any incidental, consequential, special or any other damages. Please do consult a professional where appropriate.

SBN (10) : 81-8052-268-7
ISBN (13) : 978-81-8052-268-0

All rights reserved. No part of this book may be reproduced in any form including photocopying, microfilms, photoprints, storage in any retrieval system, transmission in any permanent or temporary form, without the prior written consent of the publisher.

Printed at : Tuli Offset Printers Pvt. Ltd., New Delhi.

To
my daughter-in-law
Eram
a promising dental surgeon

Foreword

It is a matter of great pleasure for me to write the foreword for Prof. A. Halim's excellent book entitled "Anatomy of Head and Neck"—For Dental and Medical Students. Prof. Halim, a distinguished senior teacher of Anatomy has very successfully produced an attractive and easy to comprehend aid for learning anatomy of head and neck. The line drawings are accurate and appealing almost providing temptation for a quick revision of the region. The sketches depict the structures layer after layer as the student had seen them during his gross-anatomy practicals. In order that the student may be able to turn the pages and study figure after figure without requiring to reorient himself, all the illustrations have been made from the right side in a sequence from deeper to superficial strata. This provides means for reconstruction of the anatomical details and facilitates the task of learning gross anatomy of the complicated region of head and neck by the students. The diagrams are accurate and illustrate exhaustively the details. Spacing of diagrams and related text on double spread sheets further facilitates the reading.

I have no doubt that the book will be received very well by the students of gross-anatomy in the first year of medical college, by the residents in the surgical specialities and by the teachers who wish to recapitulate in a hurry before going over for a teaching assignment.

V. Bijalani M.S., PhD
Formely Head of the Department of Anatomy
All India Institute of Medical Sciences
New Delhi

Preface to the Second Edition

The success of the first edition has been most gratifying as it was well received by the dental as well as medical students. It has been said "Longer you look back the further you can look forward". It is the methodology and presentation of teaching of anatomy which is of great importance. Keeping this fact in view the format of this edition departs from the first one. The diagrams have been put within the text, instead of on double spread sheets, to facilitate reading. The positive aspect of a compact text with important structural details has been retained. Emphasis has been put on some "key structures" of a part which will be helpful in clear understanding of that region and create a reinforcement of learning. The diagrams restrict themselves to the identification of structures while the text restricts it self to important features or the region thereby completing what is essential knowledge. To make the diagrams realistic colour has been used lavishly. Colour captures a reality that is more consistent with the mode of learning and has become an increasingly important element for most of the students today.

The author hopes that students will find this second edition useful and a comprehensive study guide to the anatomy of head and neck.

A. Halim

Preface to the First Edition

For more than thirty-six years the author has been privileged to teach gross anatomy to freshmean medical students at King George's Medical College, Lucknow, and to give postdoctoral course in anatomy of the Head and Neck and other disciplines. These students have chosen specialities involving an intimate knowledge of structure within the head and neck. Not a few of them have suggested that my lecture diagrams be presented in an atlas form. Seldom does a teacher experience more gratification then when students express kind words regarding his teaching.

The preparation of this atlas on Head and Neck was also inspired by the atlases of Latc Prof. M. A. H. Siddiqi on Superior and Inferior extremities, Thorax, Abdomen and Pelvis. He did not do a volume on Head and Neck as he shifted to Surgery after his tenure as Professor and Head of Anatomy at King George's Medical College, Lucknow from 1932 to 1941. This volume has been more challenging than I expected as I wanted it to match his style but the format had to be a little different as it was desirable that the labelling and comments be more elaborate for greater usefulness for the present needs.

The subject of anatomy by its very nature is a visual one and the best means of visual recall are simple diagrams. Dissection proceeds from superficial structures but it is more educative if a reconstructive approach builds up a region from the deepest background towards the superficial aspect. A series of diagrams have been used to build a particular region. All the illustrations are from the right side for correct orientation. Diagrams and related text have been presented on the same doublespread page which facilitates reading and removes the need for cross references. The purpose of comments on the illustrations is to interpret them and hence they are not exhaustive but are sufficient to stress points and to convey what cannot be illustrated.

The atlas presents to the student of medicine and dentistry an account of anatomical facts necessary to appreciate structural organisation of the Head and Neck. I hope it will also be useful in forming an anatomical baseline upon which an Otologist, Oral surgeon, Ophthalmologist, Larynogologist or whatever, may add knowledge peculiar to the successful practice of his speciality.

A. Halim

Acknowledgements

The degree of my success in realising my intentions can be gauged only by the criticism that I invite from my students and colleagues who select this book as an aid to learning and teaching Head and Neck. During the preparation of this book I have already received both encouragement and criticism from clinical and anatomical colleagues and from medical students, for which I am most grateful.

Originally, all illustrations were drawn by me. They were redrawn in an accurate and palatable fashion by Late Mr. G.C. Das under my supervision. Mr. G.C. Das was a medical artist, in the Department of Anatomy, King Georges Medical College, Lucknow. I count myself most fortunate in having his expert assistance throughout and for his careful devotion to accuracy. His care in checking the labelling many times eliminated many errors. I cannot thank him sufficiently for his care and patience with the drawings. Any shortcomings are of course the sole responsibility of mine.

I must thank Dr. Vina Bijlani, Formerly Professor and Head, Department of Anatomy, All India Institute of Medical Sciences Delhi, for the honour she has done me in writing a Foreword for this book.

Finally this book has been made possible by the interest and support of my family. To my wife, Mahmuda, I owe a continuing debt of gratitude for her selflessness and for the true understanding of the academic way of life.

In the publication of this second edition I am grateful to Mr. Sunil Saxena, Managing Director, Ane Books Pvt. Ltd., for encouraging me to provide a revised edition. He got a very good job done in getting excellent colour diagrams out of the black and white ones of the first edition. My sincere thanks are due to all those members of staff of Ane Books Pvt. Ltd., who are involved in the production of this edition.

A. Halim

Contents

The Scalp

Chapter 1

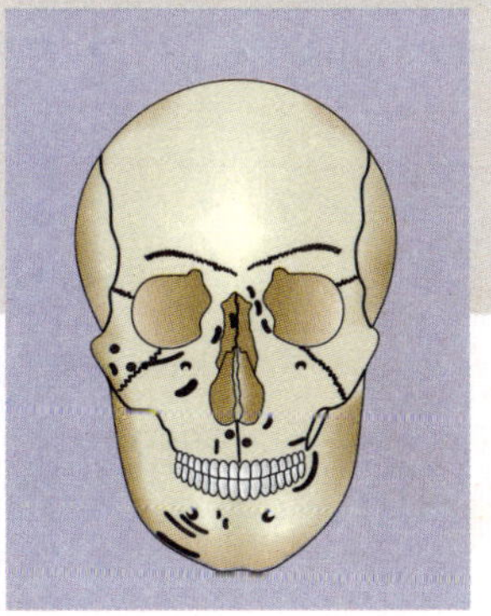

1.1 The skull viewed from above (Norma verticalis)

Note the four bones, frontal (F), two parietals (P) and occipital (O). Identify the sutures and their meeting points v.z., bregma and lambda.

The scalp covers the skull from one superior temporal line to the other at the sides and from the eyebrows to the superior nuchal lines at the back.

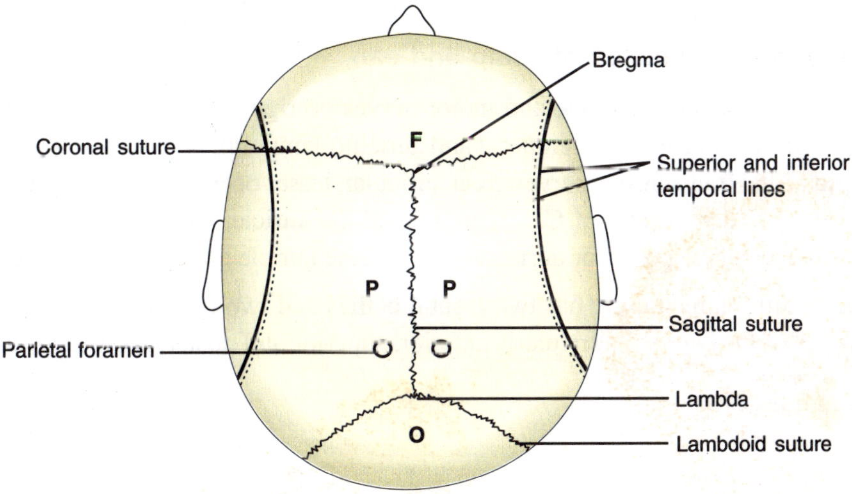

Fig. 1.1 Bones of skull as viewed from above (Norma verticalis)

1.2 Layers in the scalp

Each letter of scalp serves as a 'Memory Key' for the five layers—S (skin), C (connective tissue), A (aponeurosis), L (loose areolar tissue) and P (pericranium).

It is through the fourth layer of loose areolar tissue (L) that shearing accidents can separate the overlying layers of scalp from the subjacent pericranium (P) and bone as the first three layers are attached to each other. The fourth layer has been termed as "Dangerous area" because infection can spread in it and from there into the intracranial structures by way of emissary veins.

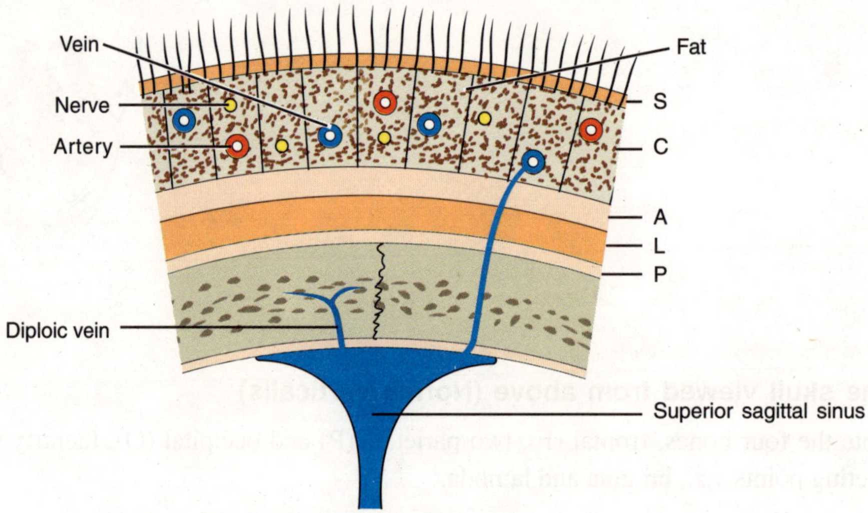

Fig. 1.2 Layers in the scalp

1.3 The nerves and muscles of scalp and ear

Note sensory nerves on left side and motor nerves on right side. Four sensory nerves supra-trochlear, supra-orbital, zygomatico-temporal and auriculo-temporal, branches of trigeminal (V), are in front of auricle; and four sensory nerves great auricular, lesser occipital, greater occipital and third occipital, branches of dorsal rami of C2, 3, are behind the auricle. One motor nerve (temporal) in front and one motor nerve (posterior auricular) behind the auricle are branches of facial nerve.

The occipito-frontalis muscle has two frontal bellies and two occipital bellies. Note the three extrinsic muscles of the ear viz., auricularis anterior, superior and posterior on each side.

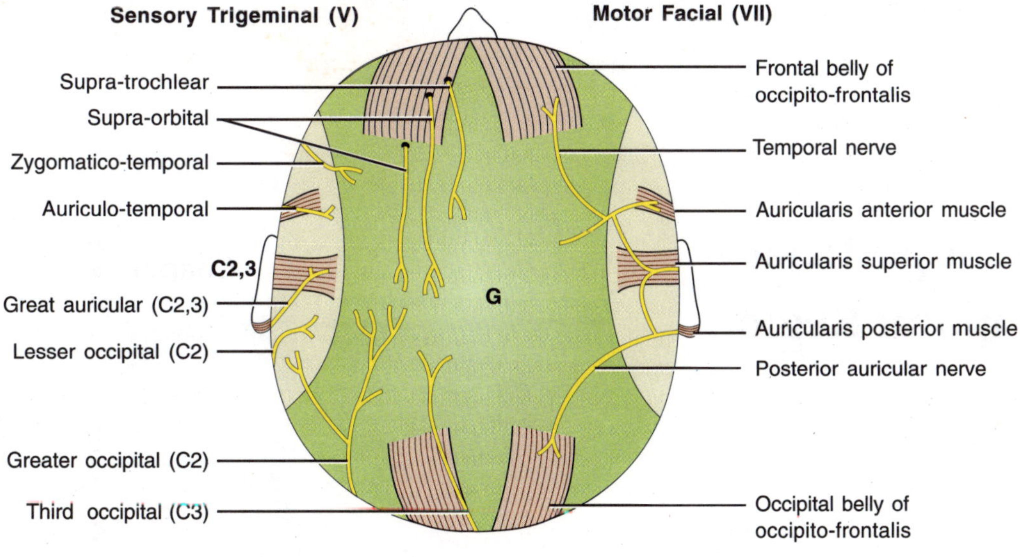

Fig. 1.3 Sensory and motor nerves of scalp. G-Galea aponeurotica

1.4 The Blood Vessels of the scalp

The arteries are shown on right side and veins on left side. The veins anastomose freely and form a network in the second layer.

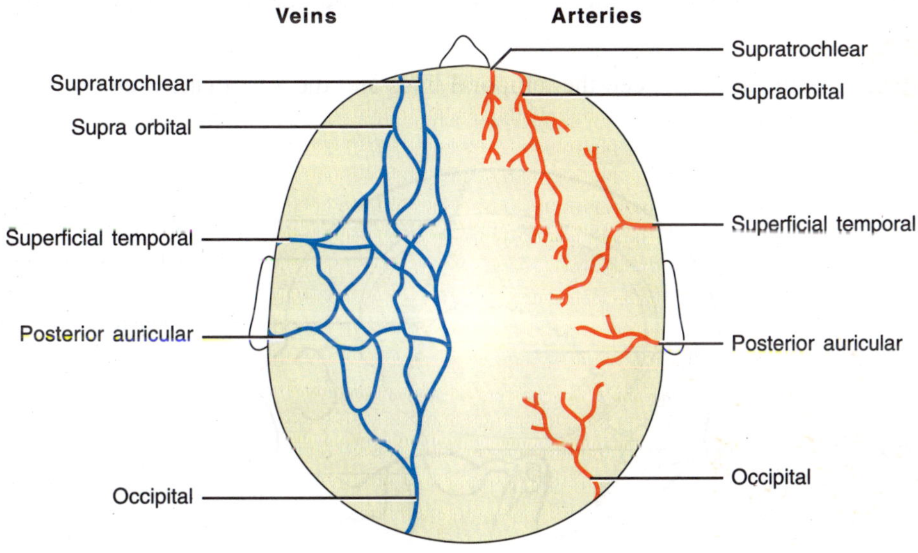

Fig. 1.4 Blood vessels of scalp

The Superficial Temporal Region

Chapter 2

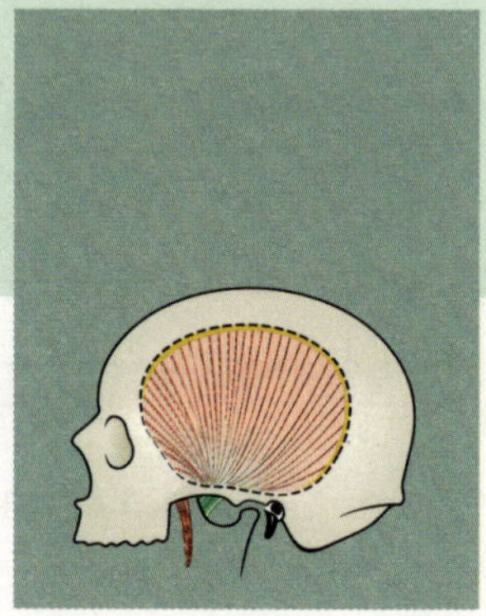

2.1 The skull viewed from the lateral side (Norma lateralis)

Four bones, parietal (P), frontal (F), temporal (T), and sphenoid (S), form the temporal fossa and meet at Pterion. Superior and inferior temporal lines are duplications of temporal line on the parietal bone.

The temple is the area between the temporal lines and the zygomatic arch.

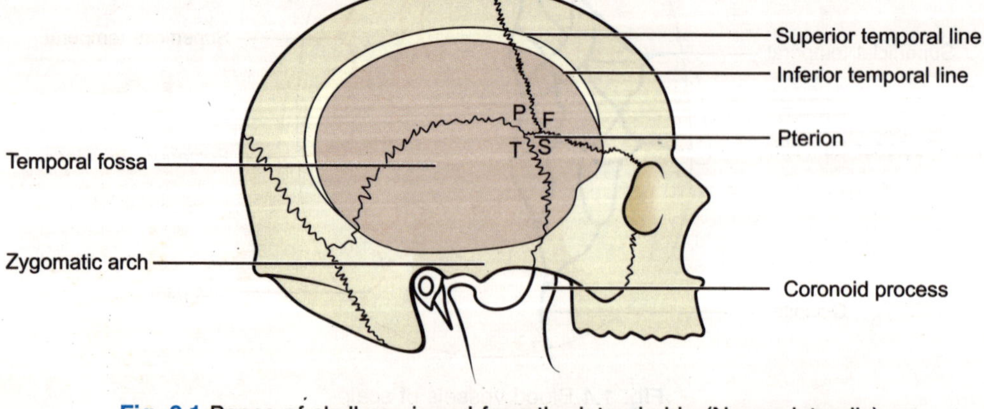

Fig. 2.1 Bones of skull as viewed from the lateral side (Norma lateralis)

2.2 The six layers of the temporal region and their relationship with the five layers in scalp

The first and second layers are the same as in the scalp, the third layer is a thin extension of epicranial aponeurosis from which the extrinsic auricular muscles arise. The fourth layer is the temporal fascia, the fifth is the temporalis muscle. The sixth or the last layer is the same as in scalp, i.e., the pericranium.

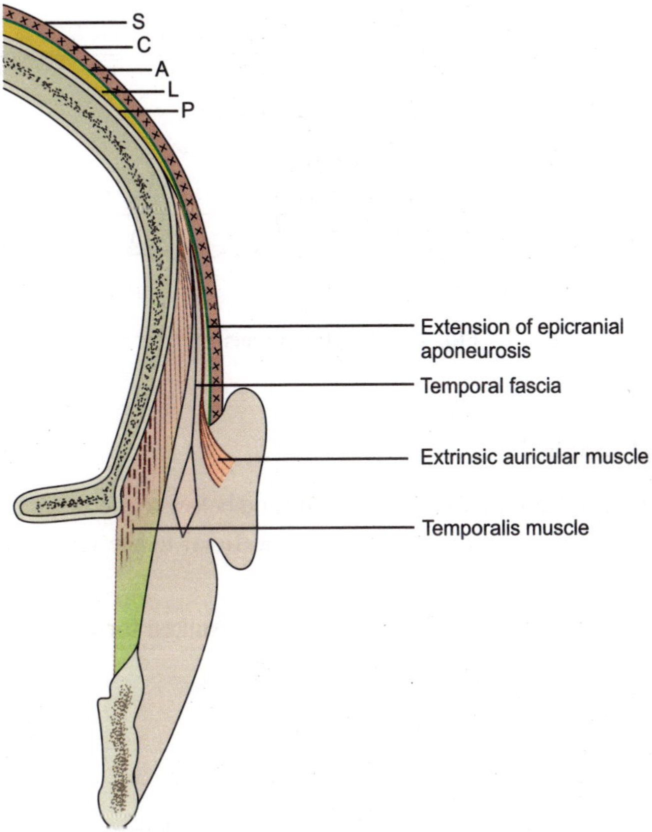

Fig. 2.2 Layers in the superficial temporal region

2.3 The temporalis muscle

It arises from the whole of temporal fossa extending upto inferior temporal line and is inserted into the coronoid process of mandible.

Nerve supply : Deep temporal nerves from the anterior division of mandibular nerve

Action : Anterior vertical fibers elevate the mandible to close the jaw, posterior horizontal fibers retract the mandible after protraction.

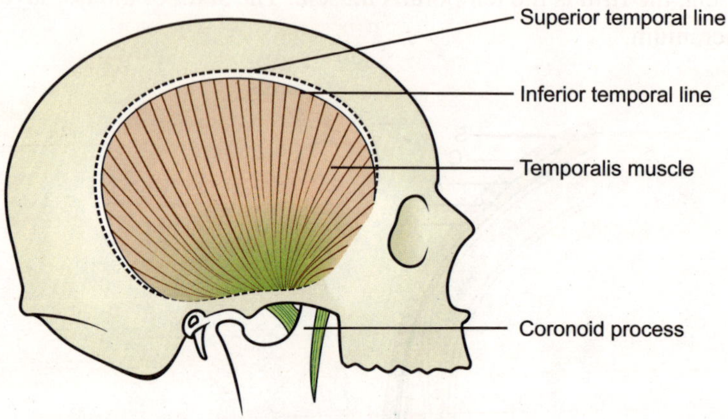

Fig. 2.3 The temporalis muscle

2.4 The temporal fascia

It is attached above to the superior temporal line and below to the zygomatic arch. The superficial temporal vessels and auriculo-temporal nerve lie superficial to the temporal fascia but the middle temporal artery pierces it.

It is exceedingly dense and so its wounds may be mistaken for wounds of the skull, because of the firmness of the wound edges to the examining finger.

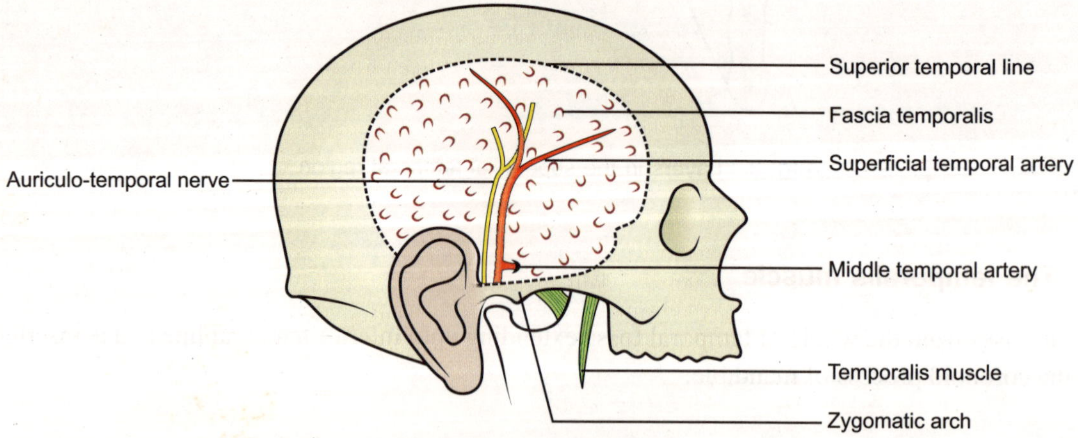

Fig. 2.4 The temporal fascia

The Face

Chapter 3

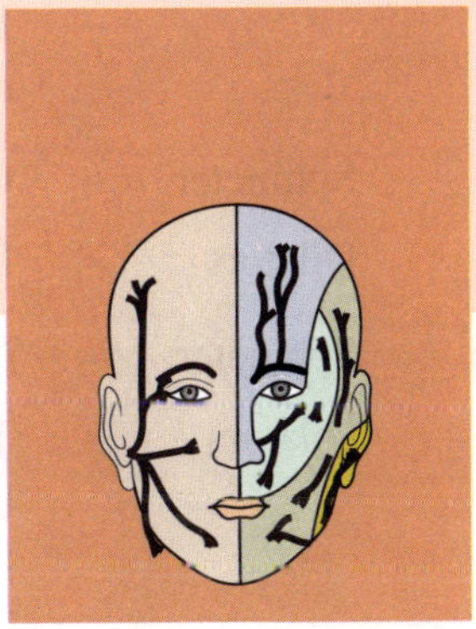

3.1 The front view of the skull (Norma frontalis)

The front view of the skull comprises the anterior part of the brain case above, and the skeleton of the face below. Study the attachments of various muscles of face.

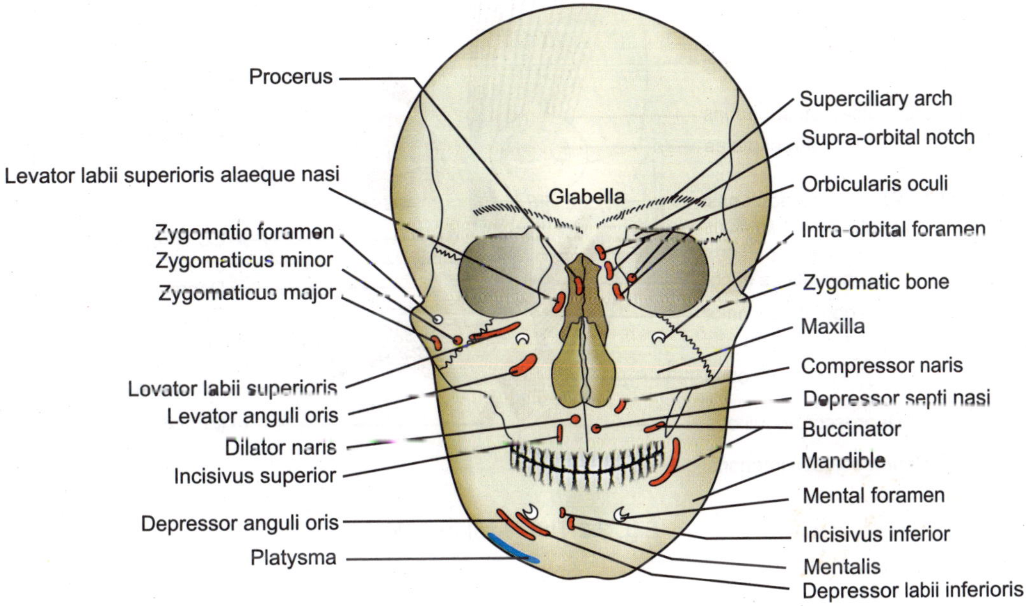

Fig. 3.1 The front view of the skull (Norma frontalis)

3.2 The facial muscles

The facial muscles are collectively known as the muscles of facial expression. There are three orifices on the face viz., orbit, nose, and mouth guarded by eyelids, nostrils, and lips. Facial muscles are arranged as sphincters and dilators.

Orbit	Sphincter	–	Orbicularis oculi
	Dilators	–	Frontal belly of occipito-frontalis
		–	Levator palpebrae superioris (which is not a muscle of facial expression)
Nose	Sphincter	–	Compressor naris
	Dilators	–	Dilator naris
Mouth	Sphincter	–	Orbicularis oris (bulk of which comes from Buccinator)
	Dilators	–	The remainder of the facial muscles which radiate outward from the lips like the spokes of a wheel viz., Levator labii superioris alaque nasi, Levator labii superioris, Levator anguli oris, Zygomaticus minor, Zygomaticus major. Risorius, Depressor anguli oris and Depressor labii inferioris.

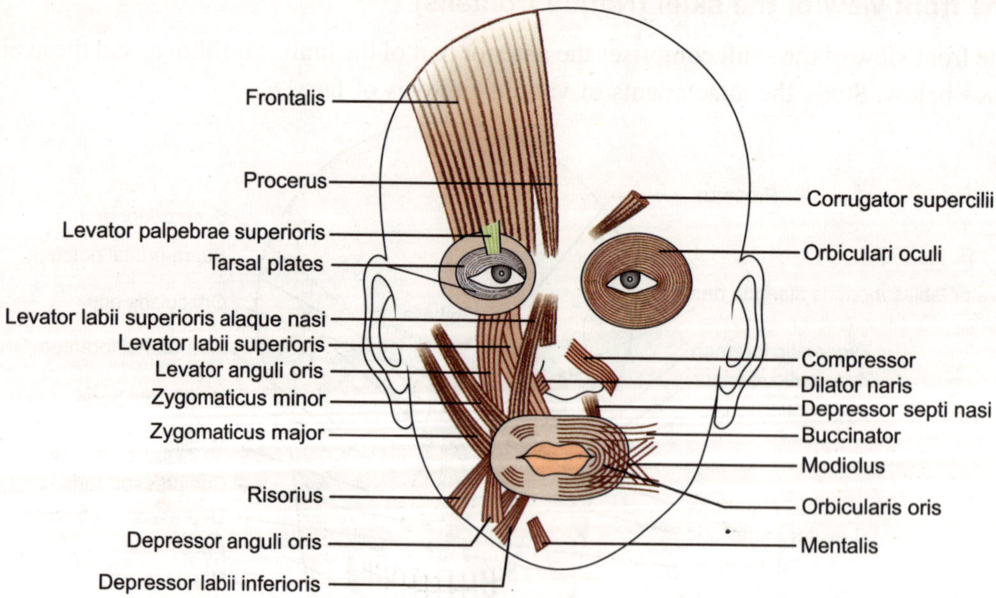

Fig. 3.2 The facial muscles

Note the muscle knot known as modiolus lying lateral to the angle of mouth. Intersecting fibres cannot slip here as they are bound together by fibrous tissue.

Wounds of face tend to gape, and require numerous stitches for the fibres attached to the skin draw the margins of the wound apart.

3.3 Origin of facial muscles from the bones in Norma lateralis

The skin is the chief insertion of facial muscles.

Make a careful study of the orbicularis oris and orbicularis oculi. The orbicularis oculi has three parts–an orbital part on and around the margins of the orbital opening, a palpebral part in the eyelids and a lacrimal part related to the lacrimal sac.

The orbicularis oris is not a simple muscle. It has intrinsic fibres of its own besides the fibres of all other muscles which converge upon the mouth.

The muscles of the nose are small and unimportant.

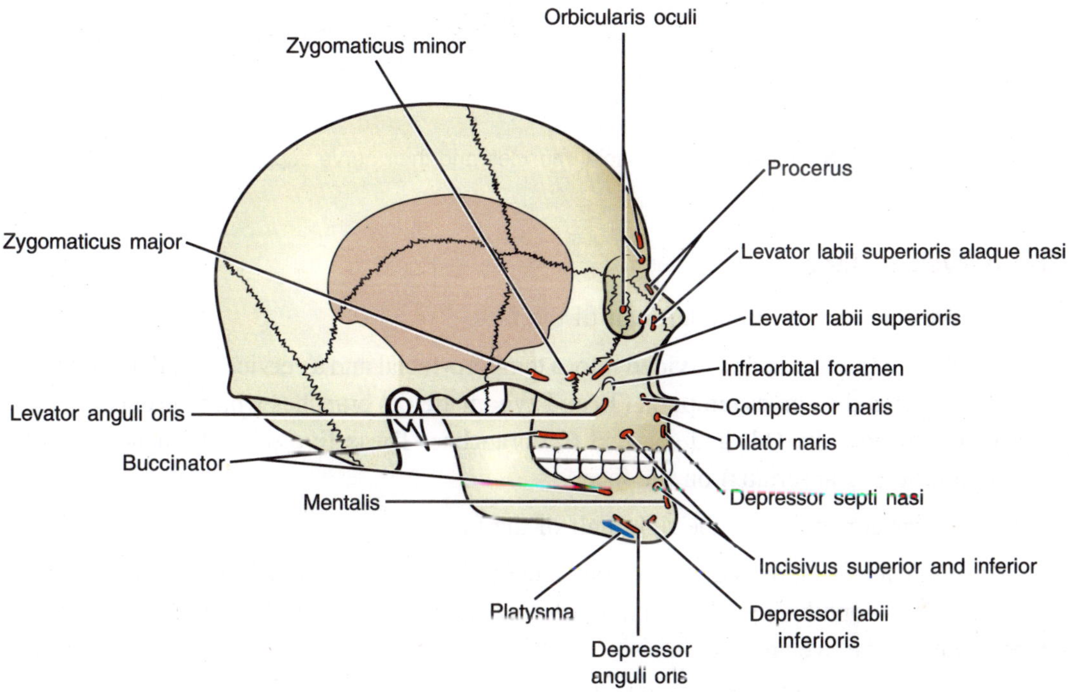

Fig. 3.3 Origin of facial muscles from the bones in Norma lateralis

3.4 Lateral view of facial muscles and their nerve supply

Note the distribution of the five branches of facial nerve, i.e., temporal (T), zygomatic (Z), buccal (B), mandibular (M) and cervical (C).

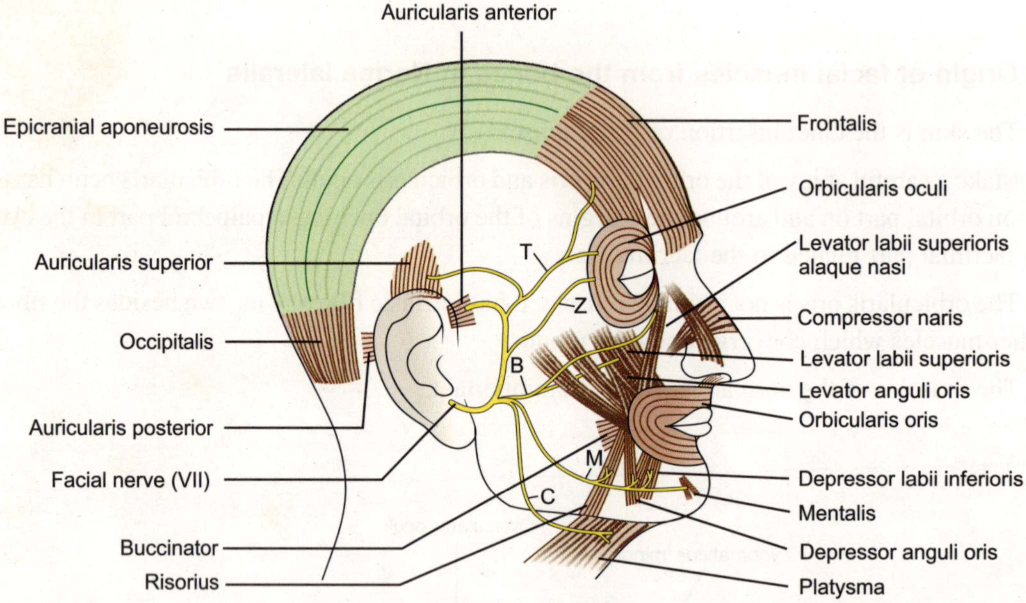

Fig. 3.4 Lateral view of facial muscles and their nerve supply

3.5 The nerves of face

Motor nerves are shown on the left half of the face.

The facial nerve (motor) is first divided into a temporo-facial and a cervice-facial division. The temporo-facial division then gives temporal (T) and zygomatic (Z) branches while the cervico-facial gives buccal (B), mandibular (M) and cervical (C) branches. These five set of branches form the goose's foot pattern (pes anserinus) on the face.

Sensory nerves are shown on the right half of the face.

The trigeminal nerve supplies the three cranial dermatomes of face by various sensory branches of its three divisions—ophthalmic (V1), maxillary (V2) and mandibular (V3). These dermatomes meet at the angles of the eye and mouth.

Supratrochlear, supraorbital, lateral palpebral, infratrochlear and external nasal are branches of ophthalmic division; zygomatico-temporal, zygomatico facial, and infra orbital are branches of maxillary division and auriculo-temporal, buccal and mental are branches of mandibular division.

The skin over the angle of mandible is supplied by great auricular nerve (C2, 3 ventral rami).

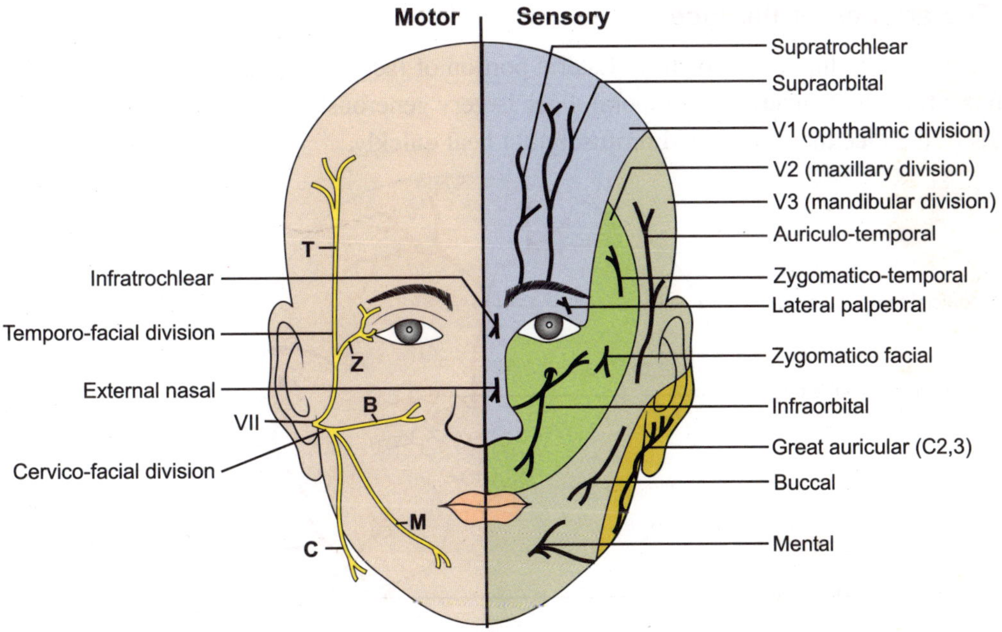

Fig. 3.5 The nerves of face (C, Cervial; B, Buccal; M, Mandibular; T, Temporal)

3.6 The cutaneous nerves of head

Note the three strips on the face supplied by the trigeminal nerve. The dermatome of mandibular division extends to the temple while great auricular nerve (C2, 3) encroaches over the angle of mandible and parotid region. The expanded part of neck behind parotid gland and much of ear and scalp behind this is supplied by branches of C2.

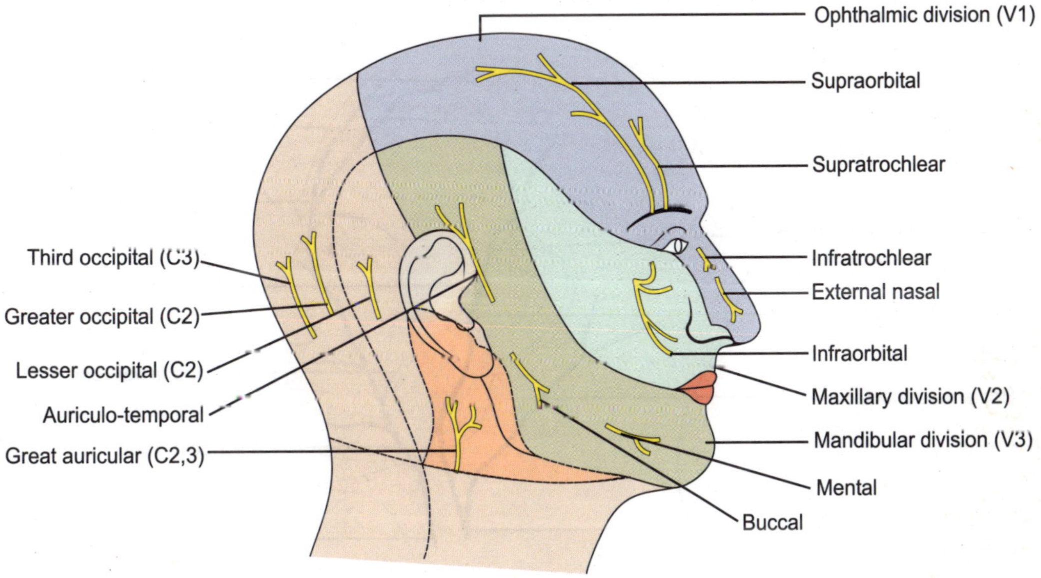

Fig. 3.6 The cutaneous nerves of head

3.7 The arteries of the face

Facial is the chief artery of face. Lateral portion of face is supplied by transverse facial artery which is a branch of superficial temporal. Face is very generously supplied with blood vessels, and wounds of the face therefore bleed profusely but heal quickly.

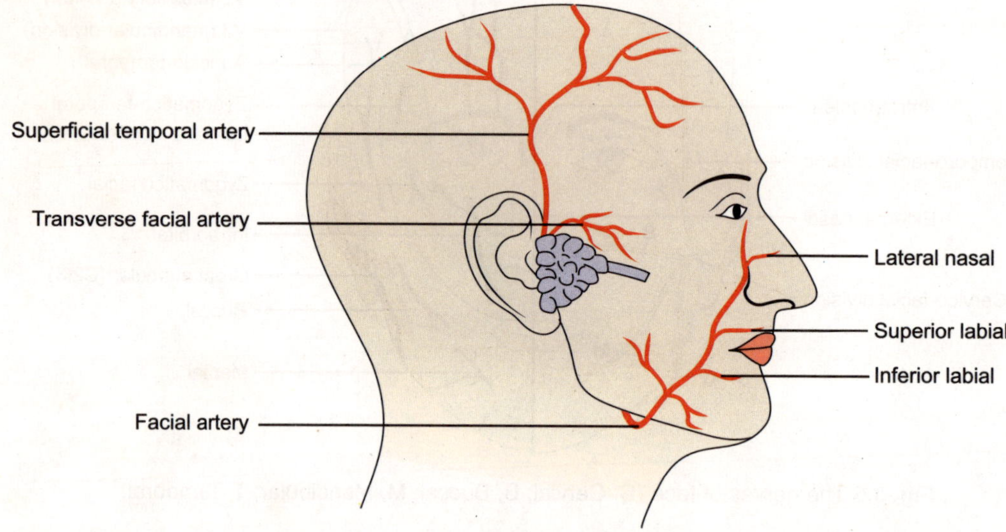

Fig 3.7 The arteries of the face

3.8 The veins of the face

Facial vein runs posteroinferiorly and has a straighter course as compared to the facial artery. It joins the anterior branch of retromandibular vein to form common facial vein. Deep facial vein connects it with pterygoid venous plexus and so the cavernous sinus.

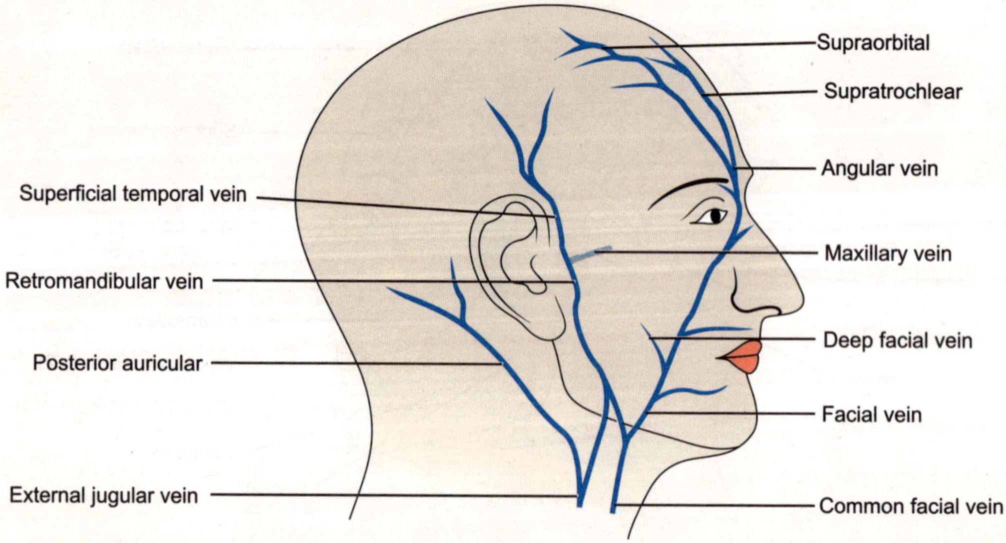

Fig. 3.8 The veins of the face

3.9 The facial expressions

Facial expressions are the side effects of functions of facial muscles.

The man seems a trifle angry. Though we have no clue what triggered his reaction (he is in fact an actor), the emotion is written all over his face. Most of us will have no trouble reading it, no matter where we come from. The classic study of psychologist Paul Ekman of the University of California, San Francisco, gives powerful support to the notion that the facial expressions of basic emotion are universal, an idea first put forth by Charles Darwin. According to Ekman, six emotions expressing anger, happiness, sadness are themselves universally evolved to prepare us to deal quickly with circumstances we believe will affect our welfare.

The diagrams in Figure 3.9 depict the skin movement produced by the muscles of facial expression to express some of the emotions.

Anger

Dilatation of anterior nasal aperture and depression of nasal septum downwards.

By—Dilator naris and depressor septi nasi.

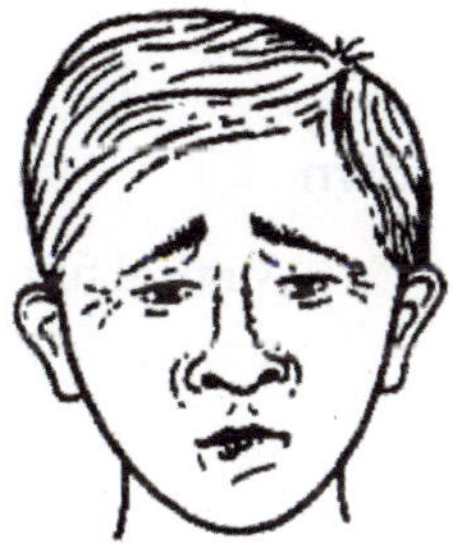

Anger

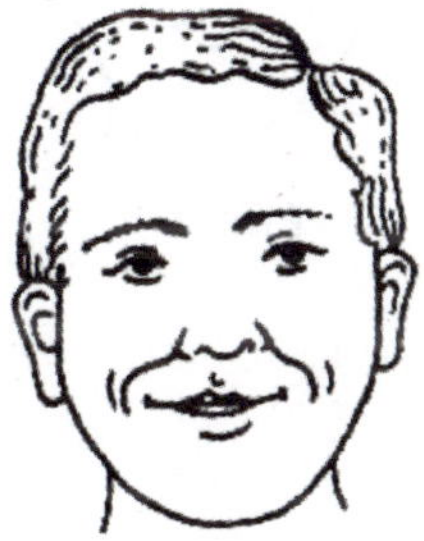

Happiness

Happiness

Drawing angle of mouth upwards and laterally.

By—Zygomaticus major.

Sadness

Production of prominent naso-labial fold, and elevation and eversion of upper lips.

By—Levator labii superioris, zygomaticus minor and levator anguli oris.

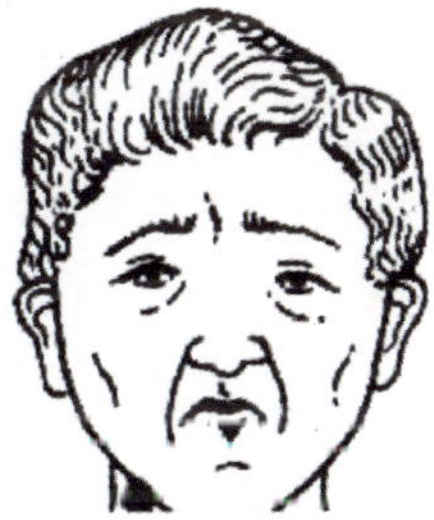

Sadness

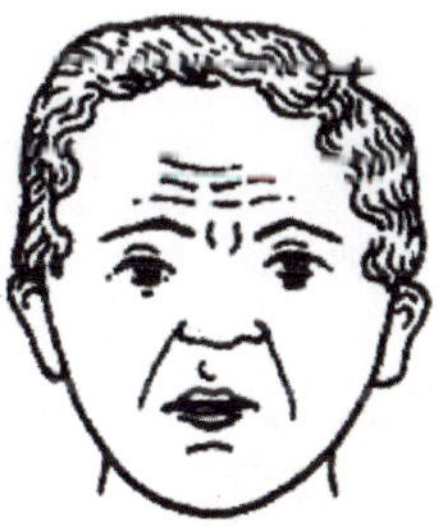

Surprise

Surprise

Transverse wrinkles on forehead by elevating eyebrows.

By—Frontalis and procerus.

Displeasure

Vertical furrow above the nose.

Elevation of nasal wing and enlargement of nostril.

By—Corrugator supercilli and levator labii superioris alaque nasi.

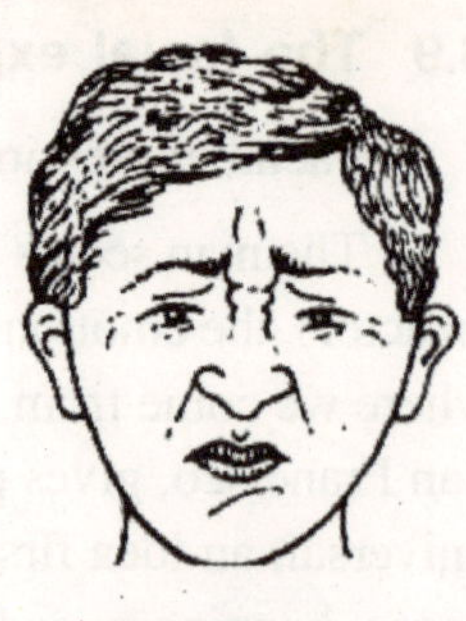

Displeasure

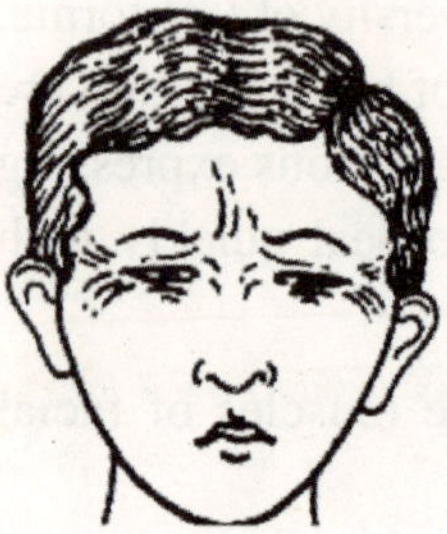

Worry

Worry

Radial folds at the lateral margin of eyelids.

By—Orbicularis oculi.

Frown

Vertical furrow above the nose by drawing the eyebrows downwards and medially.

By—Corrugator supercilli.

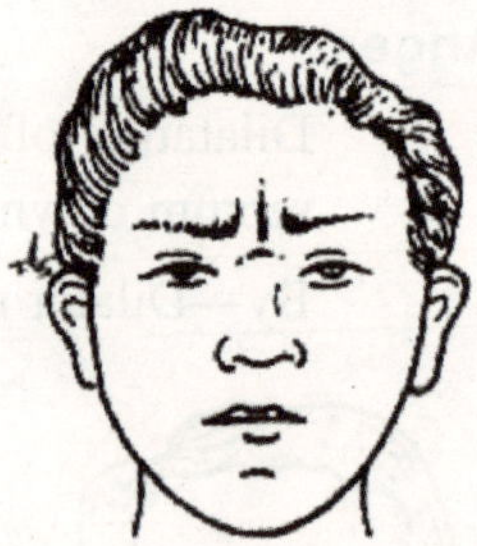

Frown

Chapter 4

The Eyelids and the Lacrimal Apparatus

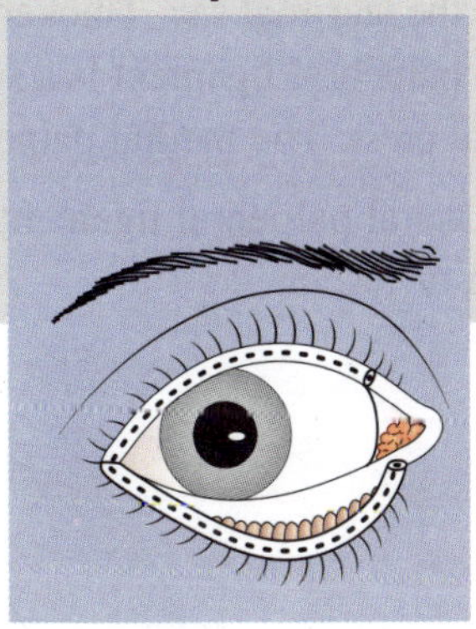

4.1 The eyeball and palpebral fissure

Eyelids are slightly everted in Figure 4.1 to show part of the conjunctival sac and other features.

The deep surface of the lower eyelid shows the tarsal glands as yellowish parallel streaks. Lacus lacrimalis is a small triangular space in the medial part of palpebral fissure; the reddish, fleshy looking elevation in its centre is the lacrimal caruncle. The plica semilunaris is a small curved fold of the conjunctiva that slightly overlaps the eyeball immediately lateral to the caruncle. The portion of the free margin of an eyelid that binds the lacus is smooth and rounded and it ends laterally in a small

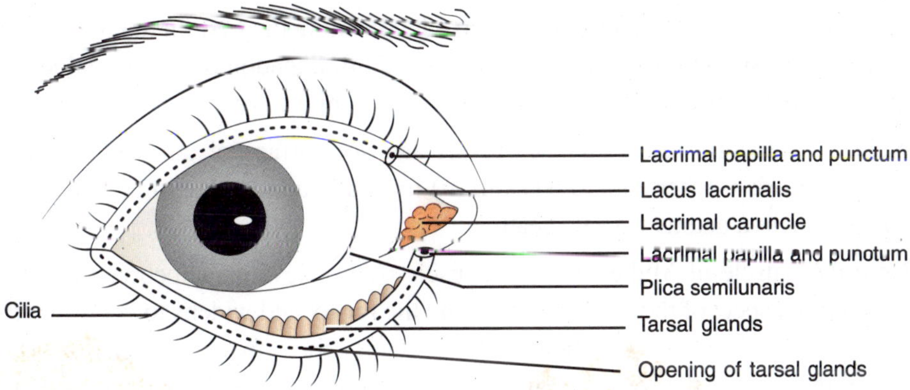

Fig. 4.1 The eyeball and palpebral fissure

eminence called the lacrimal papilla, on the summit of which is a black spot called the lacrimal punctum—the open commencement of the lacrimal canaliculus. The eyelashes or cilia project from the anterior edge of the lid margin and the tarsal glands open on the posterior edge by a row of minute apertures.

4.2 The orbital septum or palpebral fascia

The orbital septum is attached to orbital margins except at the medial side where it passes behind the lacrimal sac. Thickenings in the septum are the superior and inferior tarsal plates and the medial palpebral ligament is a strong fibrous band connecting the two tarsal plates with the anterior lacrimal crest. The medial palpebral ligament crosses in front of the lacrimal sac.

Lateral palpebral ligament is attached to the marginal tubercle (Whitnall's) behind the orbital septum or fascia.

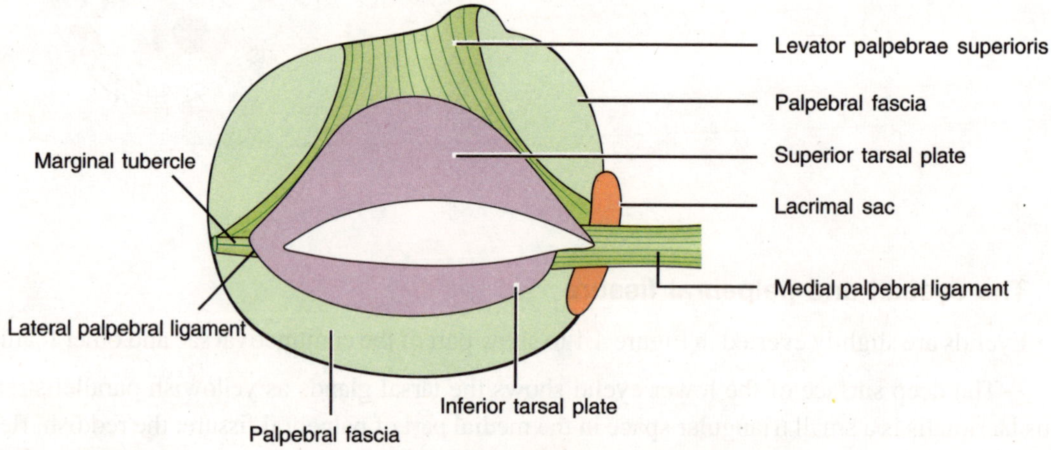

Fig. 4.2 The orbital septum or palpebral fascia

4.3 The structure of the upper eyelid as seen in section

Skin, superficial fascia and orbicularis oculi constitute the first three layers of the eyelids. The fourth layer has tarsus and palpebral fascia and in addition tendon of levator palpebrae superioris in the upper eyelid. The fifth or the deepest layer is the conjunctiva.

Note the palpebral fascia attached to the anterior surface of tarsal plate. Tendon of levator palpebrae superioris is inserted into (i) skin, (ii) front and upper edge of tarsus, and also (iii) upper fornix of conjunctiva and its fascial sheath.

Note the muscle of Muller (smooth muscle part of levator palpebral superioris), that arises from the inferior aspect of the levator just behind the fornix and widens to get inserted into the upper edge of the tarsal plate. It is supplied by sympathetic fibres from the superior cervical ganglion. Paralysis of this part of the muscle contributes to partial ptosis as in Horner's syndrome. In thyrotoxicosis, however, spasm of the muscle occurs leading to widening of the palpebral fissure.

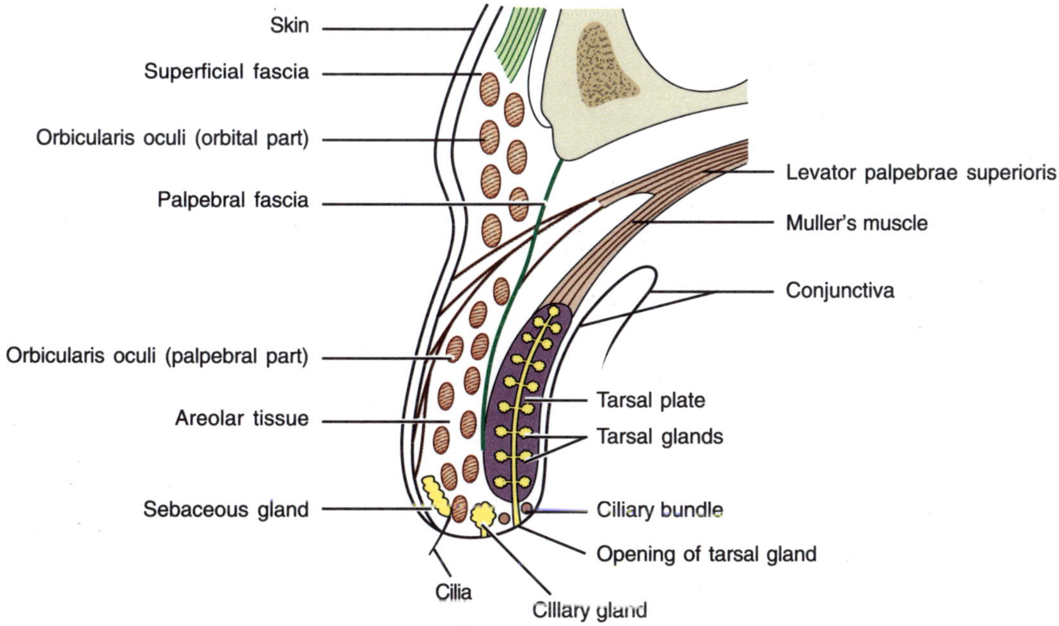

Fig. 4.3 The structure of the upper eyelid as seen in section

4.4 The lacrimal apparatus

The laerimal apparatus includes (i) lacrimal gland and its ducts, (ii) conjunctival sac, (iii) lacrimal canaliculi, (iv) lacrimal sac, (v) nasolacrimal duct, which opens into the inferior meatus of nose, and (vi) lacrimal fold, which prevents reflux from the nose.

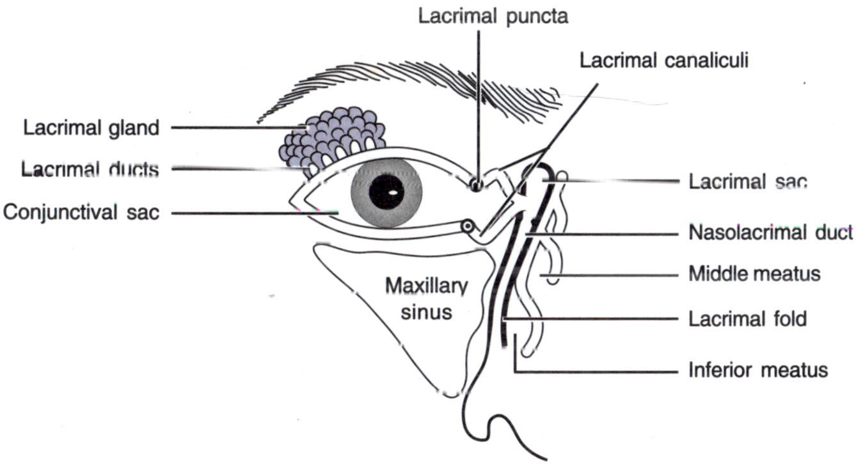

Fig. 4.4 The lacrimal apparatus

The Muscles of the Back

Chapter 5

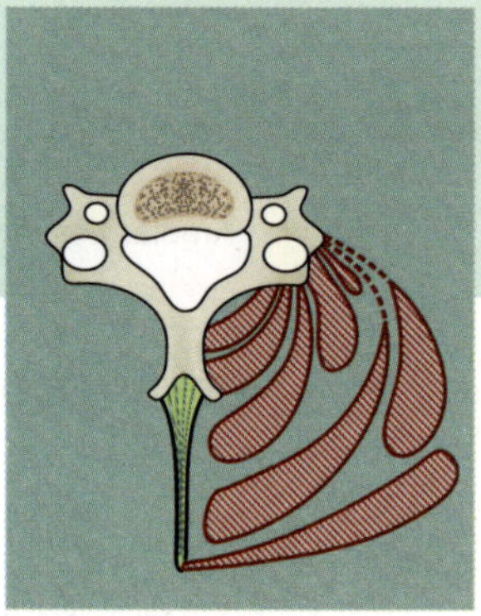

5.1 The surface anatomy of the back

Note the various bony landmarks on the posterior aspect of the skull and back of neck. Observe the position of spines from cervical seven (C7) down to lumbar five (L5). The scapula lies from T2 to T7 spines. The highest points of iliac crest lie in the interval between L3 and L4 spines—a fact important for lumbar puncture.

The muscles of the back are classified into three main groups.

Building up the muscular layers of the back.

I. Deep muscles or postvertebral muscles—responsible for maintenance of normal curves of the vertebral column.

They are subdivided into four subgroups.

(a) Interspinalis and intertransversari group—runs between spines or between transverse processes.

(b) Transverso-spinalis group—arise laterally but run towards midline.

(c) Erector spinae group—arises from midline or more laterally and runs almost longitudinally.

(d) Splenius group—arises from midline and runs laterally and upwards.

II. Intermediate muscles—associated with respiration.

(a) Serratus posterior superior
(b) Serratus posterior inferior
(c) Levator costarum

III. Superficial muscles—belong to the upper limb.

(a) Trapezius
(b) Latissimus dorsi
(c) Levator scapulae
(d) Rhomboideus minor and major

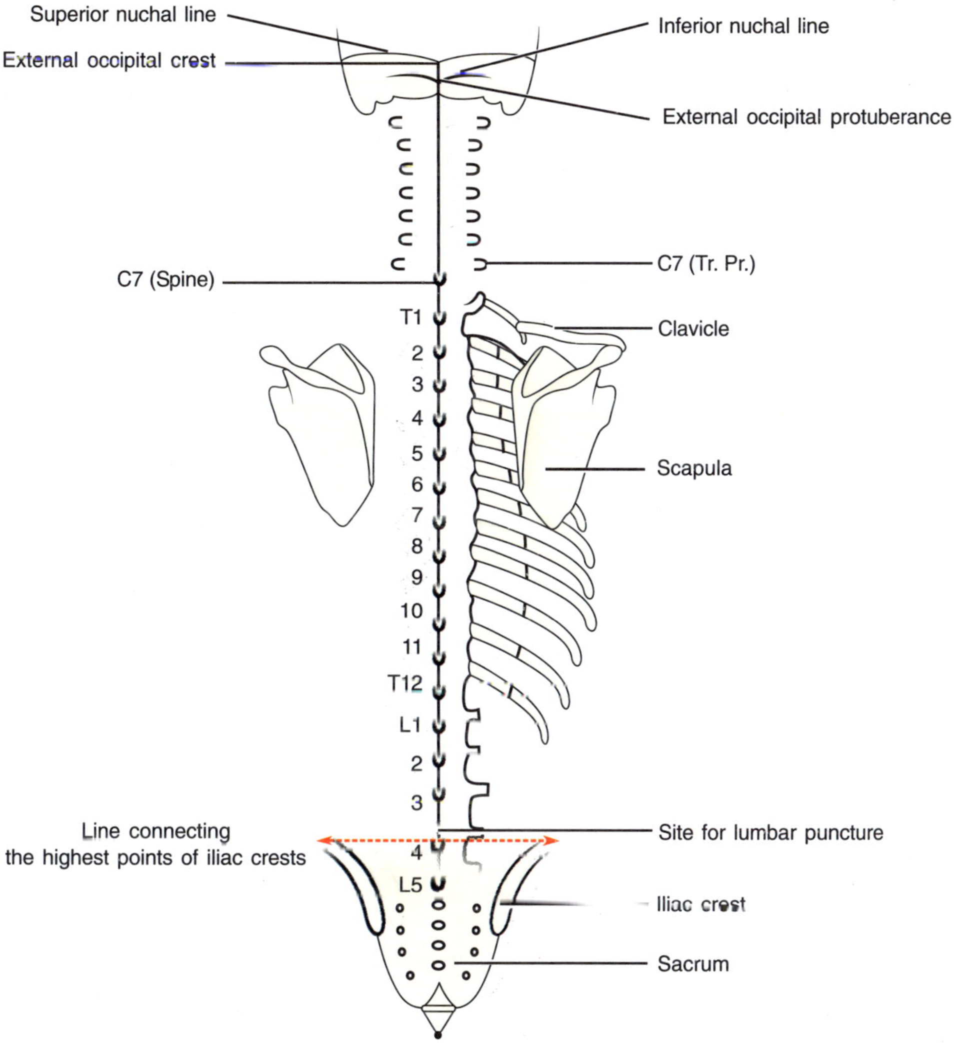

Fig. 5.1 The bony landmarks of the back

5.2 I. Deep muscles

(a) *Interspinalis and Intertransversari group*

(i) Interspinalis—between spines.
Poorly represented in thoracic region.

(ii) Intertransversari—between transverse processes.
Best developed in cervical and lumbar regions.

(b) *Transverso-spinalis group*

(i) Multifidus.
Extends from upper part of sacrum to upper part of neck (S4 to C2). Fibres slope upwards and medially as shown on the left side.

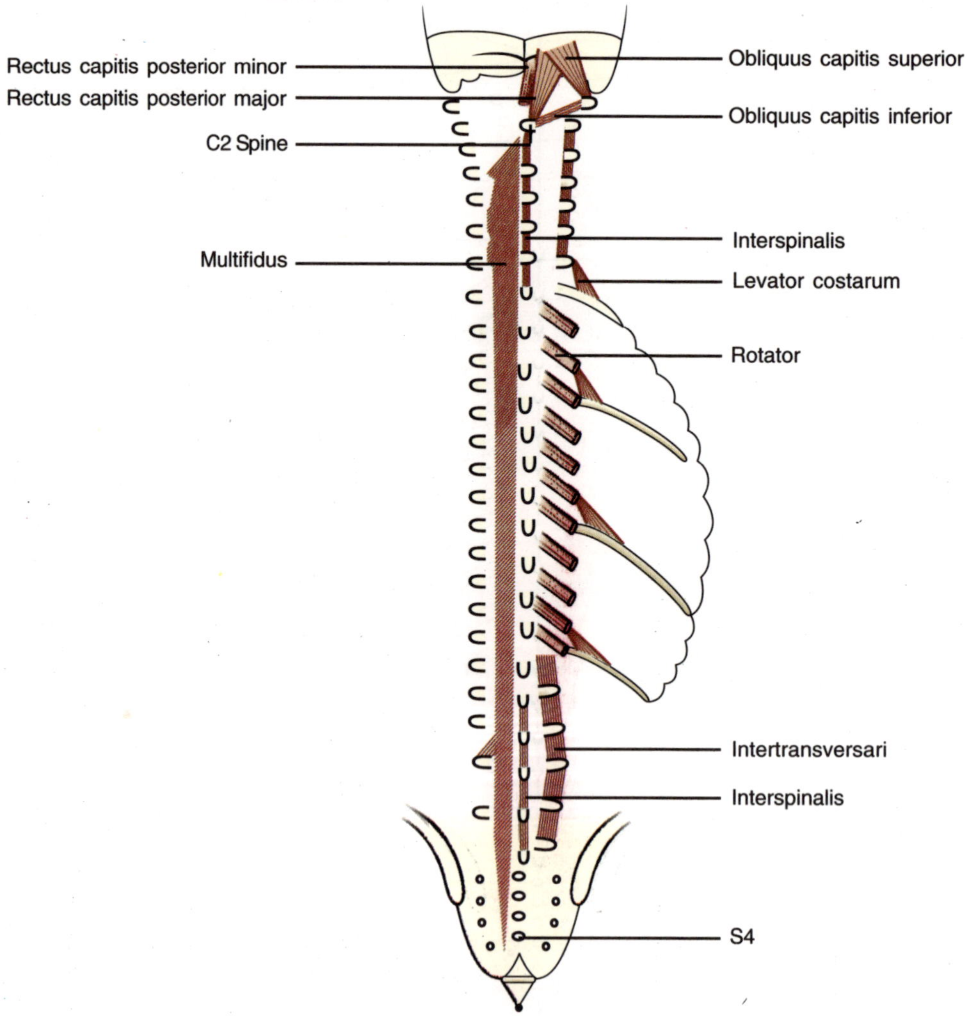

Fig. 5.2 Deep muscles—Interspinalis, intertransversari and transverso-spinalis group

(ii) Rotatores

Confined to thoracic spines. There are eleven on each side as shown on the right side. They extend from a transverse process to a lamina and in the occipital region are modified into obliquus (obliquus capitis superior and inferior) and recti (rectus capitis posterior major and minor) which form the boundaries of suboccipital triangle.

5.3 Deep muscles I *(Contd.)*

(iii) Semispinalis

The semispinalis has three parts:

- Semispinalis thoracis
- Semispinalis cervicis
- **Semispinalis capitis**

The first two are shown on the left side while semispinalis capitis which is inserted into the skull is shown on the right side. The breadth extends from spines to transverse process (equal to the breadth of thumb). **Semispinalis capitis is the only muscle in this group which is of importance as it appears in the floor of posterior triangle at its apex and also forms the roof of suboccipital triangle.**

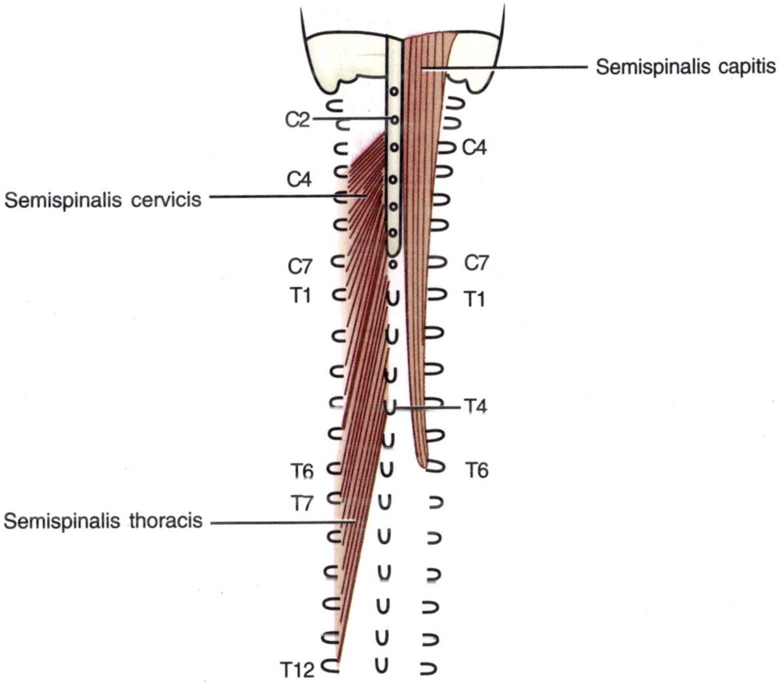

Fig. 5.3 Deep muscles—Semispinalis group

5.4 The structures exposed by the reflection of splenius group

- Semispinalis capitis
- Longissimus capitis
- Obliquus capitis superior
- Occipital artery
- Obliquus capitis inferior
- Transverse process of atlas.

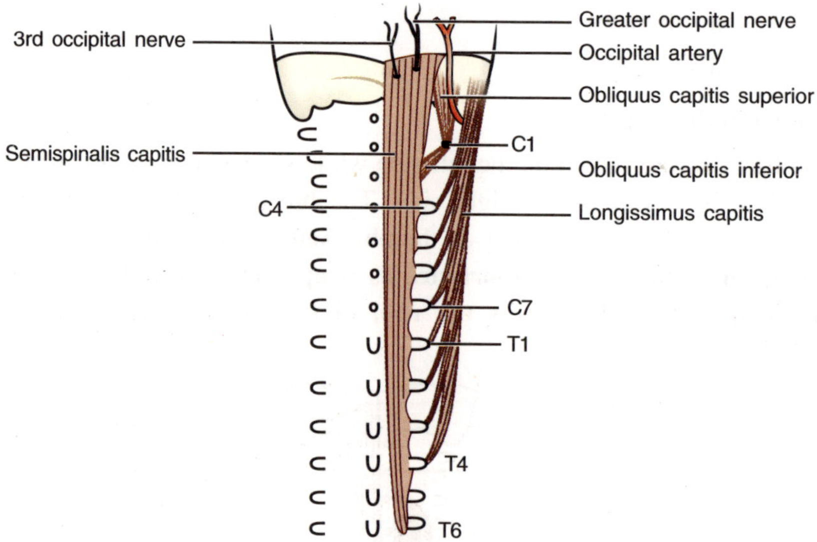

Fig. 5.4 The structures exposed by the reflection of splenius group

5.5 Deep muscles I *(Contd.)*

(c) *Erector spinae group*

It is a composite muscle and as it ascends it splits in the upper lumbar region into three vertical columns. The breadth is from the spines to the angles of the ribs (equal to the breadth of palm). Each column has three parts:

(i) Iliocostalis (lateral column). The three parts are

- Iliocostalis lumborum
- Iliocostalis thoracis
- Iliocostalis cervicis

(ii) Longissimus (intermediate column). The three parts are

- Longissimus thoracis

- Longissimus cervicis
- Longissimus capitis

Longissimus capitis is the only part inserted into skull, and its origin and insertion are shown on the right side.

(iii) Spinalis (medial column). The three parts are

- Spinalis thoracis
- Spinalis cervicis
- Spinalis capitis.

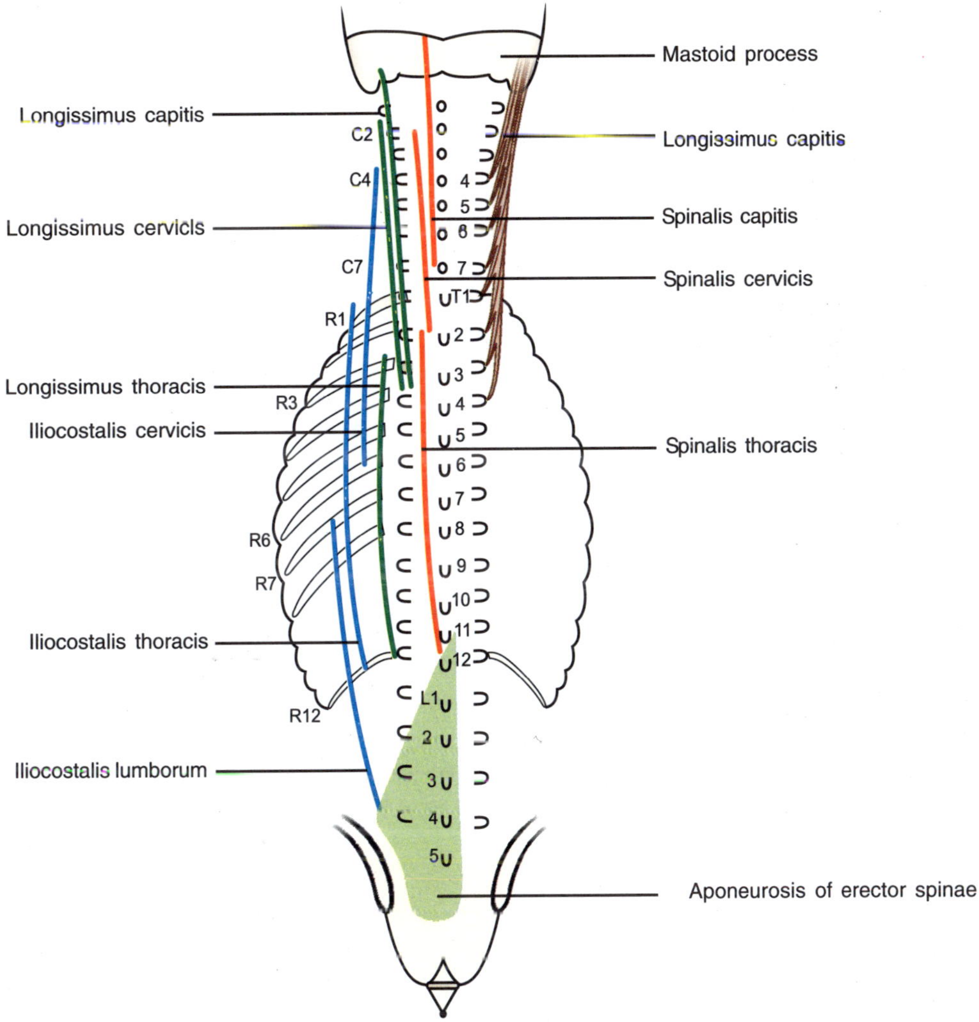

Fig. 5.5 Deep muscles—Erector spinae group

5.6 and 5.7 Deep muscles I *(Contd.)*

(d) *Splenius group*

Note its continuous origin from the ligamentum nuchae and spines of the lower cervical and upper thoracic vertebrae. It overlaps semispinalis capitis and levator scapulae and is wrapped around the neck like a bandage (splenius = bandage). It divides into

(i) Splenius cervicis (cervical part) inserted into transverse processes of upper four cervical vertebrae, which also give rise to the levator scapulae.

(ii) **Splenius capitis** (cranial part) inserted into the mastoid process and lateral part of superior nuchal line. **It is to be remembered as it forms the floor of the upper part of posterior triangle and roof of suboccipital triangle.**

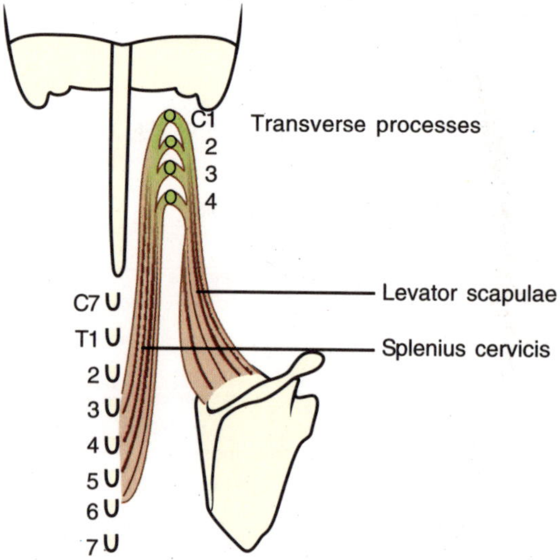

Fig. 5.6 Deep muscles—Splenius cervicis

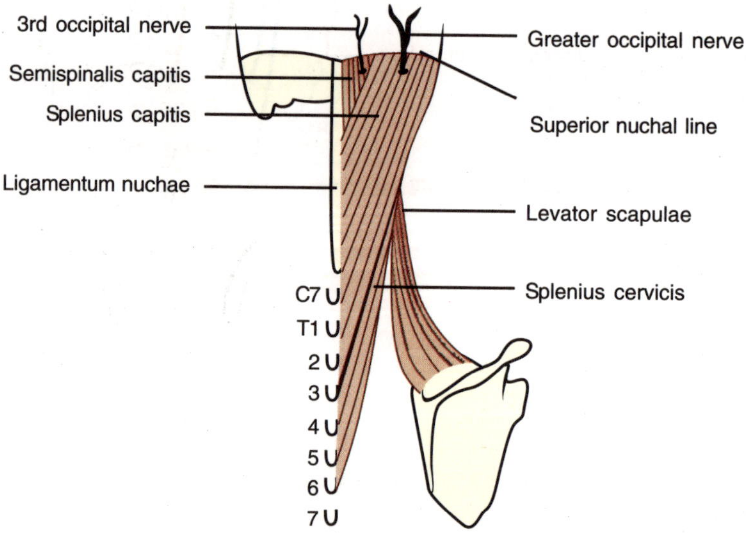

Fig. 5.7 Deep muscles—Splenius cervicis and splenius capitis

5.8 Intermediate muscles II *(Contd.)*

(i) Serratus posterior superior

It can be seen after the rhomboids are removed. Note its attachment to the second, third, fourth and fifth ribs (R2 to R5) as it raises these ribs and helps in respiration. Origin is from spines of C7 to T3.

(ii) Serratus posterior inferior

Removal of latissimus dorsi exposes this muscle and its insertion into the lower four ribs (R9 to R12). Origin is from spines of T11 to L2.

(iii) Levatores costarum

These are a series of twelve muscles, assoicated with respiration and found in the deep part of thoracic region. The first arises from transverse process of cervical seven. They are inserted into the rib below.

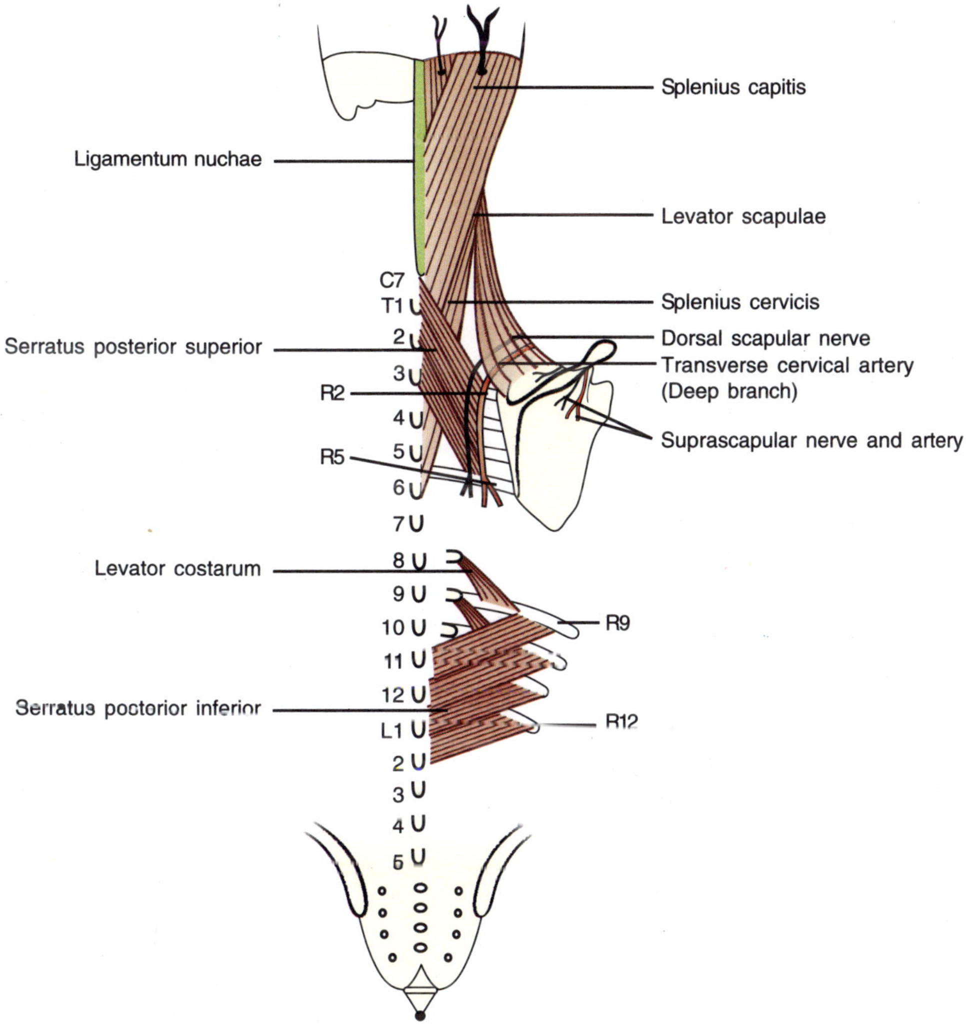

Fig. 5.8 Intermediate muscles—Serratus posterior superior and inferior, and levatores costarum

5.9 Superficial muscles III *(Contd.)*

Levator scapulae (Appears in the floor of posterior triangle)

- *Origin*
  - Tr. pr. of C1 and C2.
  - Posterior tubercles of Tr. pr. of C3 and C4.
- *Insertion*
  - Medial border of scapula from the superior angle to spine.
- *Nerve supply*
  - C3 and C4.
- *Action*
  - Elevation and medial rotation of scapula.

Rhomboideus minor and major

Rhomboideus minor

- *Origin*
  - Lower part of ligamentum nuchae.
  - Spines of C7 and T1 vertebrae.
- *Insertion*
  - Medial border of scapula at the level of root of spine.
- *Nerve supply*
  - Dorsal scapular nerve (C5).
- *Action*
  - Drawing the vertebral border of scapula medially and upwards.

Rhomboideus major

- *Origin*
  - Spines of T2, 3, 4 and 5 vertebrae.
- *Insertion*
  - Medial border of scapula from the root of the spine upto its inferior angle.
- *Nerve supply*
  - Dorsal scapular nerve (C5).
- *Action*
  - Adduction, medial rotation and elevation of scapula.

The accessory nerve (XI) accompanied by the superficial branch of transverse cervical artery is seen superficially while the dorsal scapular nerve accompanied by the deep branch of transverse cervical artery lies deep is the three muscles.

The suprascapular nerve and artery course towards suprascapular notch.

Splenius, a deep muscle, with its two parts (capitis and cervicis) is also shown related to these muscles.

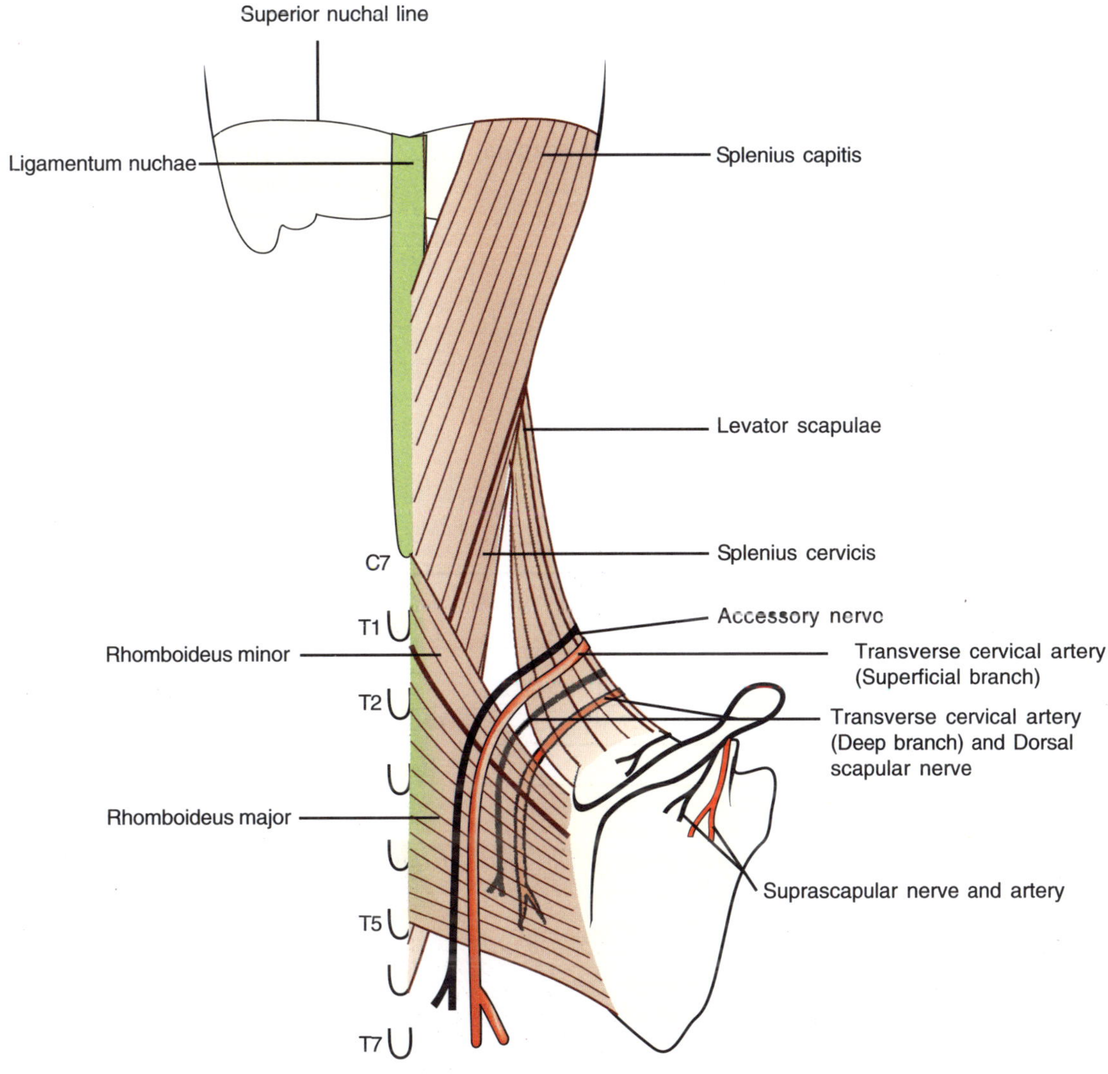

Fig. 5.9 Superficial muscles—Levator scapulae and rhomboideus major and minor

5.10 Superficial muscles III *(Contd.)*

Trapezius (Forms the posterior boundary of posterior triangle)

Origin

- Medial 1/3 of superior nuchal line.
- External occipital protuberance.
- Ligamentum nuchae.
- Spines of C7 and T1 to T12 vertebrae.

Insertion

- Lateral half of the posterior surface of clavicle.
- Medial border of acromion and the upper lip of spine of scapula.
- Tubercle at the root of spine of scapula.

Nurve supply

- Spinal part of XI.
- Branches from C3 and C4.

Action

- Rotation of scapula.

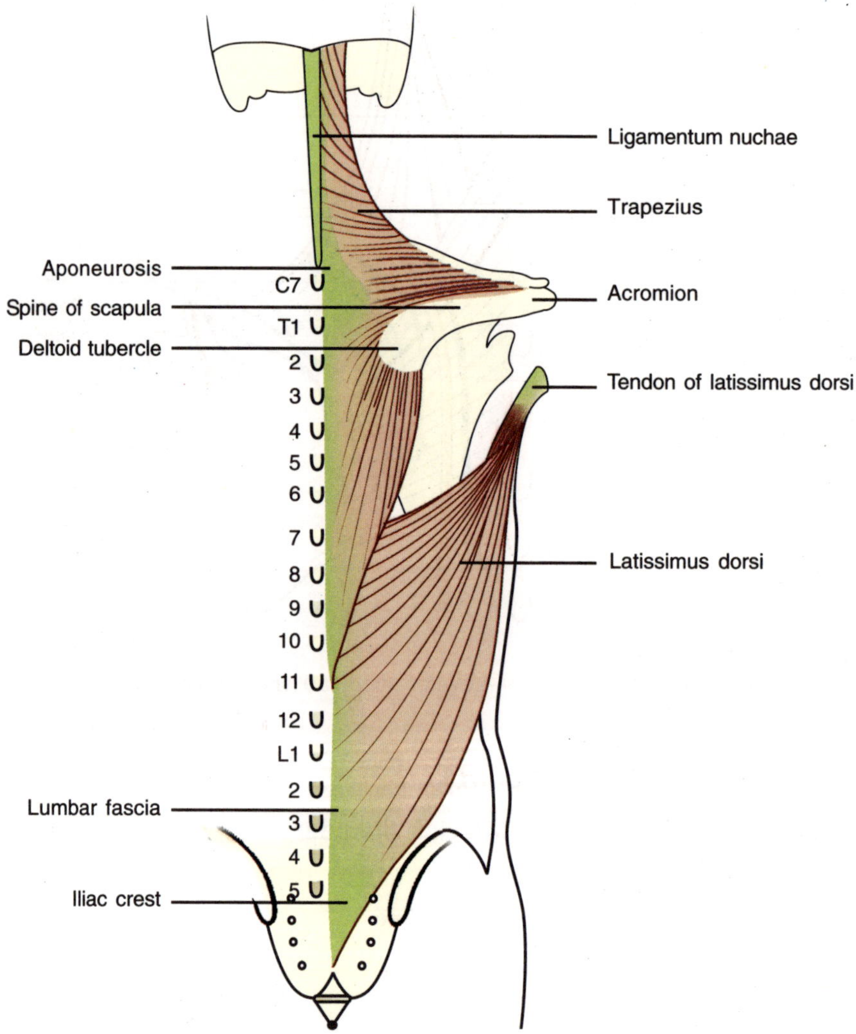

Fig. 5.10 Superficial muscles—Trapezius and latissimus dorsi

Latissimus dorsi

Origin

- Spines of T7 to L5.
- Supraspinous ligaments.
- Outer lip of posterior part of iliac crest.
- Lower three or four ribs.
- Inferior angle of scapula.

Insertion

- Floor of bicipital groove of humerus.

Nurve supply

- Nerve to latissimus dorsi (C6, 7 and 8) from posterior cord of brachial plexus.

Action

- Extension, adduction and medial rotation of arm.

5.11 A Schematic transverse section through neck

Study the various groups of muscles in the back of neck. Intermediate group of muscles are not represented. Also note that the rotatores are missing.

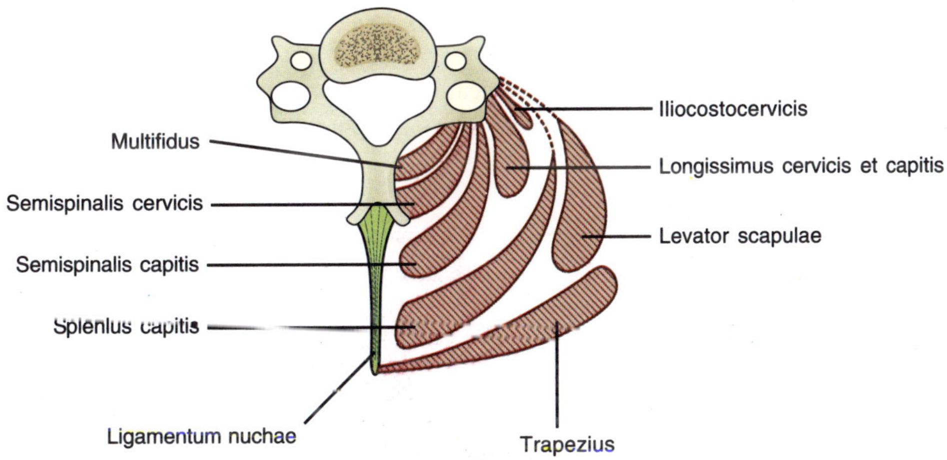

Fig. 5.11 A schematic transverse section through neck

5.12 A transverse section to show the muscles of back in thoracic region

Note that the splenius group is missing in this region.

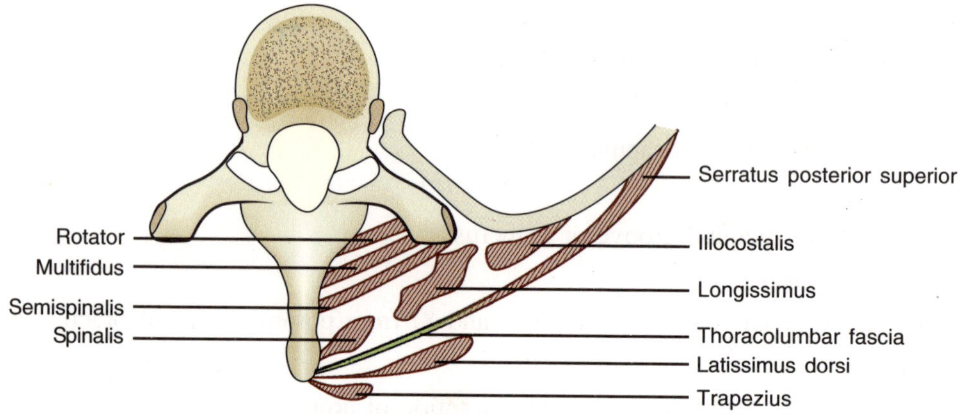

Fig. 5.12 A transverse section to show the muscles of back in thoracic region

5.13 A transverse section through lumbar region

Note the disposition of the three layers of lumbo-dorsal fascia.

Splenius group is missing and the semispinalis and rotatores are absent in this region.

The muscle mass of the erector spinae lies beneath the lumbar fascia and its upward continuation, the thoraco-lumbar fascia. In the neck, this fascia disappears and the muscle mass is covered by the splenius capitis muscle.

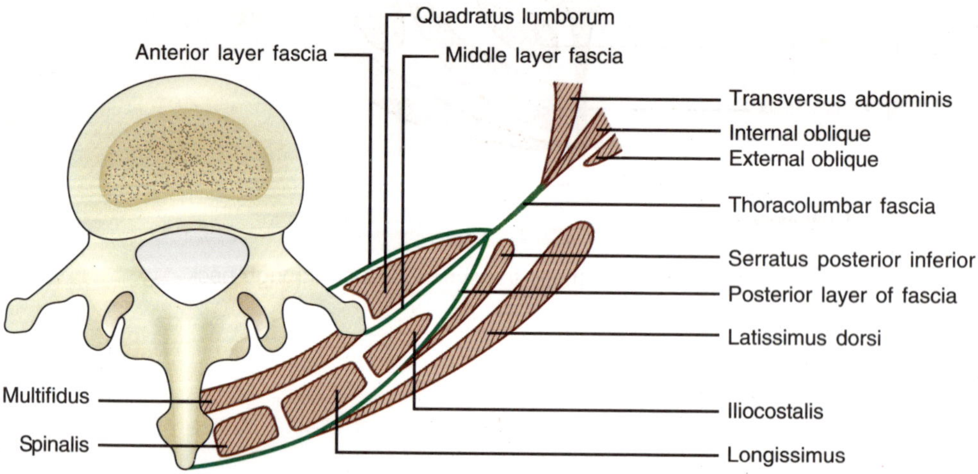

Fig. 5.13 A transverse section through lumbar region

The Back of the Neck

Chapter 6

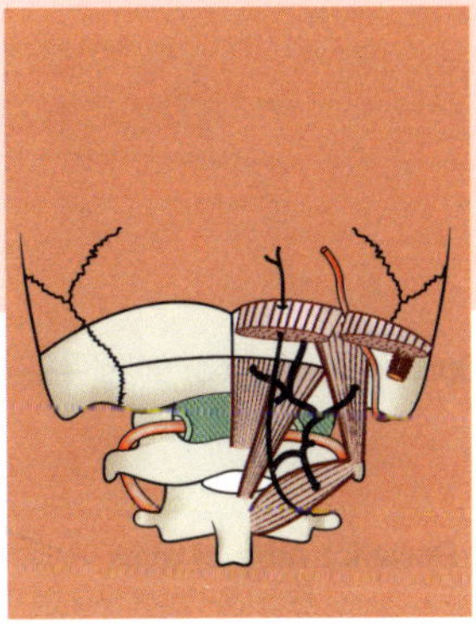

BUILDING UP THE BACK OF THE NECK

6.1 The posterior view of the skull (Norma occipitalis)

The superior nuchal line crosses the lateral aspect of the mastoid, dividing it into a smooth upper and a rough lower part. The nuchal area below the superior nuchal line is for the muscles of neck. The insertion of longissimus capitis is confined to the back of mastoid process while the two muscles above it extend to the occipital bone. Attachments on atlas and axis vertebrae should be noted.

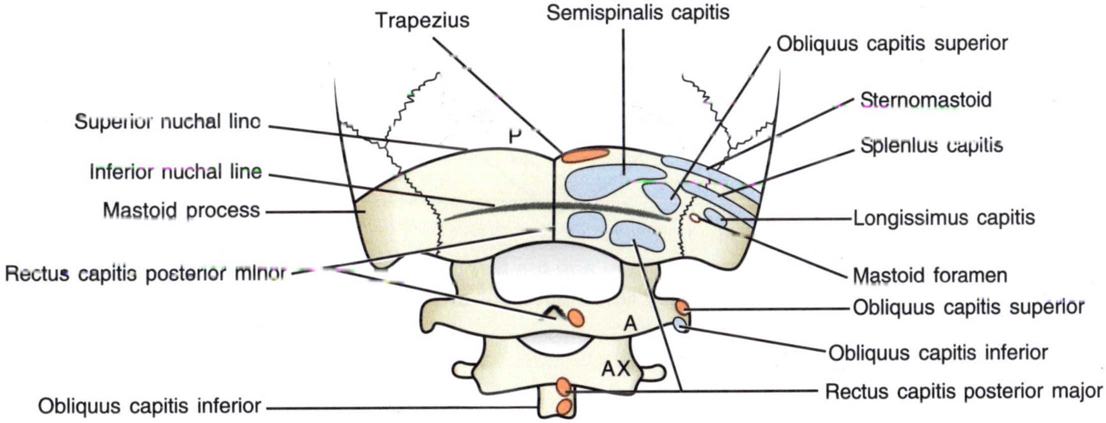

Fig. 6.1 The posterior view of the skull (Norma occipitalis)

6.2 The floor of suboccipital triangle

It is formed by two structures viz., posterior arch of atlas and posterior atlanto-occipital membrane.

The third part of the vertebral artery passes under the oblique ligament of atlas which is the unattached thickened lateral part of the lower border of the membrane.

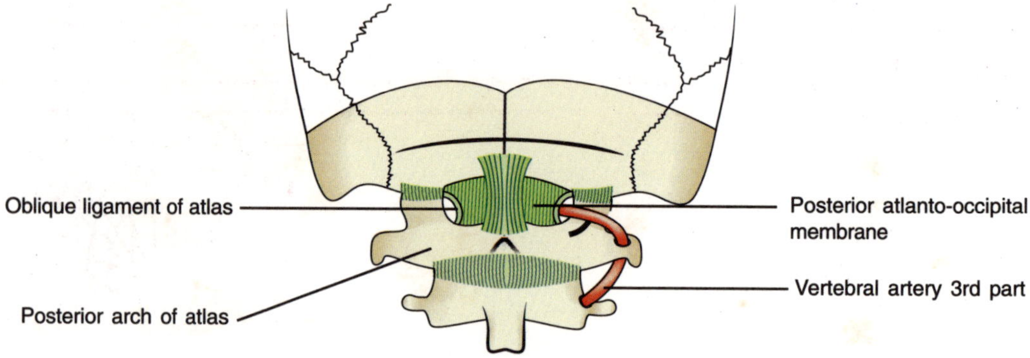

Fig. 6.2 The floor of suboccipital triangle

6.3 The third part of the vertebral artery and the first cervical nerve with its ventral and dorsal rami as they lie on posterior arch of atlas.

Note their relationship with the lateral mass of atlas.

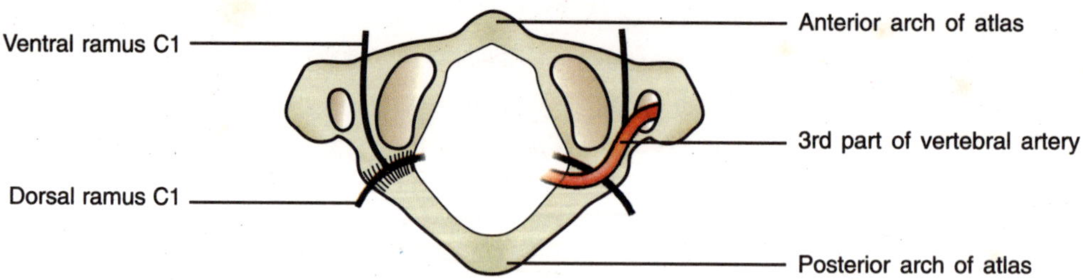

Fig. 6.3 The third part of the vertebral artery and the first cervical nerve with its ventral and dorsal rami as they lie on posterior arch of atlas.

6.4 The boundaries and contents of suboccipital triangle

The muscles of the roof viz., semispinalis capitis and splenius capitis are shown cut.

The contents are (i) the third part of vertebral artery, (ii) the dorsal ramus of first cervical nerve (suboccipital nerve), (iii) the suboccipital venous plexus and (iv) the tough fibrous tissue mingled with fat.

The suboccipital nerve breaks up into (i) five musclar branches, and (ii) one communicating branch to greater occipital nerve.

Boundaries:

- Medially : Rectus capitis posterior major reinforced by rectus capitis posterior minor
- Below and laterally : Obliquus capitis inferior
- Above and laterally : Obliquus capitis superior

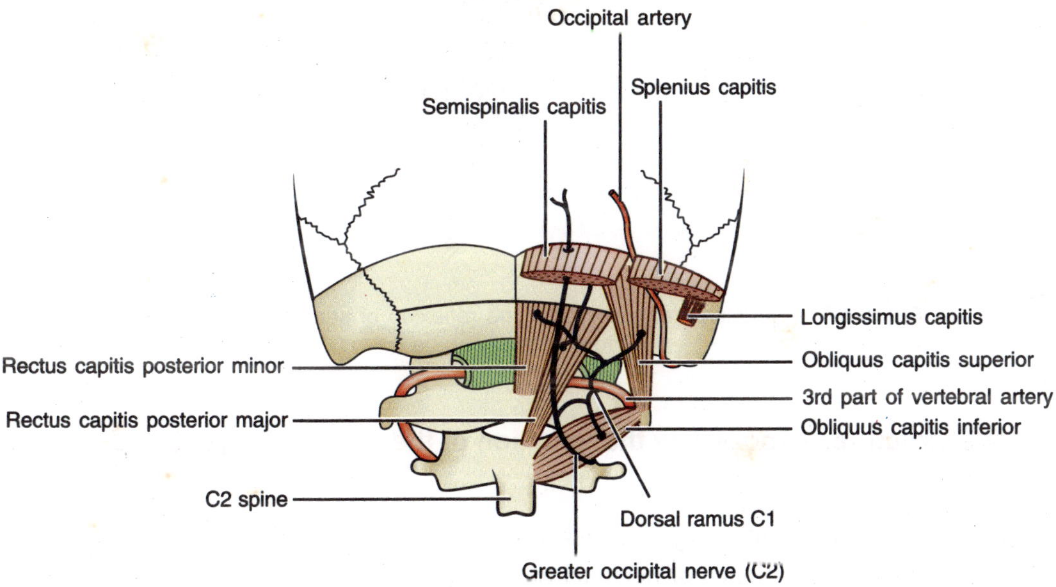

Fig. 6.4 The boundaries and contents of suboccipital triangle

6.5 The structures exposed after the reflexion of semispinalis capitis and logissimus capitis

Multifidus can be seen below the second cervical spine and suboccipital muscles and related structures above this spine.

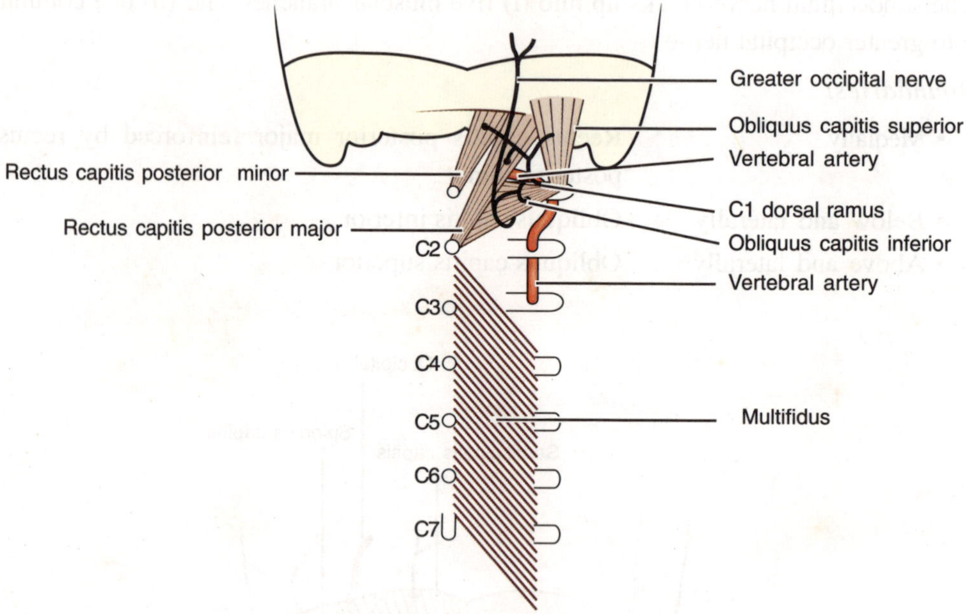

Fig. 6.5 The structures exposed after the reflexion of semispinalis capitis and logissimus capitis

6.6 The structures exposed by the reflexion of the splenius capitis and the removal of underlying fat

Note the deep cervical artery a branch of costocervical trunk anastomosing with the deep branch of the descending branch of occipital artery in the dense fascia under semispinalis capitis. Superficial to the muscle is the anastomosis between the superficial branch of the descending branch of occipital artery with the ascending branch of the transverse cervical artery. This anastomosis around semispinalis capitis is ultimately between external carotid and subclavian arteries.

6.7 The structures exposed by the removal of sternomastoid and trapezius from the back of the neck

Parts of semispinalis capitis and levator scapulae are seen above and below the splenius, respectively. Semispinalis is pierced by two nerves and one artery abelled in Figure 6.6 while levator scapulae is crossed by one nerve and one artery. Rhomboidei cover lower part of splenius.

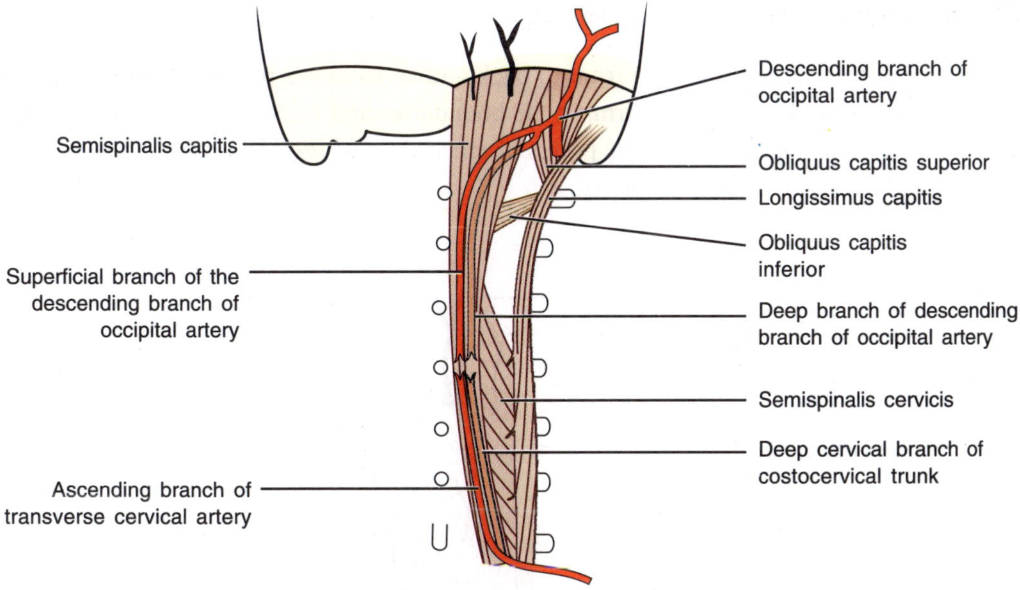

Fig. 6.6 The structures exposed by the reflexion of the splenius capitis and the removal of underlying fat. Arterial an astomosis around semispinalis capitis is to be noted

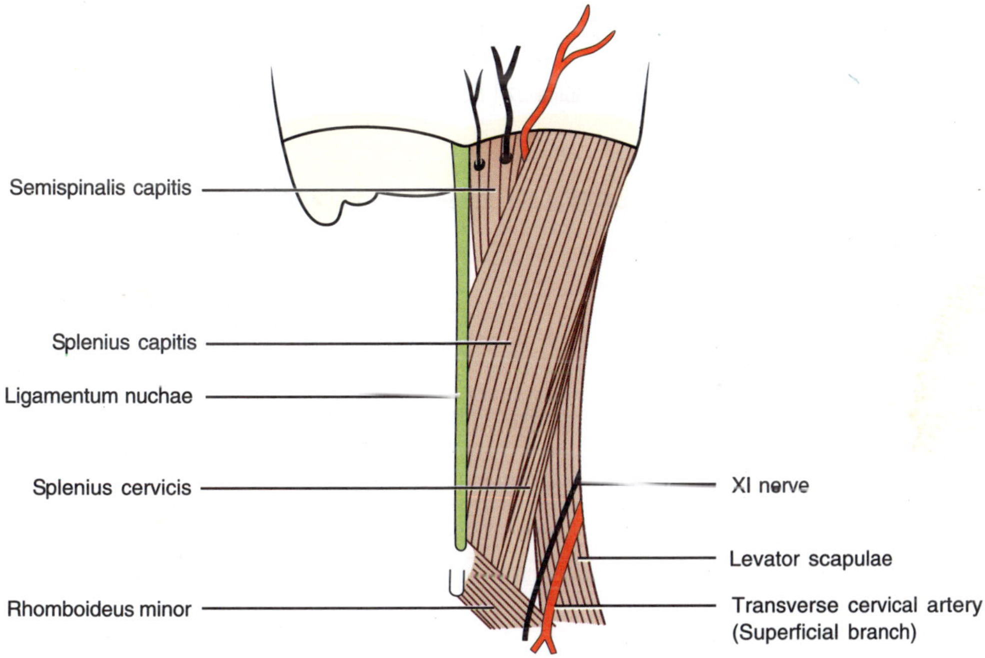

Fig. 6.7 The structures exposed by the removal of sternomastoid and trapezius from the back of the neck

6.8 The superficial structures of the back of the neck

The posterior triangle spirals from front to back and so its upper part faces backwards and is seen at the back of neck. The muscles forming the boundaries and floor of the posterior triangle in this part can easily be recognised. Note the points of emergence of lesser occipital, greater occipital and third occipital nerves and occipital artery.

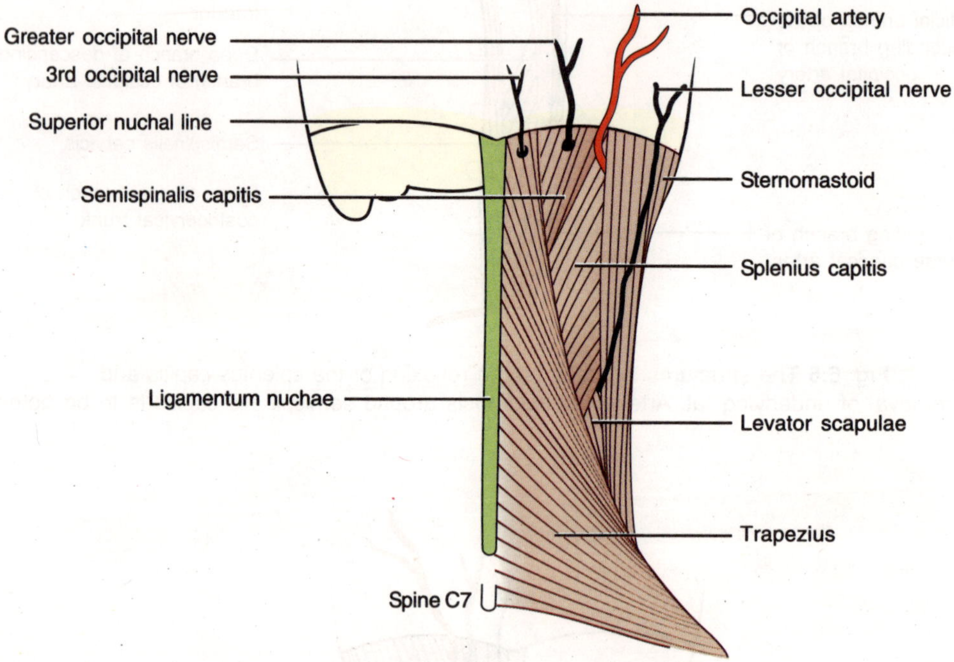

Fig. 6.8 The superficial structures of the back of the neck

The Brachial Plexus

Chapter 7

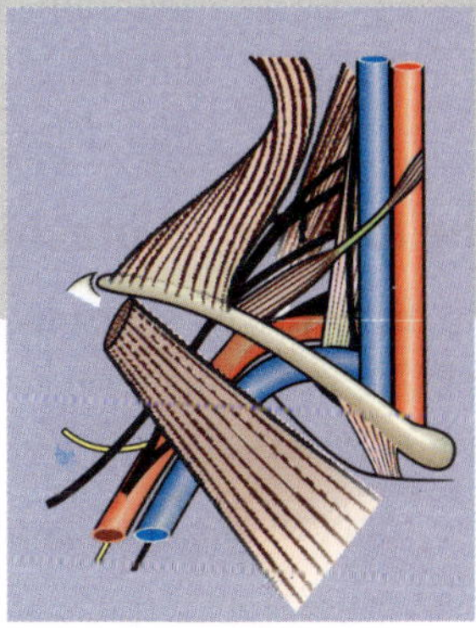

BUILDING UP THE RELATIONS OF SUPRACLAVICULAR PART OF BRACHIAL PLEXUS

7.1 The parts of brachial plexus

Roots – The ventral rami of C5, 6, 7, 8 and T1 with variable contribution from C4 and T2.

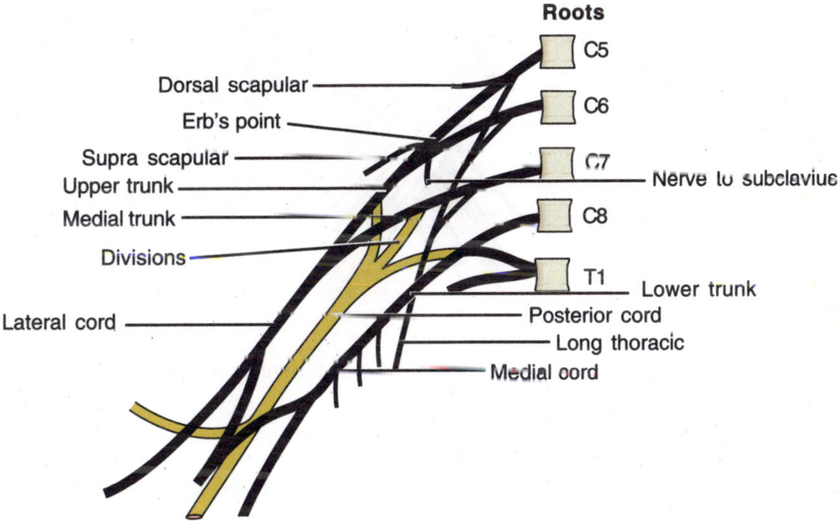

Fig. 7.1 The parts of brachial plexus

Trunks	–	C5 and C6 join to form the upper trunk, C7 forms the middle trunk and C8 and T1 join to form the lower trunk.
Division	–	Each trunk splits into an anterior and a posterior division.
Cords	–	The three posterior divisions unite to form the posterior cord. The upper two anterior divisions form the lateral cord. The lower anterior division forms the medial cord.
Branches	–	They are given off from roots, trunks and cords as can be studied from the diagram. Four branches of brachial plexus which lie in the neck have been labelled viz., dorsal scapular, long thoracic from the roots, and suprascapular and nerve to subclavicle from the trunks.

7.2 The location of brachial plexus

The first rib, the scalenus medius and the calvicle have been shown to indicate that the roots and trunks lie in the neck on scalenus medius muscle, the divisions are behind the clavicle and the cords are in the axilla.

The roots of the plexus lie behind the scalenus anterior and the lower trunk is posterior to subclavian artery.

The cords of the plexus are related to the axillary artery covered by pectoralis minor and major muscles in the axillary region.

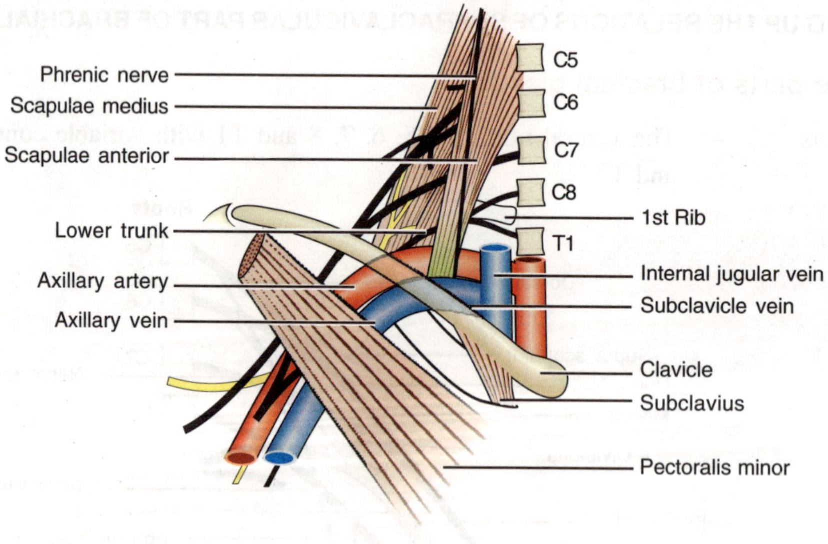

Fig. 7.2 The location of brachial plexus

7.3 The brachial plexus and omohyoid muscle

The cartoid sheath lies on scalenus anterior and is crossed by the common tendon of omohyoid while the inferior belly covers the lower trunk of brachial plexus at a lower level and forms the superior boundary of the subclavian triangle.

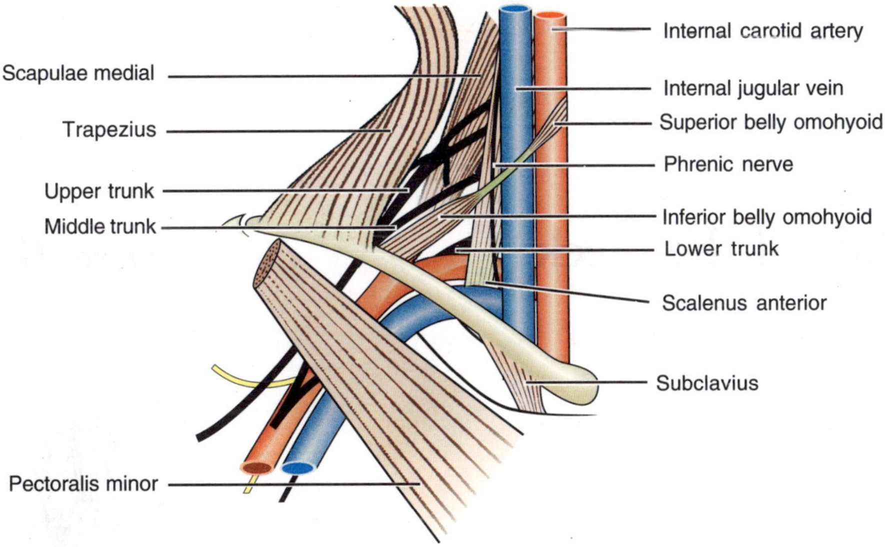

Fig. 7.3 The brachial plexus and omohyoid muscle

7.4 The subclavian or omoclavicular triangle

Sternomastoid covers the anterior relations of scalenus anterior. The third part of subclavian artery lies in a triangle bounded by inferior belly of omohyoid, posterior border of calvicular head of sternomastoid and intermediate third of calvicle.

Deltoid and pectoralis major below the clavicle form a small delto-pectoral triangle.

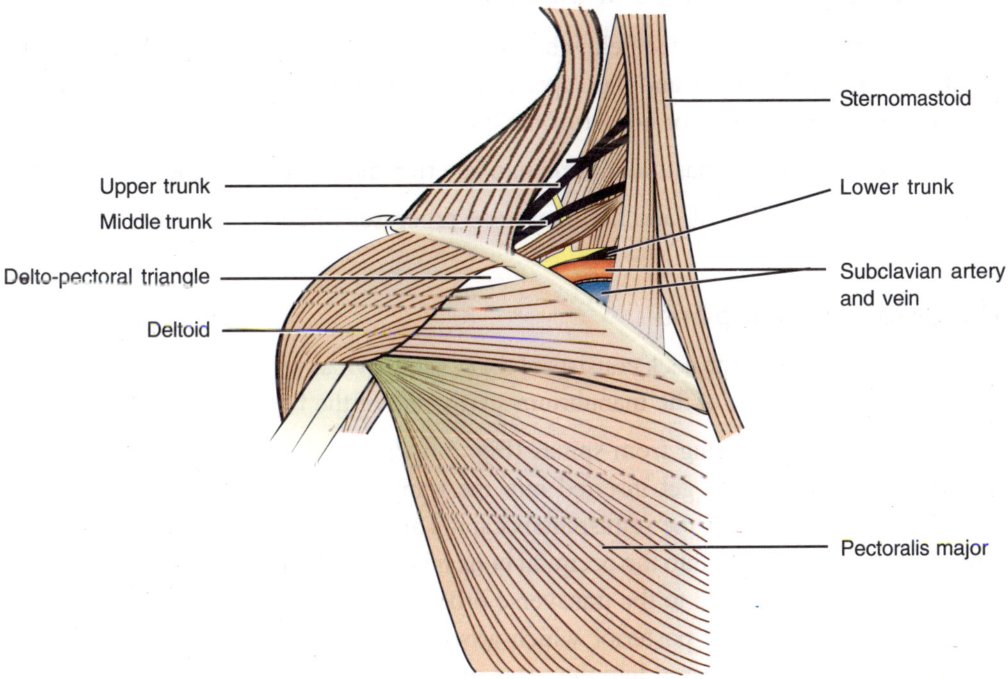

Fig. 7.4 The subclavian or omoclavicular triangle

The Side of the Neck

Chapter 8

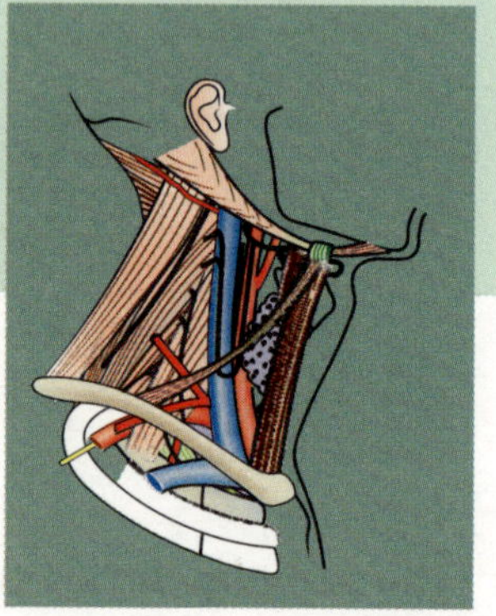

BUILDING UP THE POSTERIOR TRIANGLE

8.1 The boundaries of the side of the neck

The side of the neck is bounded below by the clavicle, above by the lower border of the body of mandible, the mastoid process and the superior nuchal line. It extends anteriorly to the median plane and posteriorly to the anterior border of the trapezius.

It is divided by the sternomastoid muscle into anterior and posterior triangles.

Note the position of first rib and the transverse processes of cervical vertebrae (C1 to C7) to the side of the neck.

8.2 The deep muscular plane

The bony framework of the neck consists of the seven cervical vertebrae and may be considered to include the superior surface of the manubrium sterni, and of the first rib.

The splenius cervicis arising from spines (Fig. 5.6 *Refer* page 24) winds from the back and passes upwards and laterally to get inserted into the transverse processes of upper four cervical vertebrae (C1 to C4). Above it is the semispinalis capitis arising from transverse processes (Fig. 5.3 *Refer* page 21) which is inserted into the occipital bone near the mid line. Portions of obliquus capitis inferior and superior are attached to the transverse process of the first cervical vertebra. Below the splenius cervicis is the scalenus posterior which arises from the posterior tubercles of transverse processes of C4 to C6 and is inserted into the outer surface of the second rib behind the tubercle for first digitation of serratus anterior.

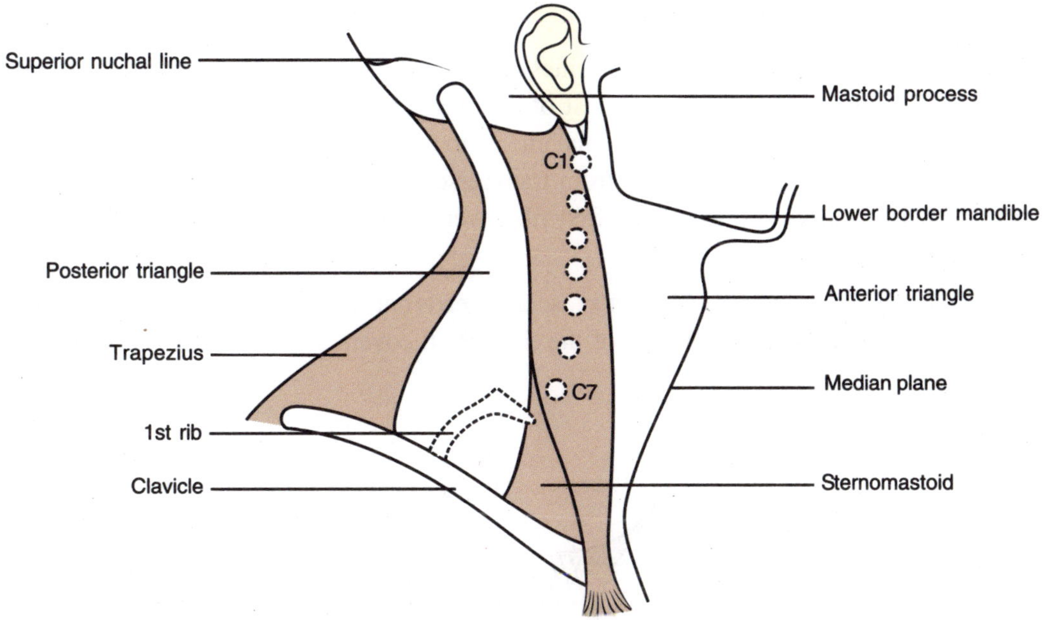

Fig. 8.1 The boundaries of the side of the neck

The neck of the first rib is related to sympatetic chain, first posterior intercostal vein, superior intercostal artery and first thoracic nerve from medial to lateral side.

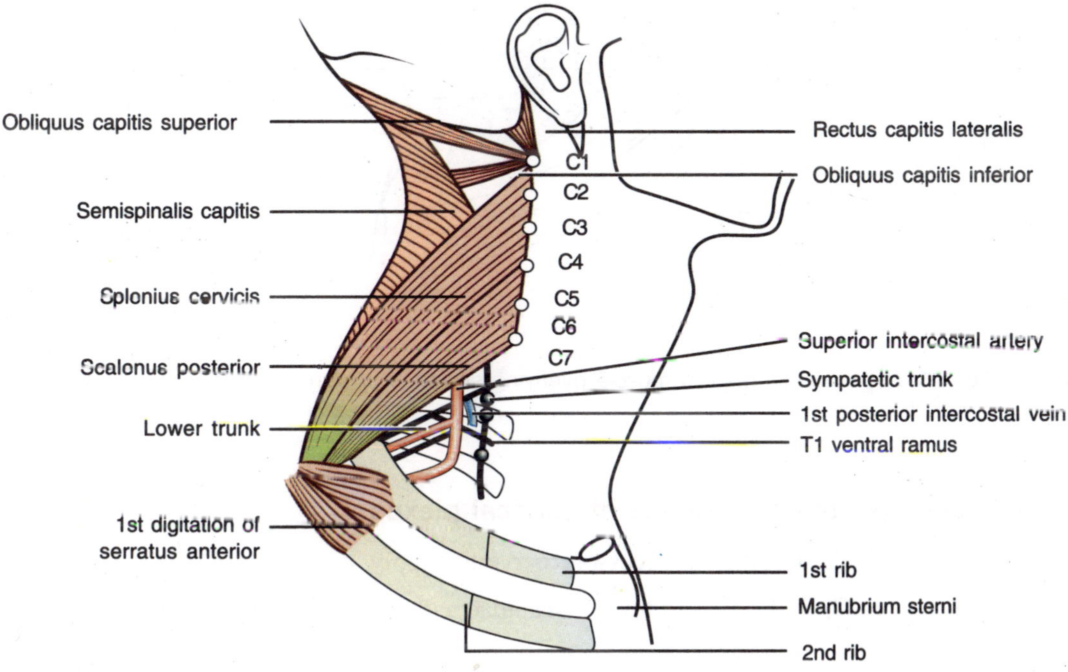

Fig. 8.2 The deep muscular plane

8.3 The scalenus medius muscle

The splenius capitis arising from the spines and ligamentum nuchae and inserted into mastoid process (Fig. 5.7 *Refer* page 24) covers most of semispinalis capitis. The levator scapulae covers most of splenius cervicis since both have attachments to transverse processes of C1 to C4 (Fig. 5.6 *Refer* page 24). Scalenus medius arising from transverse processes of C2 to C7 and inserting into the posterior part of upper surface of the first rib covers part of levator scapulae and most of the scalenus posterior.

The supra-pleural membrane (Sibson's fascia) spreads out like a fan from the transverse process of C7 to get attached to the inner border of the first rib. It covers the lateral part of upper thoracic aperture.

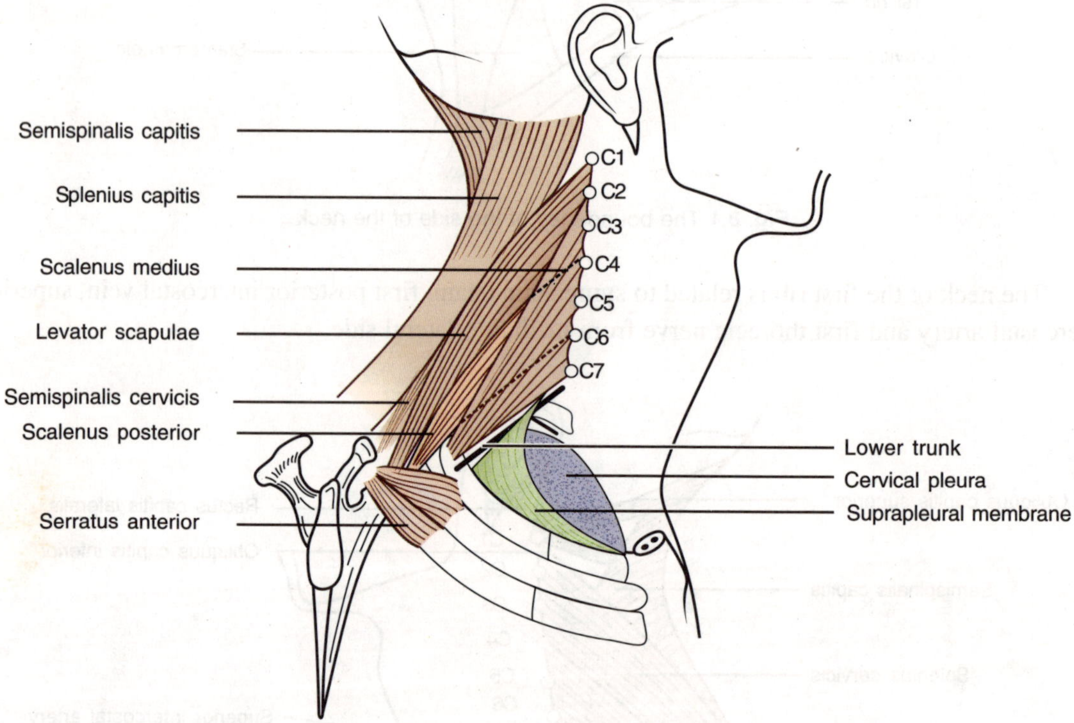

Fig. 8.3 The scalenus medius muscle overlying scalenus posterior and levator scapulae

8.4 The deep posterior branches of cervical plexus

Branches from C2 accompany accessory nerve to supply sternomastoid.

Branches from C3 and C4 go to levator scapulae and also accompany the accessory nerve to supply the trapezius.

Branches from C3 to C7 supply the scalenus medius (not shown).

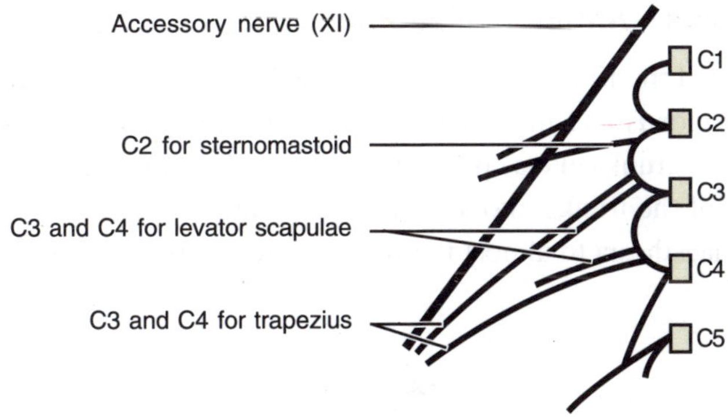

Fig. 8.4 The deep posterior branches of cervical plexus

8.5 Branches of brachial plexus in the neck

There are four nerves.

From the roots:

(i) The dorsal scapular nerve (C5)

(ii) The long thoracic nerve (C5 and C7)

From the trunks:

(i) The suprascapular nerve (C5, 6)

(ii) The nerve to subclavius (C5, 6)

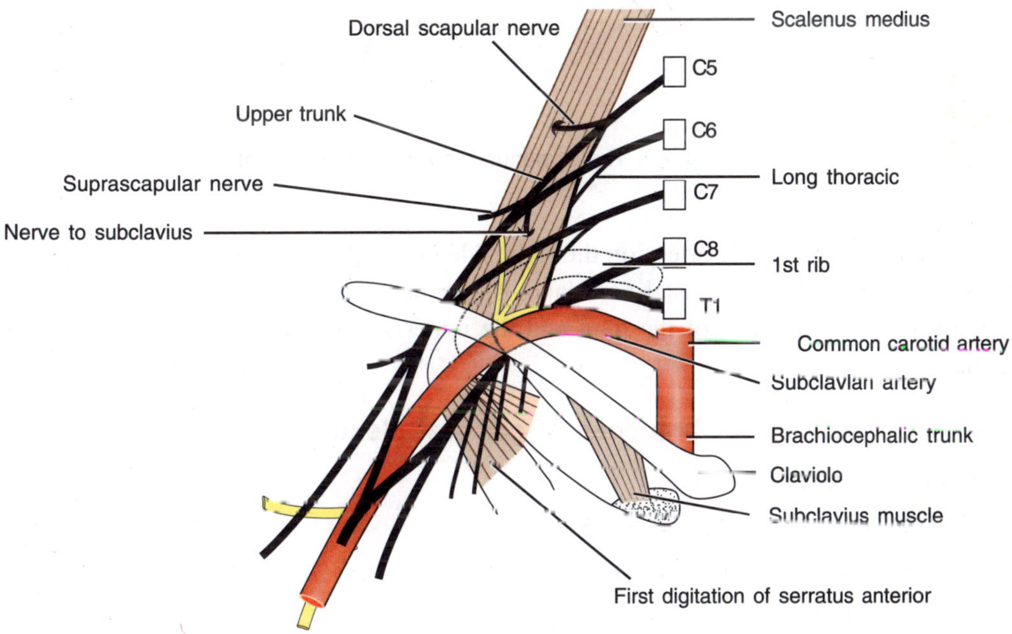

Fig. 8.5 Branches of brachial plexus in the neck: only roots and trunks with their branches are in the neck

8.6 The scalenus medius—Anterior relations

The accessory nerve and the first loop of cervical plexus lie on levator scapulae. The second and third loops of cervical plexus and the three trunks of brachial plexus lie on scalenus medius muscle. By the grouping of the trunks into a compact bundle, the lower trunk is in actual contact with the first rib. This grouping of the trunks into a compact bundle as they cross the first rib makes it simple to secure surgical anaesthesia to almost the whole upper limb by blocking the plexus in this area.

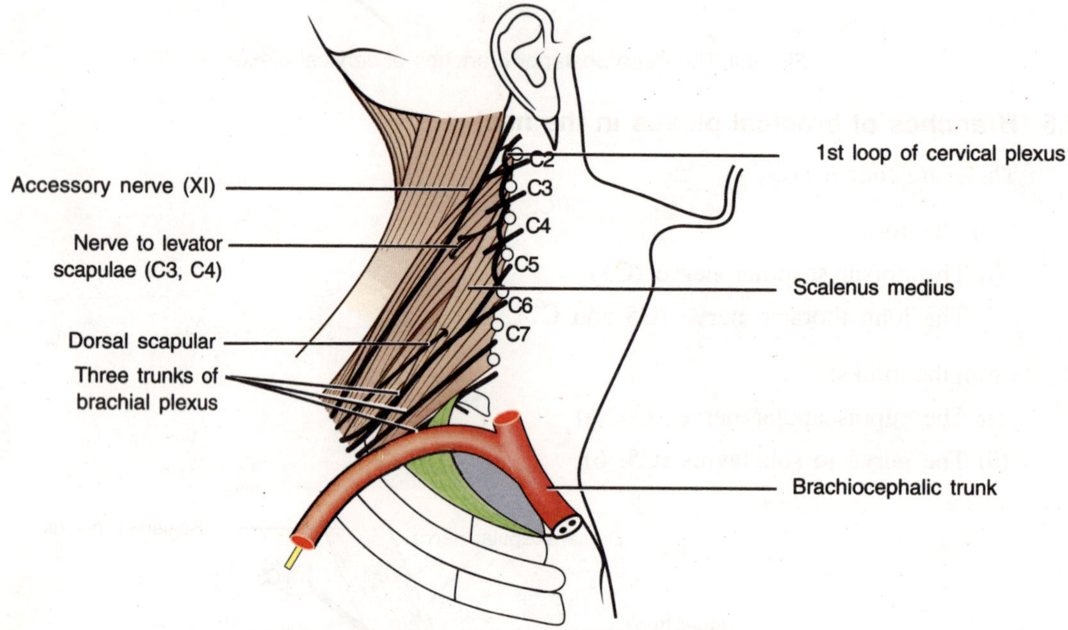

Fig. 8.6 The scalenus medius—Anterior relations

The brachio-cephalic artery on the right side enters the neck from just behind the junction of the sternum with the first costal cartillage. The subclavian artery describes an arch as it passes laterally to cross the apex of the lung and the upper surface of the first rib in front of scalenus medius.

8.7 The deep anterior branches of cervical plexus

These are as follows:

(i) Phrenic nerve (C3, 4 and 5)

(ii) Communicans hypoglossi (C1)

(iii) Superior (C1) and inferior (C2, 3) roots of ansa cervicalis

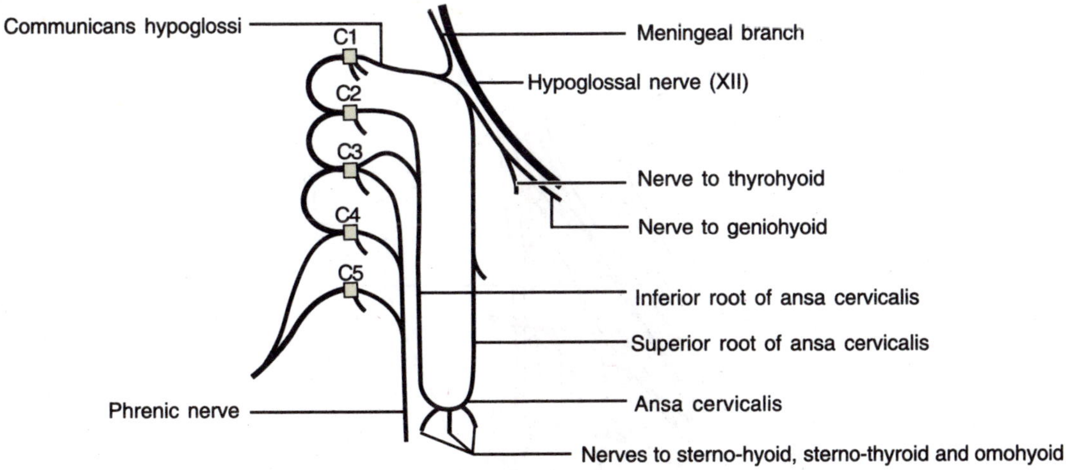

Fig. 8.7 The deep anterior branches of cervical plexus

8.8 The scalene triangle

The scalene triangle is formed between the scalenus medius and scalenus anterior muscles with the scalene groove on the upper surface of the first rib as the base. In the scalenus anterior syndrome, the muscle compresses the subclavian artery and the brachial plexus against the first rib on the fibrous prolongation of the cervical rib.

Scalenus anterior is the key muscle of the root of the neck. Its posterior relations are:

- medial part of scalenus medius
- second part of subclavian artery
- anterior rami of lower cervical nerves
- anterior ramus of first thoracic nerve
- costo-cervical trunk from the second part of subclavian artery

Its medial relations are

- Vertebral artery and thyrocervical trunk from first part of subclavian artery
- Neck of the first rib with its anterior relations (sympathetic trunk, first posterior intercostal vein, superior intercostal artery and ascending branch from T1)
- Common carotid artery

Its lateral relations are

- trunks of brachial plexus
- third part of subclavian artery

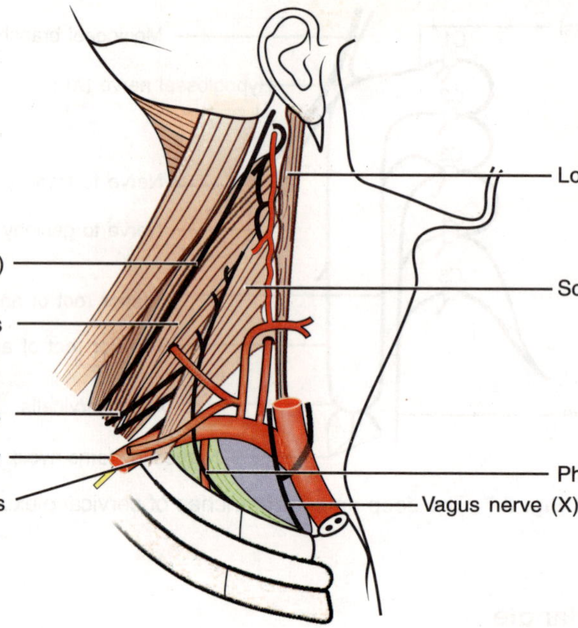

Fig. 8.8 The scalene triangle

8.9 The scalenus anterior—Anterior relations

The scalenus anterior includes the following

- Phrenic nerve
- Ascending cervial artery
- Transverse cervical artery
- Suprascapular artery
- Carotid sheath with contents
- Clavicular head of sternomastoid.

The muscle arises from the anterior tubercles of typical cervical vertebrae (C3 to C6) and is inserted into the medial margin of the first rib posterior to the subclavian vein. The phrenic nerve descends obliquely from its lateral to medial border anterior to it behind the prevertebral fascia. It is crossed horizontally by the transverse cervical and suprascapular vessels in front of the fascia. The ascending cervical artery runs upwards medial to the phrenic nerve.

The cervical part of sympathetic trunk lies on the transverse processes between the scalenus anterior laterally and longus capitis and cervicis medially. The middle ganglion encircles the inferior

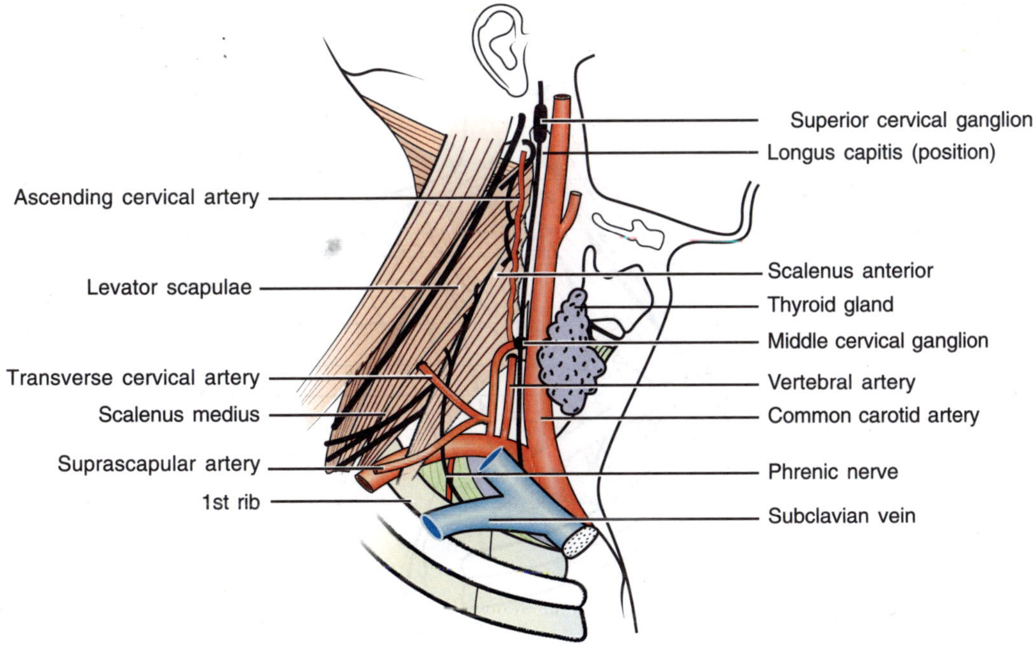

Fig. 8.9 The scalenus anterior—anterior relations

thyroid artery. The common carotid artery lies first in front of the dome of the pleura, then in front of transverse process of C7 but at a distance from it, and finally rests immediately in front of the transverse processes of C6 to C4.

The first part of the vertebral artery lies with its accompanying vein behind the common carotid artery before it enters the foramen transversarium of C6. It is crossed by inferior thyroid artery which passes behind common carotid artery towards the deep aspect of the lower pole of thyroid gland.

The internal thoracic artery runs down on the dome of pleura towards the first costal cartilage and it crosses from medial to lateral side by the phrenic nerve.

8.10 The scalenus anterior—Anterior relations *(Contd.)*

The vagus nerve lies on scalenus anterior between the common carotid artery and the internal jugular vein. It crosses the inferior thyroid artery and subclavian artery in quick succession, finally taking up a position lateral to the brachiocephalic artery. The inferior and superior roots of ansa cervicalis lie anterior to internal jugular vein and common carotid artery, respectively.

Inferior belly of omohyoid passes over the brachial plexus and joins the common tendon which links it to the superior belly deep to sternomastoid.

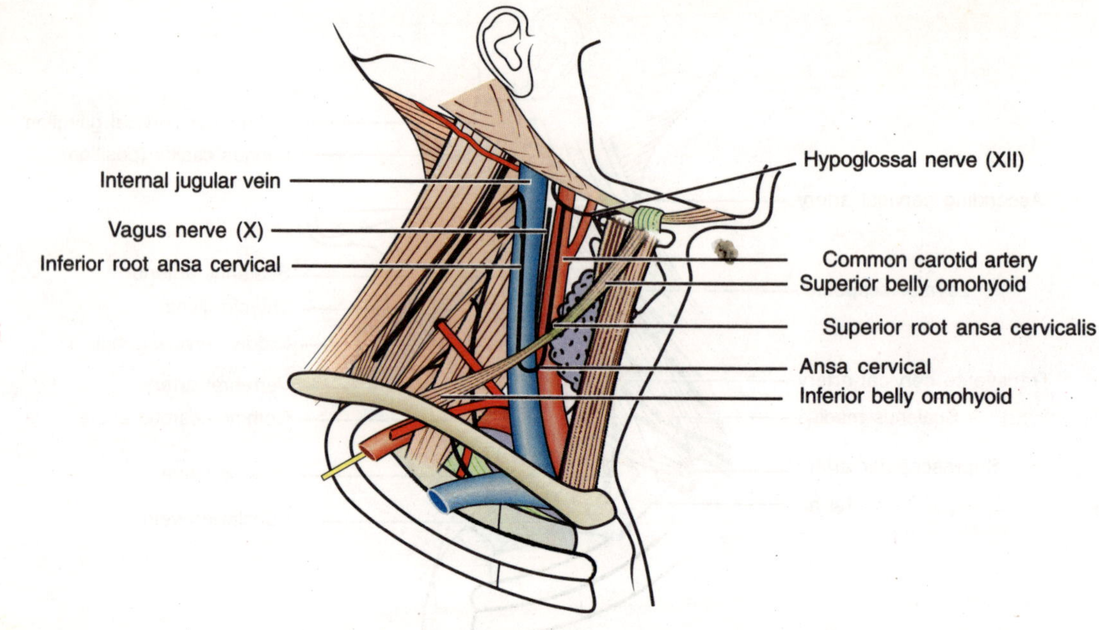

Fig. 8.10 The scalenus anterior—anterior relations (Contd.)

8.11 Reconstruction of the posterior triangle

The anterior and posterior boundaries are formed after trapezius and sternomastoid are positioned. Study the contents of the triangle thus formed.

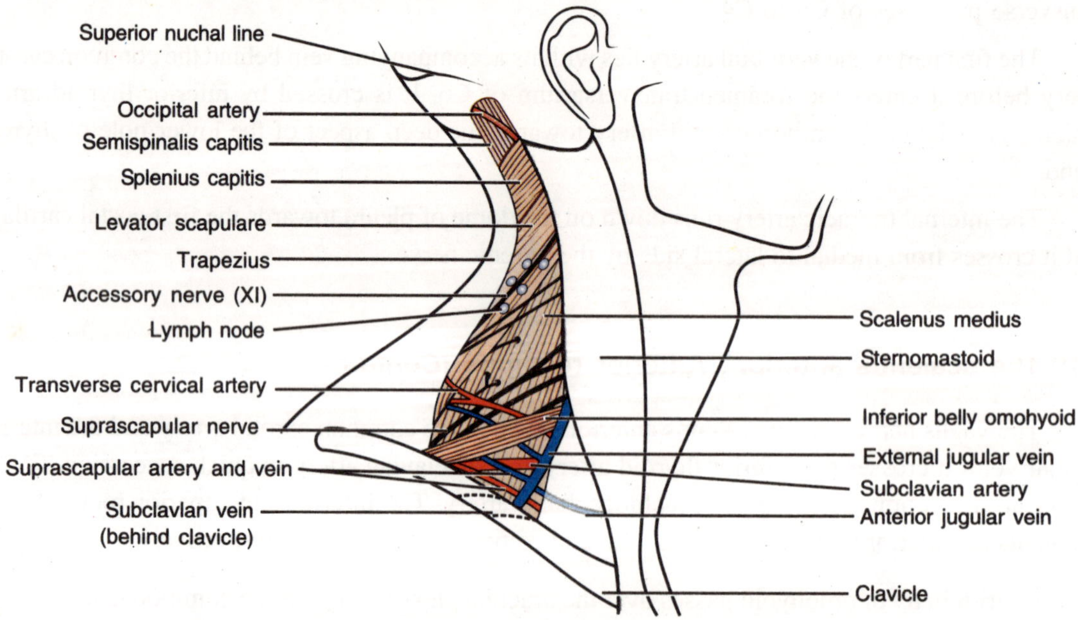

Fig. 8.11 Reconstruction of the posterior triangle by positioning trapezuis and sternomastoid over Fig. 8.10

8.12 The sternomastoid bed

Identify all the structures deep to sternomastoid. In general it can be said that deep to the upper half of the muscle lies the cervical plexus and deep to its lower part lies the carotid sheath over the scalenus anterior muscle with its other relations.

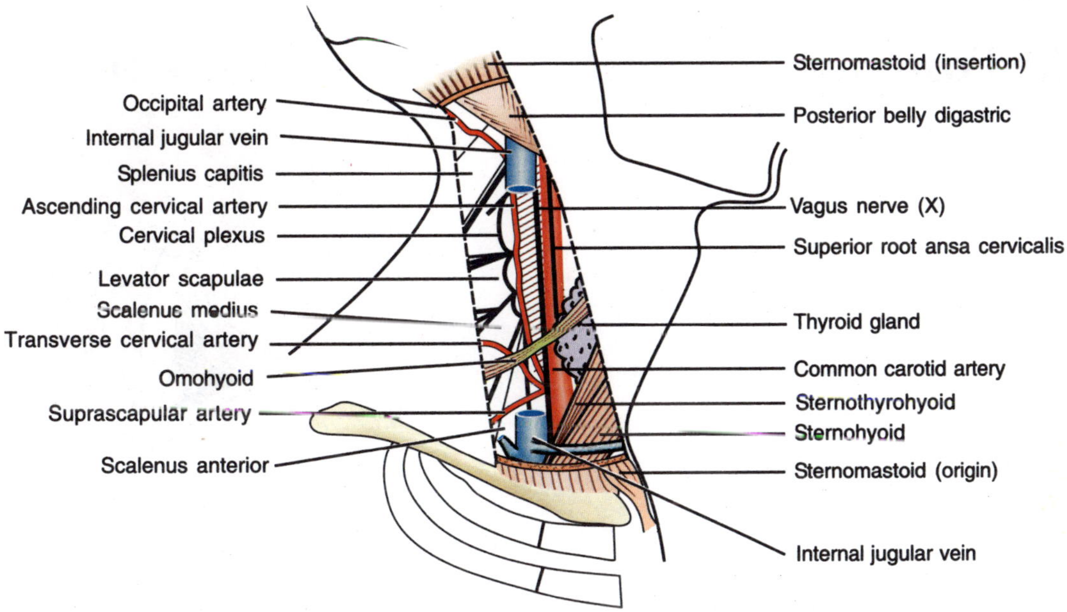

Fig. 8.12 The sternomastoid bed

The Posterior Triangle

Chapter 9

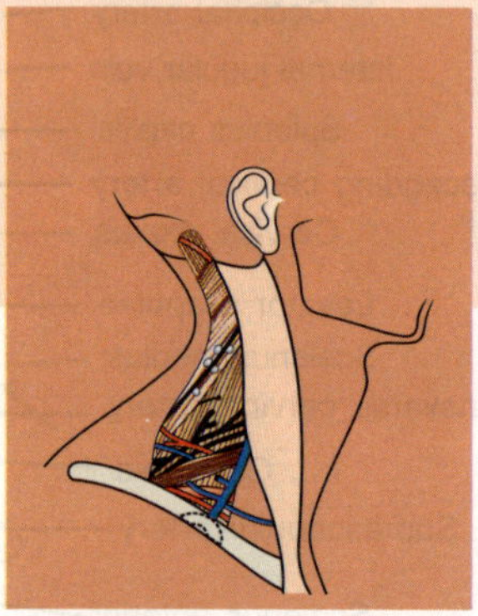

POSTERIOR TRIANGLE FROM SUPERFICIAL STRUCTURES TO DEEPER CONTENTS

9.1 and 9.2 The posterior triangle—Superficial structures

Note the platysma, the cutaneous branches of cervical plexus and the external jugular vein.

Cervical plexus is formed by the upper four cervical nerves (C1 to C4) each of which divides into upper and lower branches except C1. The first cervical nerve joins the upper branch of C2, then the adjoining upper and lower branches fuse, and the lower branch of C4 joins C5 in the formation of brachial plexus. It lies deep to internal jugular vein and sternomastoid muscle in the upper part of the neck.

The four cutaneous branches of cervical plexus emerge at the middle of the posterior border of sternomastoid by piercing the investing deep fascia.

The external jugular vein is formed behind the angle of mandible by the junction of the posterior branch of the retromandibular vein with the posterior auricular vein. It passes vertically downwards in the superficial fascia, deep to the platysma, and pierces the investing fascia 2–3 cm above the calvicle.

The platysma is seen as a broad flat sheet that extends from the deep fascia of the chest to the inferior border of the mandible. It is a part of panniculus carnosus.

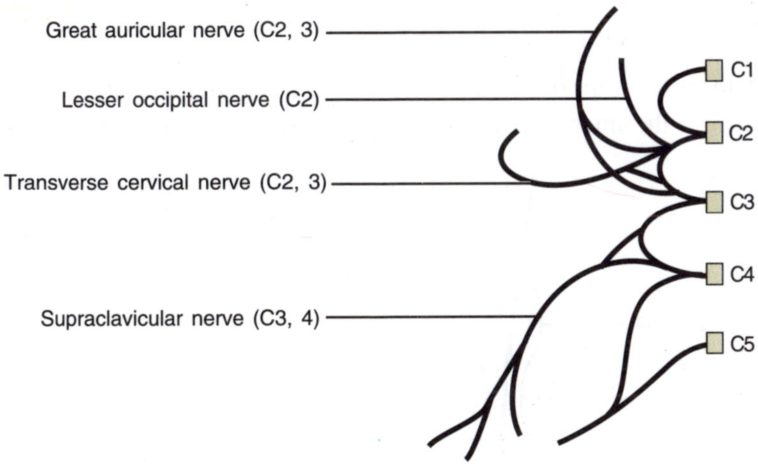

Fig. 9.1 Cutaneous branches of cervical plexus in the posterior triangle

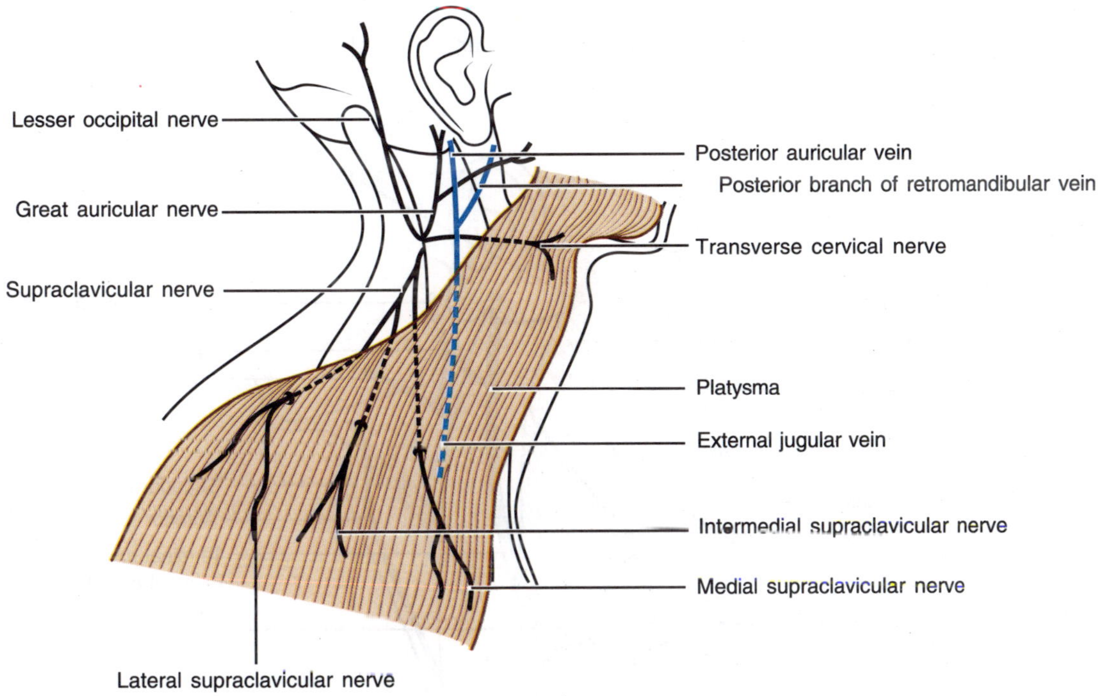

Fig. 9.2 The posterior triangle—Superficial structures

9.3 and 9.4 The posterior triangle—Roof

It is formed by the investing layer of deep fascia.

The fascia encloses the trapezius and sternomastoid and forms the superficial covering of the triangle. It extends from the intermediate third of the clavicle to the superior nuchal line and is

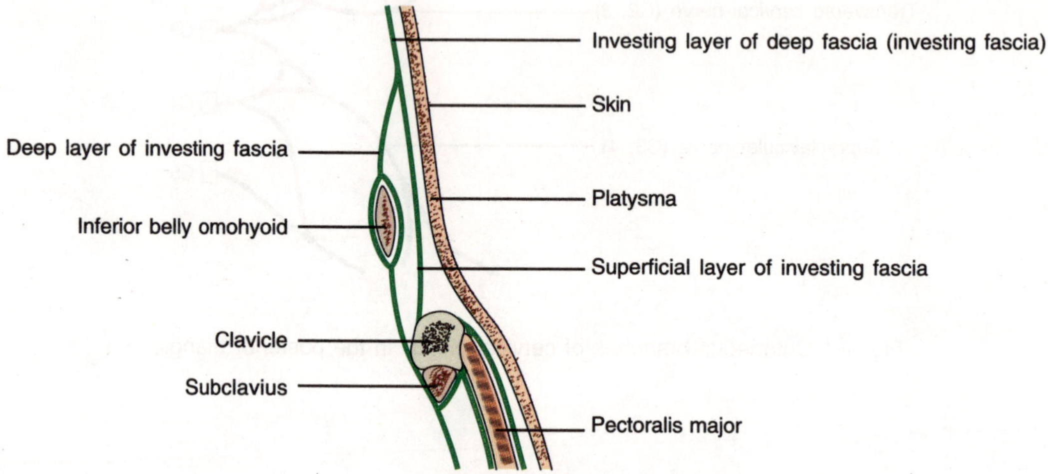

Fig. 9.3 The posterior triangle—Roof

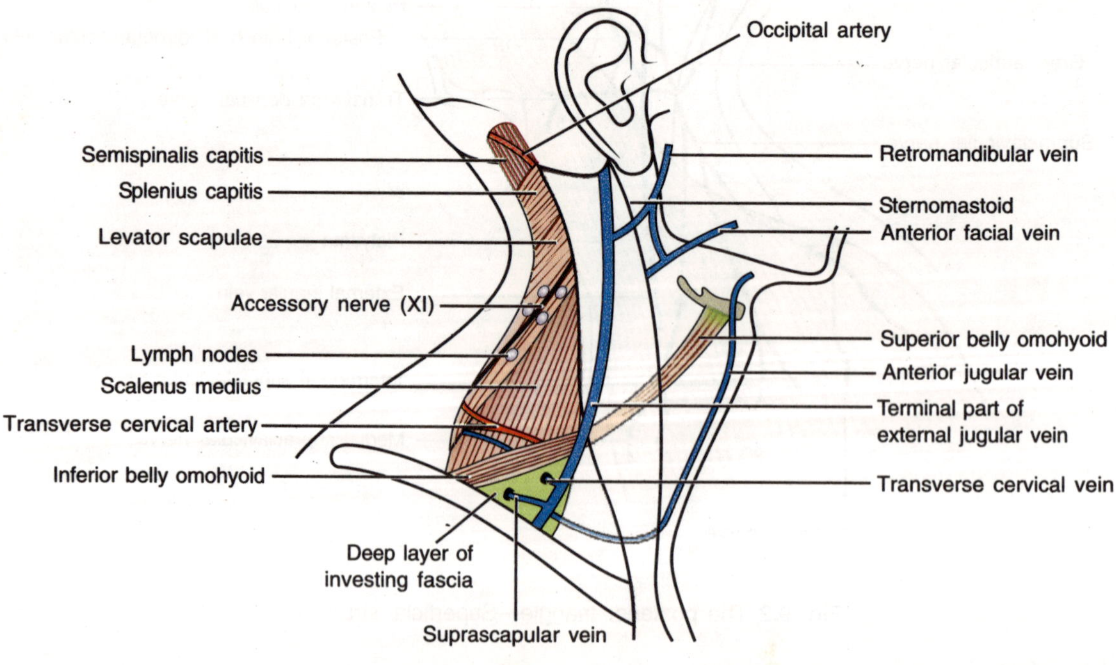

Fig. 9.4 The posterior triangle—Roof

pierced by the cutaneous nerves and external jugular vein. It splits inferiorly. The superficial layer fuses with the clavicle. The deep layer splits to enclose the inferior belly of omohyoid muscle, and passes down behind the clavicle to its lower surface and holds the muscle in position. This sling thus forms a roof for the subclavian or omoclavicular triangle. The gap between the two layers extends medially deep to the sternomastoid, and contains the terminal portions of external jugular and transverse cervical veins and the suprascapular vessels behind the clavicle. The external jugular vein pierces the superficial layer 1 inch above the clavicle, then descends between the two layers and finally pierces the deep layer to end in the subclavian vein which is wholly behind the clavicle.

The accessory nerve is embedded in the investing fascia and lies among the lymph nodes of the posterior triangle.

9.5 The posterior triangle—Boundaries and floor

Boundaries:

Anterior	–	posterior border of sternomastoid
Posterior	–	anterior border of trapezius
Inferior (base)	–	intermediate third of clavicle
Superior (apex)	–	superior nuchal line

Floor from above:

- Semispinalis capitis
- Splenius capitis
- Levator scapulae

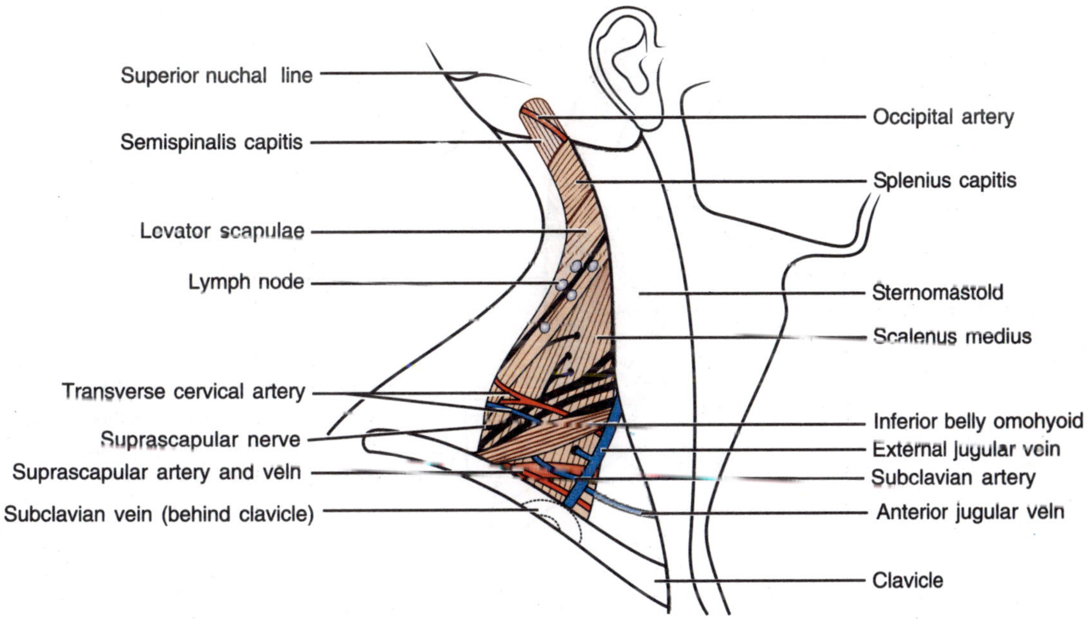

Fig. 9.5 The posterior triangle—Boundaries and floor

– Scalenus medius and
– Sometimes first digitation of serratus anterior

The prevertebral fascia lying infront of the scalenus anterior and medius muscles is known as scalene fascia. It covers the muscles of the floor of posterior triangle and lies in front of cervical plexus, branchial plexus and subclavian artery. As the latter two emerge from behind the scalenus anterior, they take with them a prolongation of this fascia to form the axillary sheath. No such sheath surrounds the axillary and subclavian veins as they lie in front of the prevertebral fascia.

The inferior belly of the omohyoid subdivides the posterior triangle into an upper large omotrapezius area (occipital triangle), containing the occipital artery near the apex, and a lower small omoclavicular area (subclavian triangle), containing the subclavian artery near the base.

The lower or deep portion of the posterior triangle is of great surgical importance since it forms a communicating region between the root of the neck and axillary and mediastinal areas.

9.6 The posterior triangle—Contents

The contents of the posterior triangle are as follows:

(i) Muscle : Inferior belly of omohyoid
(ii) Veins : External jugular, transverse cervical and suprascapular veins
(iii) Arteries : Occipital, subclavian, transverse cervical and suprascapular arteries

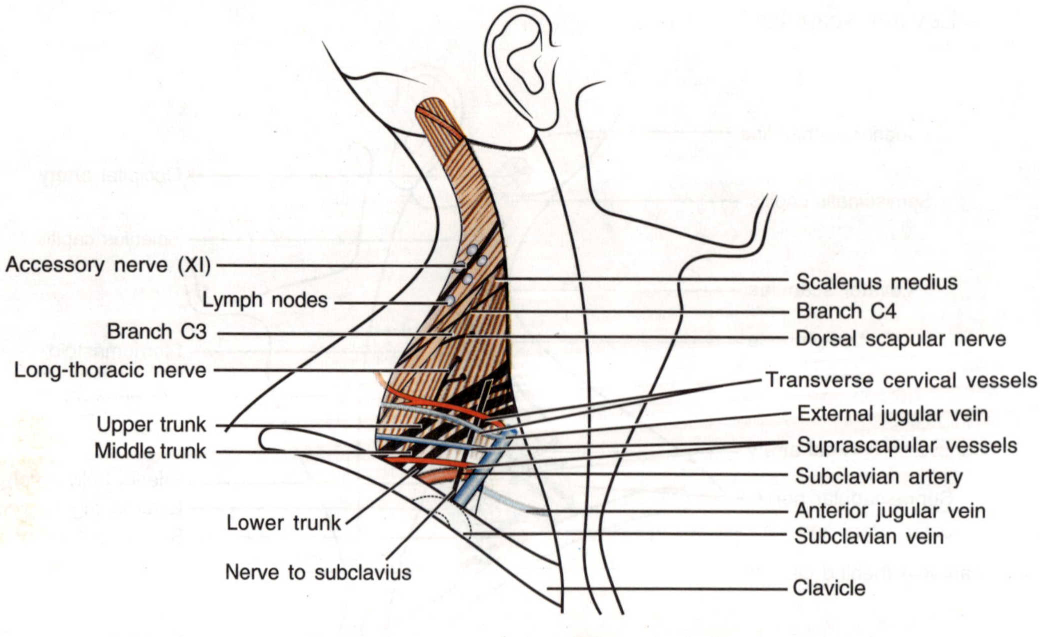

Fig. 9.6 The posterior triangle—Contents (Inferior belly of omohyoid is not shown)

(iv) Nerves : Branches of cervical and brachial plexus and the accessory nerve (XI)

(v) Lymph nodes

The contents should be studied above and below the inferior belly of omohyoid. The structures in subclavian triangle have been exposed by the removal of the inferior belly of omohyoid along with its fascial sling. Note the nerve to subclavius running in front of brachial plexus, subclavian artery and subclavian vein, to enter the back of subclavius muscle.

9.7 The sternomastoid: Deep relations of clavicular head

The clavicular head has been cut close to the clavicle and reflected forwards to expose the scalenus anterior muscle which lies under it and therefore does not belong to the posterior triangle.

In the root of the neck the scalenus anterior is a guide post to which reference has to be made in the description of other structures. Note the phrenic nerve descending over it vertically. Crossing the muscle transversely from above downwards are the inferior belly of omohyoid, the transverse cervical artery, the suprascapular artery, the anterior jugular vein and the subclavian vein.

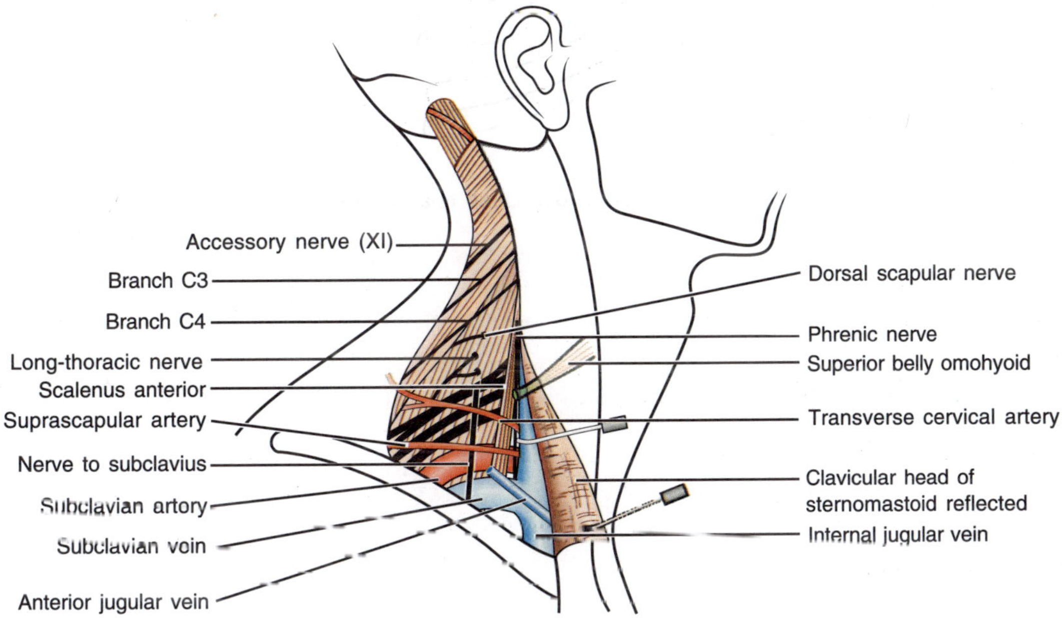

Fig. 9.7 The sternomastoid: Deep relations of clavicular head

9.8 The sternomastoid: Deep relations of both heads

The whole sternomastoid has been removed to show the bed of the muscle with internal jugular vein intact. Note the slender inferior root of ansa cervicalis (C2, C3) curving forward on the lateral surface of the vein. It joins the superior root (C1) from the hypoglossal nerve to form a loop called the ansa cervicalis (C1, C2 and C3) at the level of lower part of larynx to supply sternohyoid, sternothyroid and omohyoid muscles.

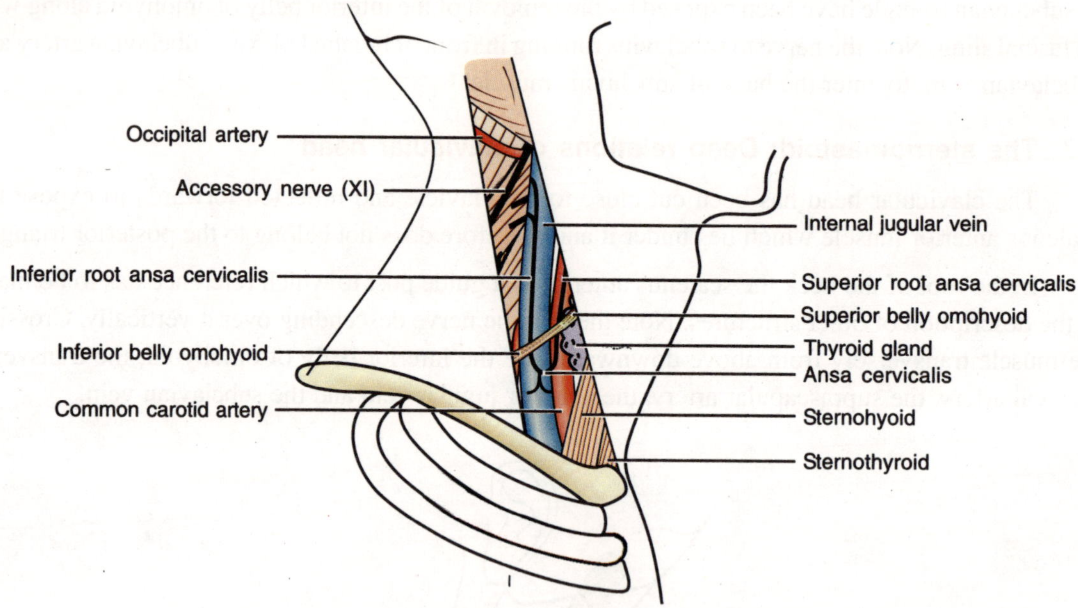

Fig. 9.8 The sternomastoid: Deep relations of both heads

The Anterior Triangle

Chapter **10**

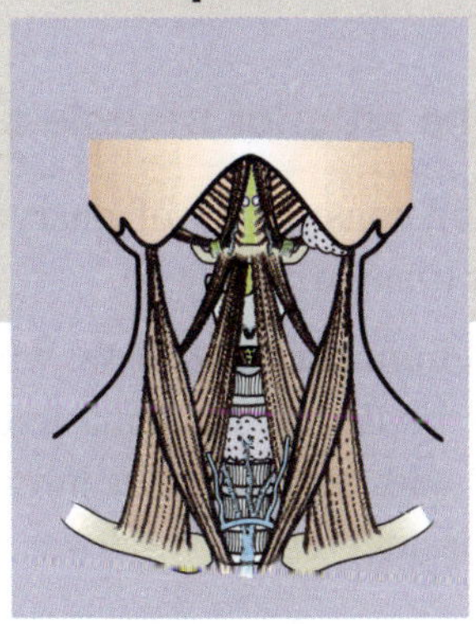

10.1 The anterior triangle: Subdivisions

The anterior triangle is bounded anteriorly by the midline, above by the mandible and posteriorly by the anterior border of strenomastoid. It is subdivided into the following:

(i) The submental triangle in the midline—bounded by the two anterior bellies of digastric on the sides and hyoid bone below. Only half of it is included in one anterior triangle.

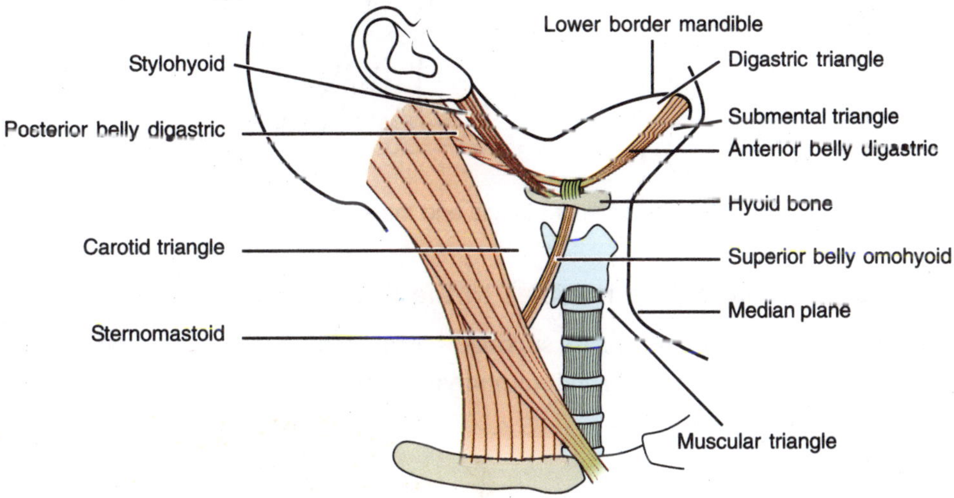

Fig. 10.1 The anterior triangle: Subdivisions

(ii) The digastric triangle—bounded by the anterior belly in front, posterior belly of digastric and strylohyoid behind and lower border of mandible above. The triangle is a part of submandibular region.

(iii) The carotid triangle—bounded by anterior border of sternomastoid posteriorly, posterior belly of digastric superiorly and super belly of omohyoid inferiorly.

(iv) The muscular triangle—bounded by anterior border of sternomastoid posteriorly, by superior belly of omohyoid above and by the median line anteriorly.

10.2 The anterior triangle and the side wall of pharynx

The constrictors of pharynx and mylohyoid are the muscles on which the contents of the anterior triangle mainly lie.

Retromandibular fossa, which is bounded anteriorly by ramus of mandible and posteriorly by anterior border of sternomastoid, is the boundary region between the head and neck. It is allied closely with structures in infratemporal fossa and is in vital connection with structures in the sternomastoid region.

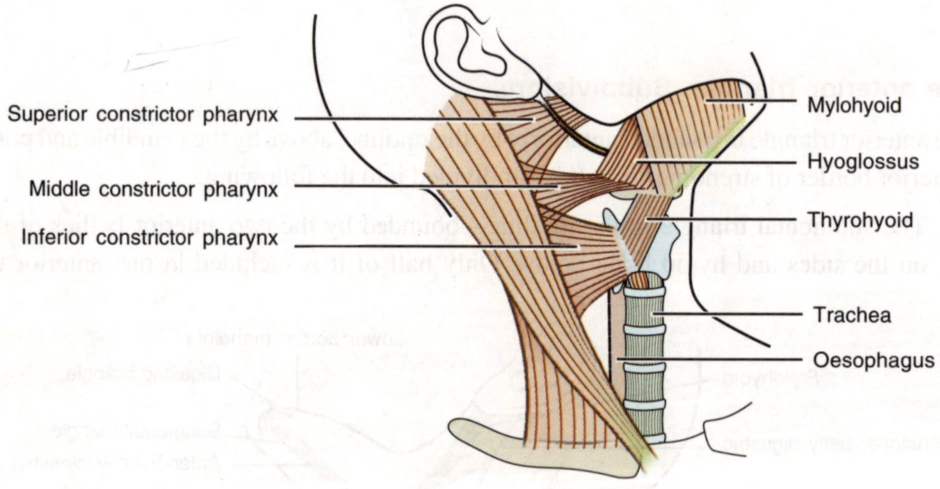

Fig. 10.2 The anterior triangle and the side wall of pharynx

10.3 The anterior triangle: The muscles in the floor of its various subdivisions

Note that the infrahyoid muscles are supplied segeme tally by the ventral rami of the upper three cervical nerves: Thyrohyoid (C1) and sternothyroid, sternohyoid and qmohyoid (C1, C2, C3) from above downwards, respectively.

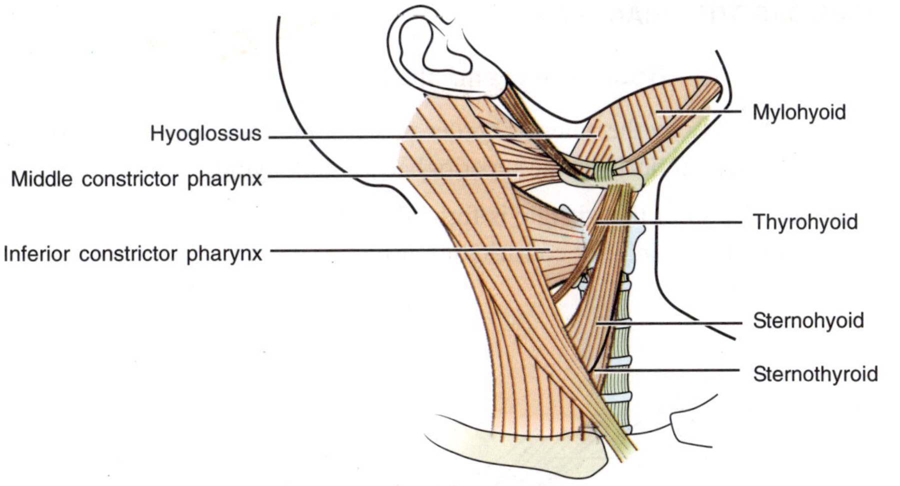

Fig. 10.3 The anterior triangle: The muscles in the floor of its various subdivisions

10.4 The median region of the front of the neck

Note the submental triangle in the suprahyoid region which contains submental lymph nodes and commencement of anterior jugular veins.

In the infrahyoid region in the midline below hyoid bone, the structures from above downwards are median thyrohyoid ligament, laryngeal prominence, cricothyroid ligament, cricoid cartilage, first ring of trachea, isthmus of thyroid gland, jugular arch and inferior thyroid veins.

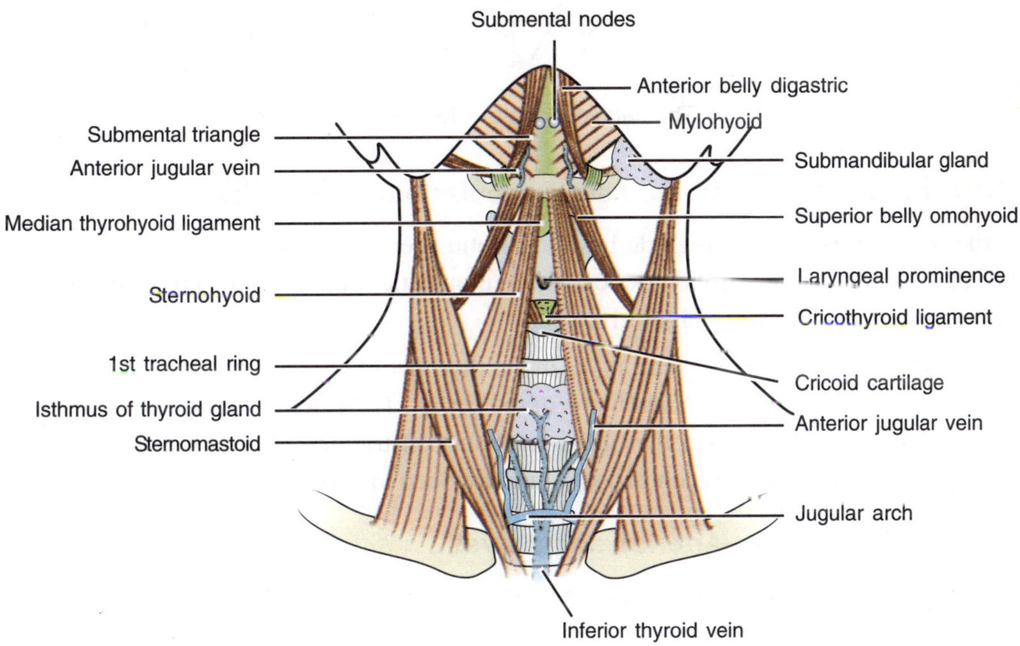

Fig. 10.4 The median region of the front of the neck

BUILDING UP THE CAROTID TRIANGLE

10.5 The carotid triangle—Boundaries and floor

It is bounded posteriorly by the anterior border of sternomastoid, above by posterior belly of digastric and stylohyoid and inferiorly by the superior belly of omohyoid.

The floor or medial wall of the triangle is formed by the hyoglossus and thyrohyoid muscles anteriorly and by the middle and inferior constrictor muscles of pharynx posteriorly.

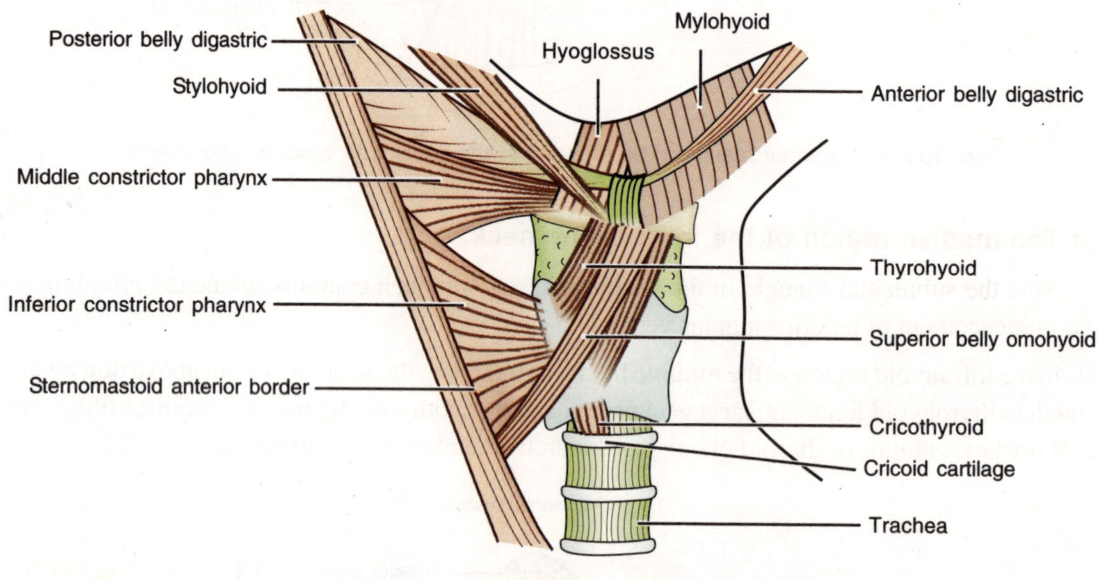

Fig. 10.5 The cartoid triangle—Boundaries and floor

10.6 The carotid triangle and the neurovascular bundle of neck

In the posterior part of the triangle lies the carotid sheath which encloses the internal jugular vein, the vagus nerve and the carotid arteries. The sympathetic trunk is on the posteromedial wall of the sheath and so is not shown in Figure 10.6.

The internal laryngeal nerve (sensory) is in the thyrohyoid interval and pierces the thyrohyoid membrane and supplies the mucous membrane of the larynx. The external laryngeal nerve (motor) is at a lower level and supplies the cricothyroid and inferior constrictor muscle of the pharynx. Both are branches of superior laryngeal branch of vagus and lie deep to carotid arteries.

10.7 The carotid triangle—Arteries and nerves

The external carotid artery arises at the level of upper border of thyroid cartilage and ascends along the side of the pharynx, anteromedial to internal carotid artery. It gives off most of its branches viz., superior thyroid, ascending pharyngeal, lingual, facial and occipital in the carotid triangle.

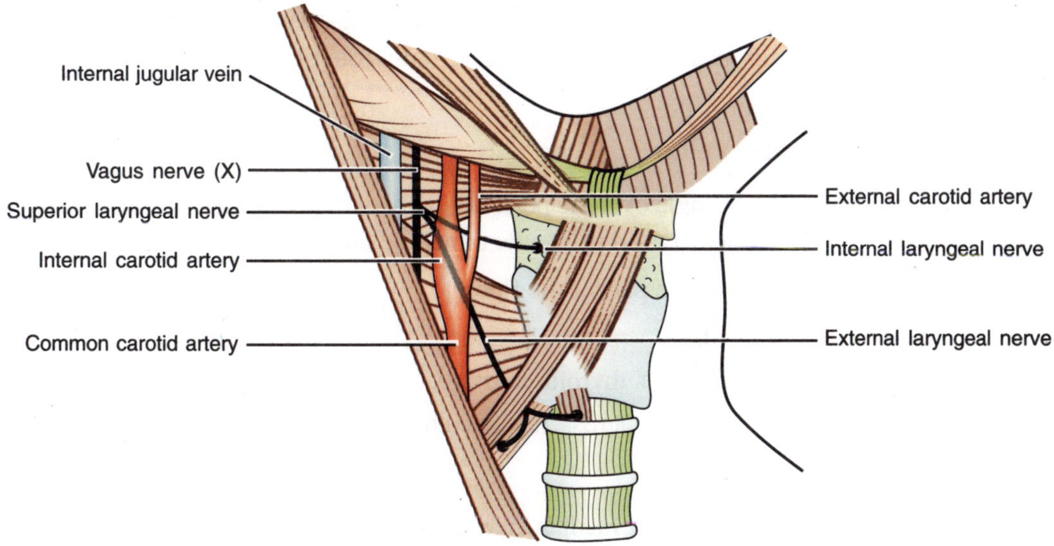

Fig. 10.6 The carotid triangle and the neurovascular bundle of neck

The accessory nerve (XI) runs posteroinferiorly usually superficial to internal jugular vein across the upper angle of the triangle.

The hypoglossal nerve (XII) appears at the lower border of posterior belly of digastric, curves forward round the root of the occipital artery and crosses internal and external carotid arteries and

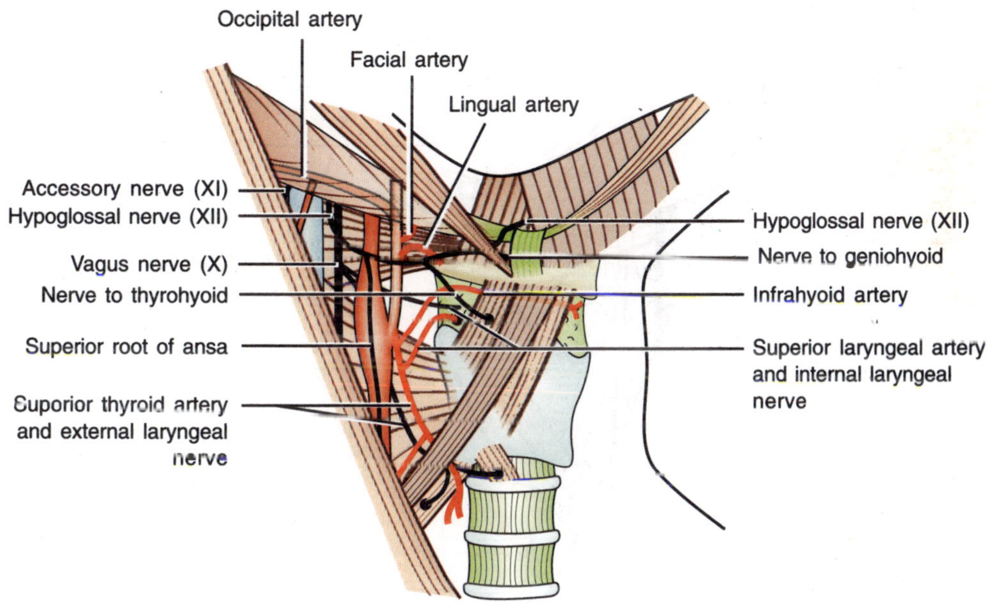

Fig. 10.7 The carotid triangle—Arteries and nerves

loop of lingual artery to disappear deep to the posterior belly of digastric. In the triangle it gives also to the superior root of ansa cervicalis (C1) and the nerve to thyrohyoid (C1).

10.8 The carotid triangle—Veins

The facial vein enters the triangle over the posterior belly of digastric and joins internal jugular vein. The lingual vein and superior thyroid vein enter either the internal jugular vein or facial vein.

Inferior constrictor forms a large part of the floor.

Origin: Side of cricoid cartilage

- Oblique line of the lamina of thyroid cartilage.
- Fine tendonous band thrown across the cricothyroid.

Insertion:

- Fibrous raphe in the posterior median line of the pharynx.

Relations: Laterally

- Thyroid gland.
- Common carotid artery.
- Stemothyroid.

The internal laryngeal nerve and the laryngeal branch of superior thyroid artery run to the thyrohyoid membrane in between its upper border and the inferior constrictor. The external laryngeal nerve pierces its lower part. The recurrent laryngeal nerve and the laryngeal branch of inferior thyroid artery ascend deep to its lower border.

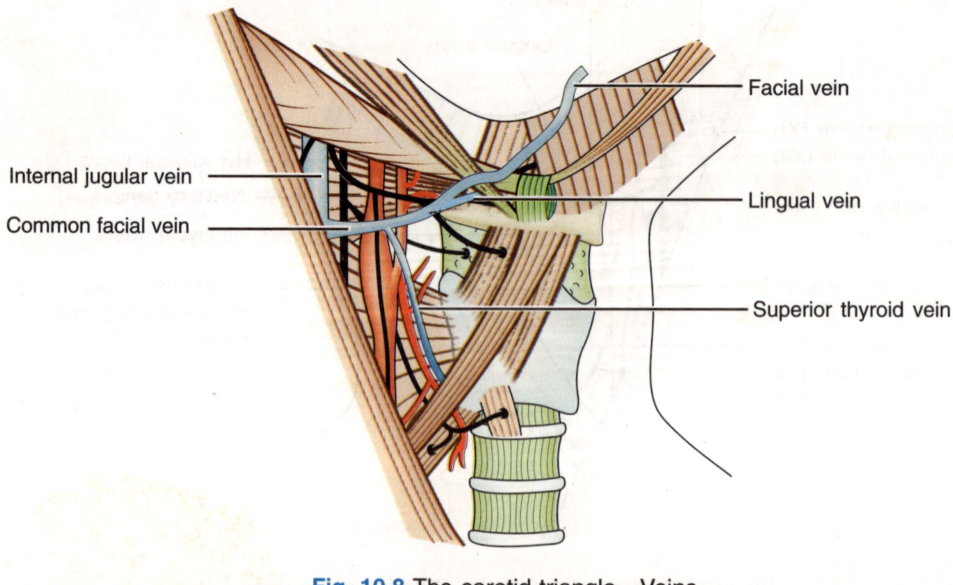

Fig. 10.8 The carotid triangle—Veins

The Cranial Cavity

Chapter 11

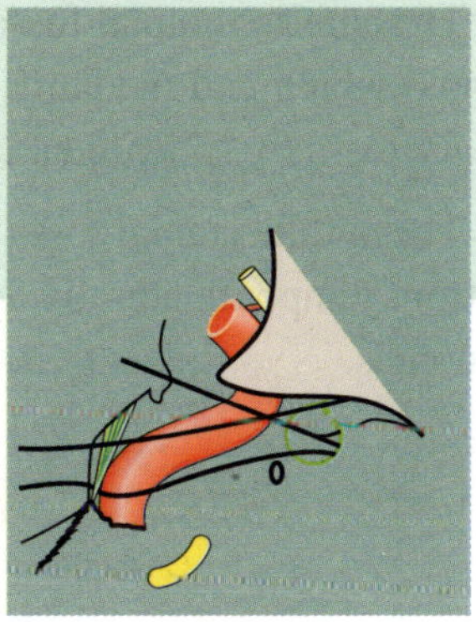

11.1 The skull cap or calvaria

The skull cap forms the roof of the cranial cavity. Internal surface shows coronal, sagittal and lambdoid sutures. In the median plane is sagittal groove lodging superior sagittal sinus by the side of

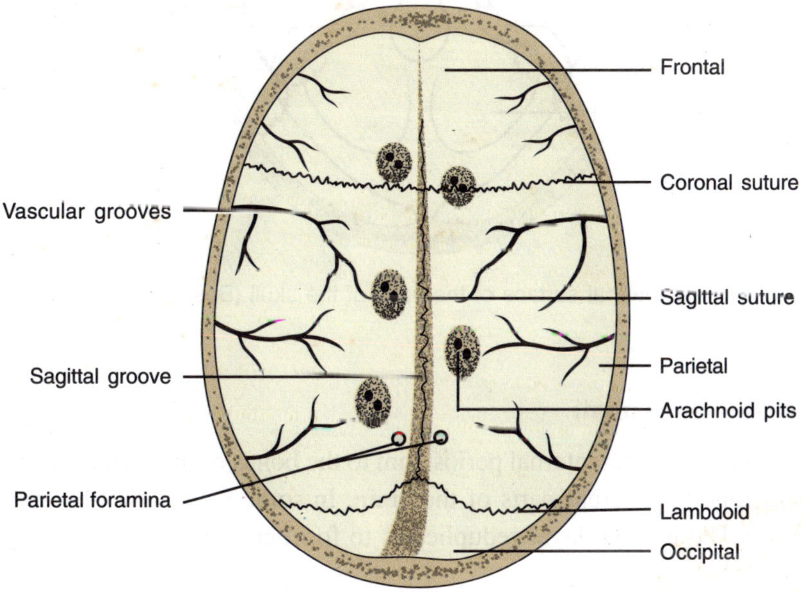

Fig. 11.1 The skull cap or calvaria

which are arachnoid pits. The parietal foramina lie near the posterior part of sagittal suture. Numerous vascular grooves for meningeal vessels and impressions for gyri of brain are present.

11.2 The internal surface of the base of skull (Basis cranii interna)

The internal surface is divisible into three large fossae viz., anterior, middle and posterior cranial fossae, each extending from one side to the other.

The anterior cranial fossa is separated posteriorly from the middle fossa by the lesser wings of sphenoid which end medially in anterior clinoid processes. In the midline it is separated from the pituitary fossa by sphenoidal crest.

The middle cranial fossa is separated posteriorly from the posterior fossa by the superior border of petrous temporal laterally and dorsum sellae medially which has posterior clinoid processes at its lateral ends.

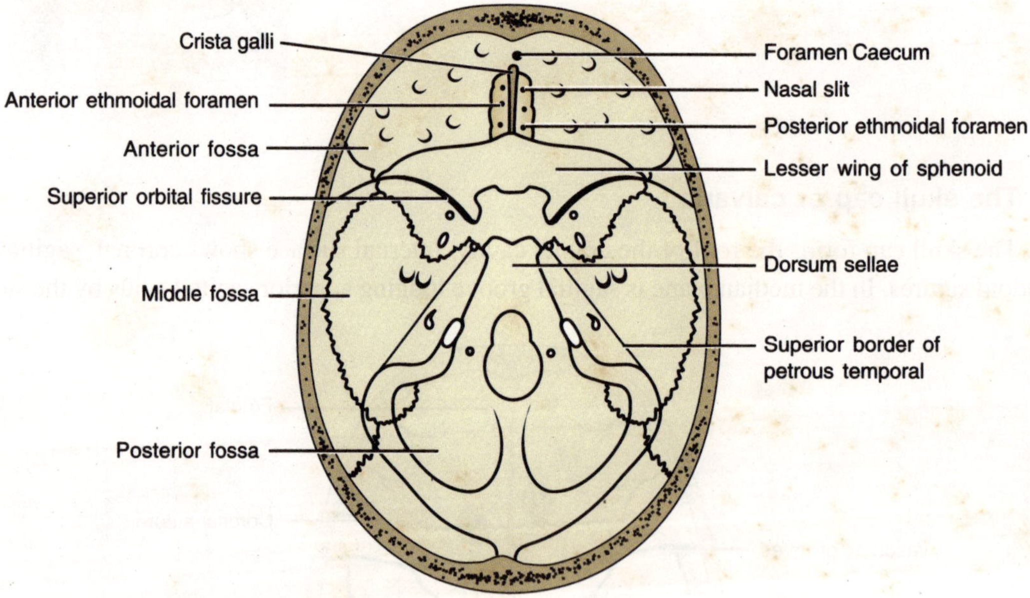

Fig. 11.2 The internal surface of the base of the skull (Basis cranii interna)

11.3 The duramater encephali

The external layer acts as an internal periosteum to the bones of the cranial cavity. The internal layer protects and supports different parts of the brain. In some places the two layers separate to form venous sinuses. The internal layer reduplicates to form curtains between parts of brain or to enclose venous sinuses.

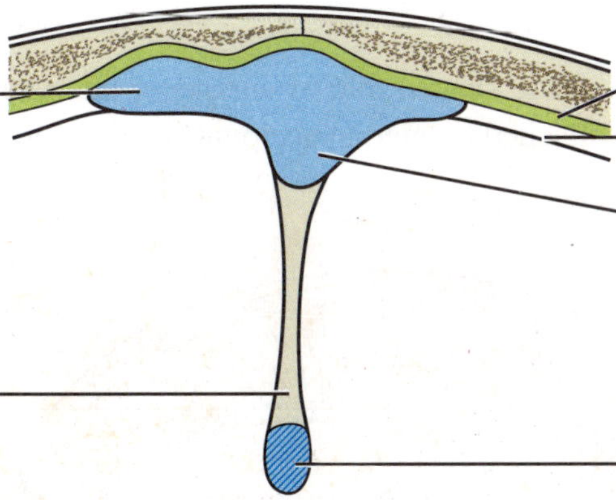

Fig. 11.3 The duramater encephali

11.4 The falx cerebri, tentorium cerebelli and diaphragma sellae

The falx cerebri is a sickle-shaped reduplication of internal layer of duramater which intervenes between medial surfaces of two cerebral hemispheres. The superior sagittal sinus runs along its upper attached border, the inferior sagittal sinus along its lower free border and the straight sinus along its line of attachment to tentorium cerebelli.

The tentorium cerebelli is a semilunar reduplication of internal layer of duramater which roofs in the posterior cranial fossa and intervenes between the cerebellum and occipital lobes of the brain. It is attached from the apex of one petrous temporal bone to the other along its upper borders and horizontally along the inner surface of each side of the skull to the internal occipital protuberance. The superior petrosal sinus runs in its attachment to petrous temporal bone and the transverse sinus runs in its attachment to the inner surface of the skull. Its free margin is U-shaped and can be traced to anterior clinoid processes after binding the tentorial notch for the passage of midbrain.

The diaphragma sellae is the fold roofing over the pituitary fossa with an aperture for infundibulum.

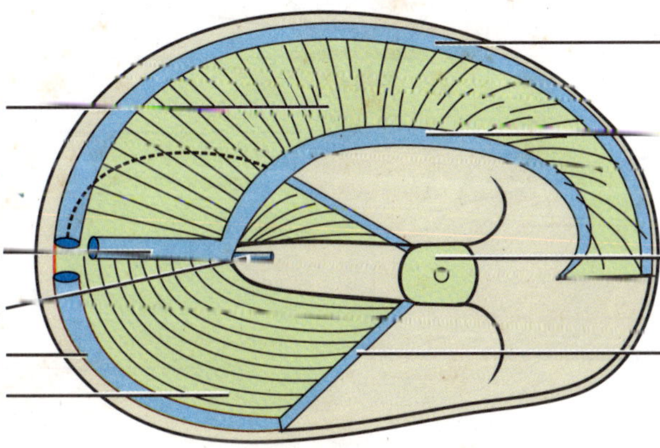

Fig. 11.4 The falx cerebri, tentorium cerebelli and diphragma sellae

11.5 The falx cerebelli

The falx cerebelli is a small sickle-shaped fold of duramater intervening posteriorly between the two halves of cerebellum. It is attached to internal occipital crest posteriorly and to the tentorium cerebelli superiorly.

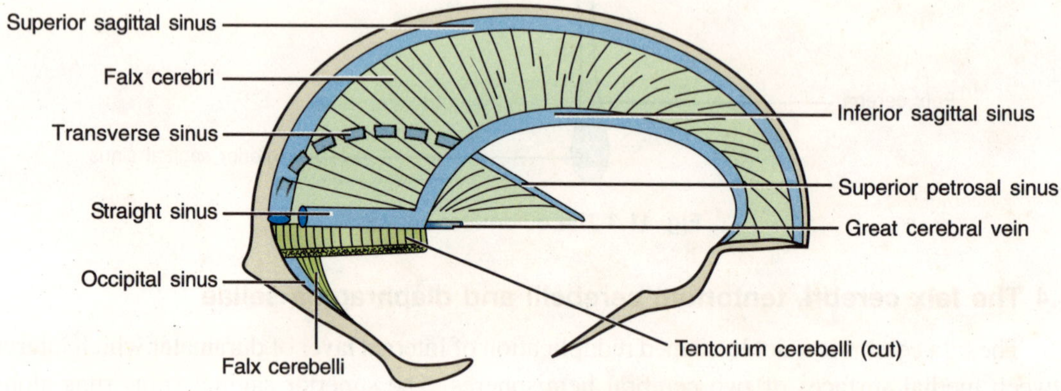

Fig. 11.5 The falx cerebelli as seen in sagittal section

11.6 The tentorium cerebelli—superior view

The straight sinus is usually continued as left transverse sinus while the superior sagittal sinus turns to right to form the right transverse sinus.

Each transverse sinus joins the superior petrosal sinus to form a sigmoid sinus.

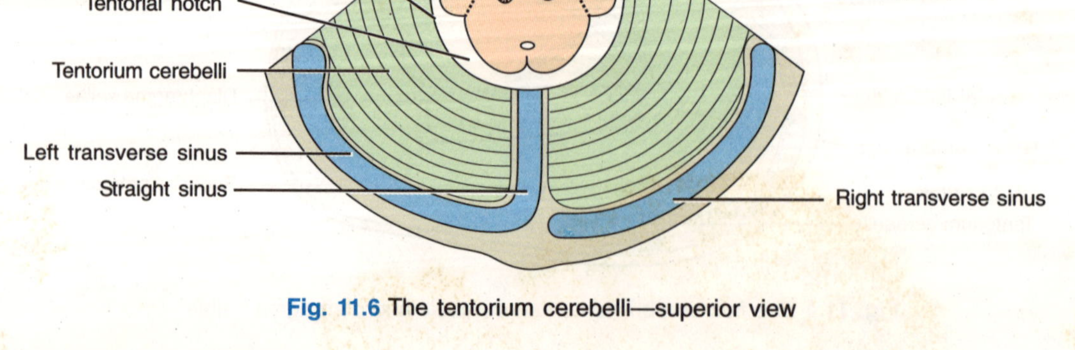

Fig. 11.6 The tentorium cerebelli—superior view

11.7 The venous sinuses of the posterior cranial fossa

The sigmoid sinus commences ast the termination of the transverse sinus and forms a deep groove on the inner surface of the mastoid bone. It curves downwards and then forwards to the posterior margin of the jugular foramen. It receives the superior petrosal sinus at its upper end and the occipital sinus at its lower end.

The posterior cranial fossa is formed in small part by the petrous temporal bone and mainly by the occipital bone. The foramen magnum is prominent in the midline of the fossa. On either side of the margin of this foramen is the hypoglossal canal.

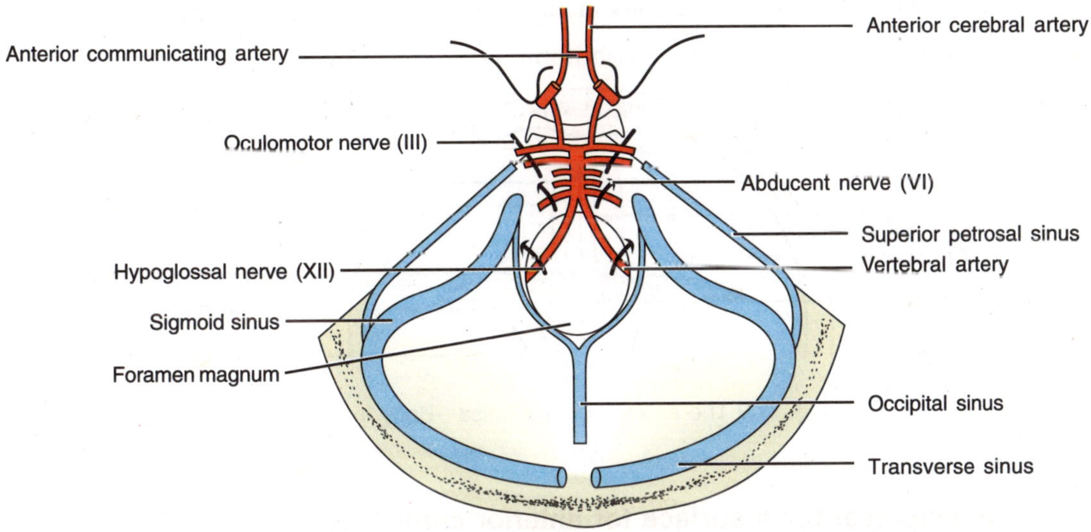

Fig. 11.7 The venous sinuses of the posterior cranial fossa

11.8 The confluence of sinuses

The posterior part of the cranial cavity behind the plane passing through the posterior part of foramen magnum is shown. The superior sagittal sinus, the straight sinus and two transverse sinuses may meet in the confluence of sinuses at the internal occipital protuberance.

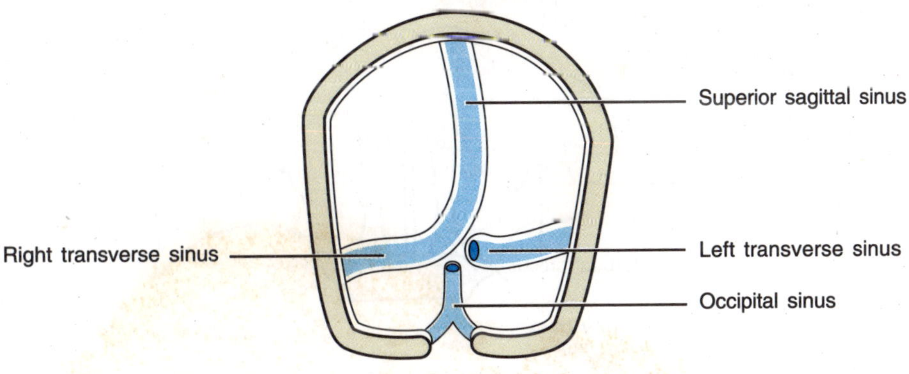

Fig. 11.8 The confluence of sinuses

The occipital sinus is a long and narrow sinus. One end joins the beginning of the transverse sinus at the internal occipital protuberance and from there it first descends in the falx cerebelli and then curves around the margin of the foramen magnum to join the sigmoid sinus near its termination.

11.9 The anterior cranial fossa—Bony features

The anterior carnial fossa is floored mainly by the orbital plates of the frontal, but behind these plates are the lesser wings of sphenoid and between them is the cribriform plate of the ethmoid.

In the median plane is the frontal crest and crista galli for the attachment of falx cerebri with foramen caecum in between. The jugum sphenoidale connects the two lesser wings. The sharp posterior border of lesser wing ends medially in the anterior clinoid process.

Note the smaller foramina related to cribriform plate.

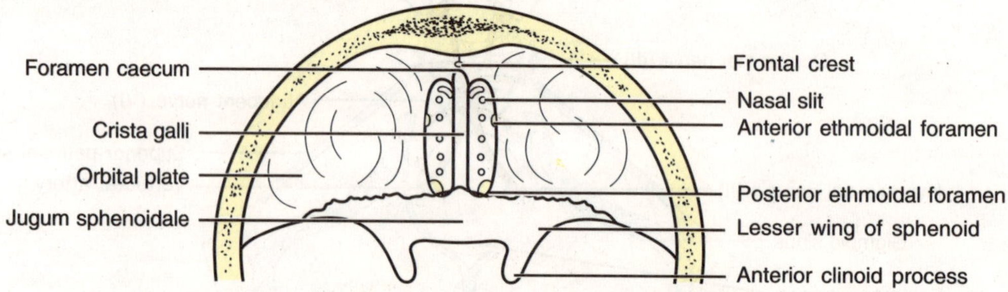

Fig. 11.9 The anterior cranial fossa—Bony features

11.10 The reciprocal brain surface for anterior cranial fossa

The olfactory bulbs and tracts are supported by the cribriform plate. The orbital surface of the cerebral hemisphere lies on the orbital plate of frontal.

Fractures of the anterior cranial fossa may damage the olfactory bulb and lead to blood and cerebrospinal fluid leaking into the nose and the orbit.

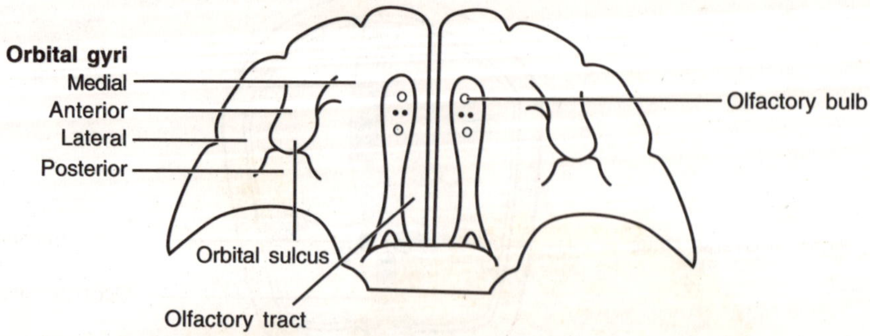

Fig. 11.10 The reciprocal brain surface for anterior cranial fossa

11.11 The middle cranial fossa—Bony features

The middle cranial fossa has the shape of a butterfly with a small median 'body' and two lateral concave 'wings'.

(i) The median 'body' has optic canal; sella turciea (Turkish Saddle) which has three parts; tuberculum sellae—pommel of the saddle; hypophyseal fossa—seat of the saddle; dorsum sellae—back of the saddle, with posterior clinoid processes at lateral angles.

Note the carotid groove on the side of the body of sphenoid.

(ii) The lateral wings are formed by

(a) The greater wing of sphenoid with a crescent made up of following seven foramina of which the first four are always present: Superior orbital fissure; foramen ovale; foramen rotundum; foramen spinosum; foramen lacrimalis; foramen vesalii (emissary sphenoidal foramen); canaliculus innominatus.

(b) The squamous part of temporal bone has only one feature—groove for middle meningeal artery and its branches.

(c) The petrous part of temporal bone has seven features.

The trigeminal impression for trigeminal ganglion; the arcuate eminence produced by anterior semicircular canal; the two hiatuses—for greater and lesser petrosal nerves; the two grooves—for the above two nerves; the remains of petro-squamosal fissure; the legmen tympani root of middle ear; the roof of internal carotid canal.

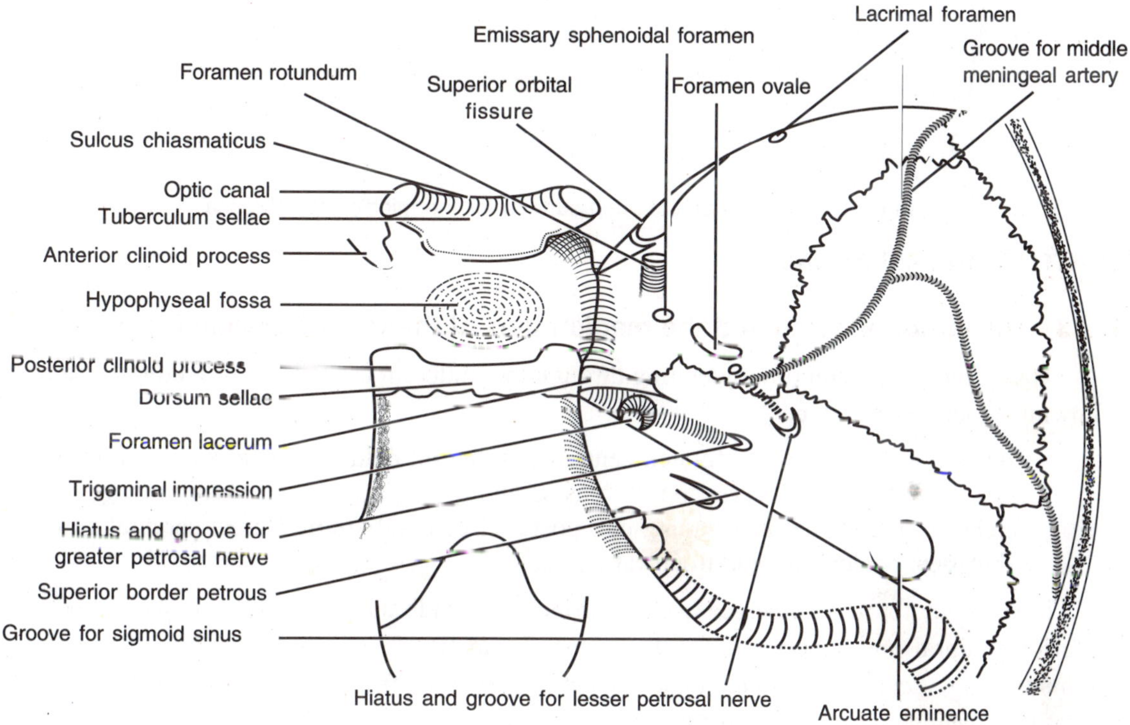

Fig. 11.11 The middle cranial fossa—Bony features

Also present in the middle cranial fossa is the foramen lacerum bounded by the body of the sphenoid, the attachment of the greater wing, the apex of petrous temporal bone and the basi-occiput.

11.12 The reciprocal brain surface for the middle cranial fossa

The interpeduncular fossa, adjacent regions and circle of Willis are related to the median part of the fossa.

The inferior surface of the temporal lobe is related to the lateral part of the fossa. Identify the structures in Figure 11.12.

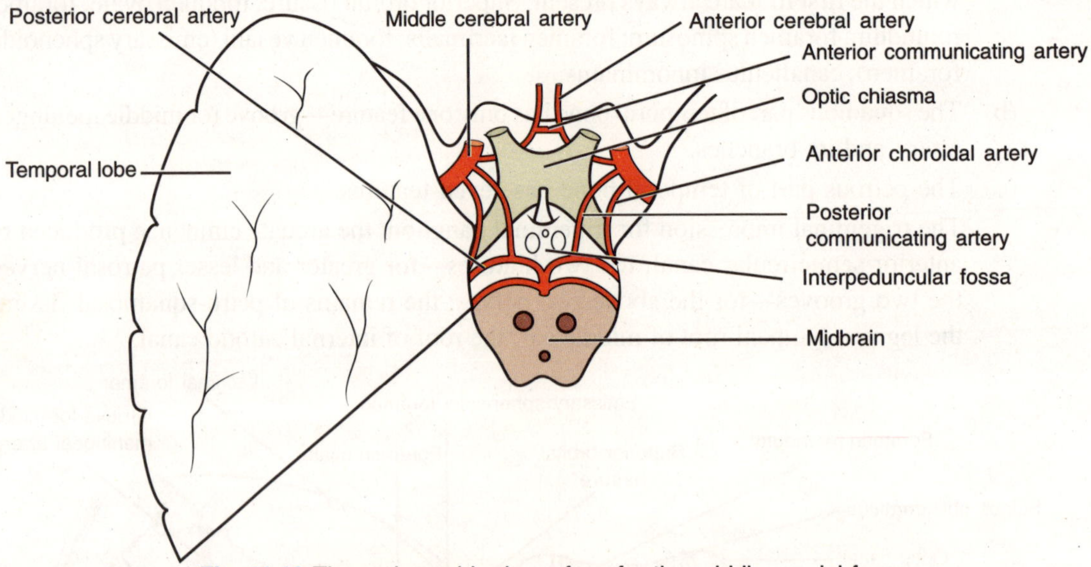

Fig. 11.12 The reciprocal brain surface for the middle cranial fossa

CONTENTS AND RELATIONS

11.13 The tentorial notch and the median part of the middle cranial fossa

After removal of cerebrum by cutting through the midbrain at the level of tentorial notch, the following structures are seen.

> The diaphragma sellae perforated centrally by the infundibulum; the arteries forming the circle of Willis; optic nerves, optic chiasma and optic tracts; basilar artery giving superior cerebellar arteries before dividing into posterior cerebral arteries; great cerebral vein with tributaries; oculomotor and trochlear nerves.

The oculomotor nerve emerges from the front of the midbrain, passes antero-laterally between posterior cerebral and superior cerebellar arteries and lies below and lateral to the posterior communicating artery. It crosses the under aspect of optic tract from medial to lateral side and then pierces the triangular area of duramater in the roof of cavernous sinus. Uncus lies above and lateral to it.

The trochlear nerve emerges from the dorsal surface of lower midbrain, curves forward round the side of it and passes anteriorly between the posterior cerebral and superior cerebellar arteries. It is medial to and below the free margin of tentorium cerebelli and pierces it through a small aperture hidden under the free margin where it crosses the petrous temporal.

The trigeminal ganglion, maxillary nerve and temporal pole form lateral relations of cavernous sinus.

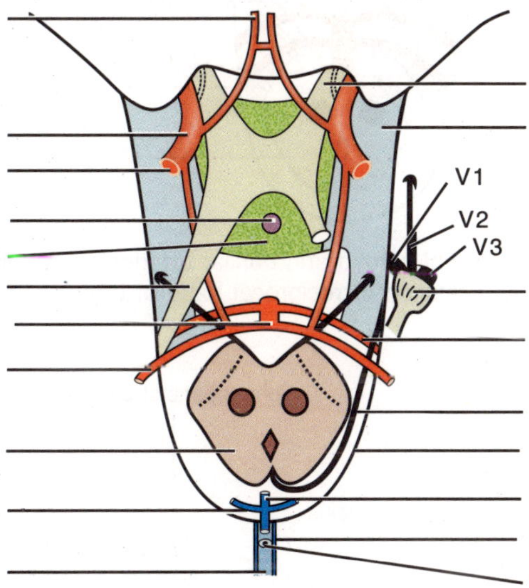

Fig. 11.13 The tentorial notch and the median part of the middle cranial fossa

11.14 The internal carotid and basilar arteries with their branches in relation to reciprocal base of brain, i.e., interpeduncular fossa

Note the three superior relations of cavernous sinus viz., the internal carotid artery, optic tract and the uncus.

11.15 The cavernous sinus—Extent and connections

The cavernous sinus extends from medial end of superior orbital fissure to the apex of petrous temporal. The connections are as follows:

Anteriorly	–	Ophthalmic veins and spheno-parietal sinus
Posteriorly	–	Superior and inferior petrosal sinuses
Medially	–	Intercavernous sinuses
Superiorly	–	Superficial middle cerebral vein and inferior cerebral veins
Inferiorly	–	Emissary vein passing through foramen of Vesalius, foramen ovale and Carotid canal connects it with pharyngeal venous plexus

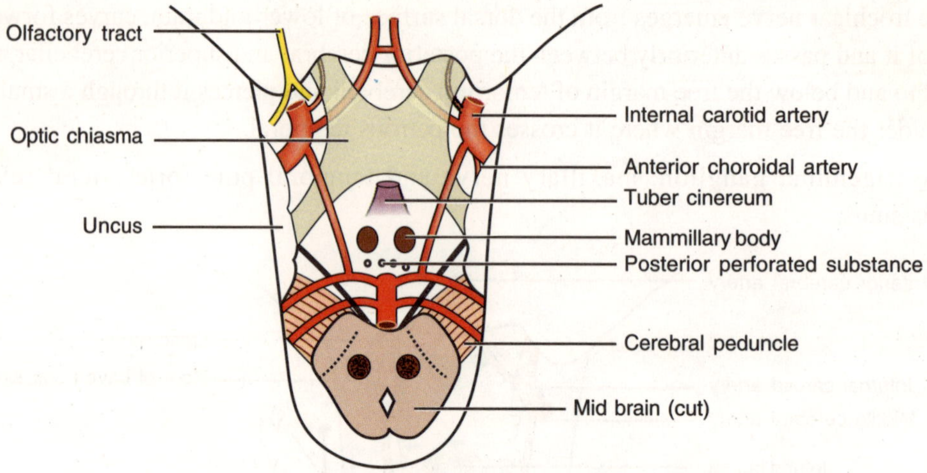

Fig. 11.14 The internal carotid and basilar arteries with their branches in relation to reciprocal base of brain

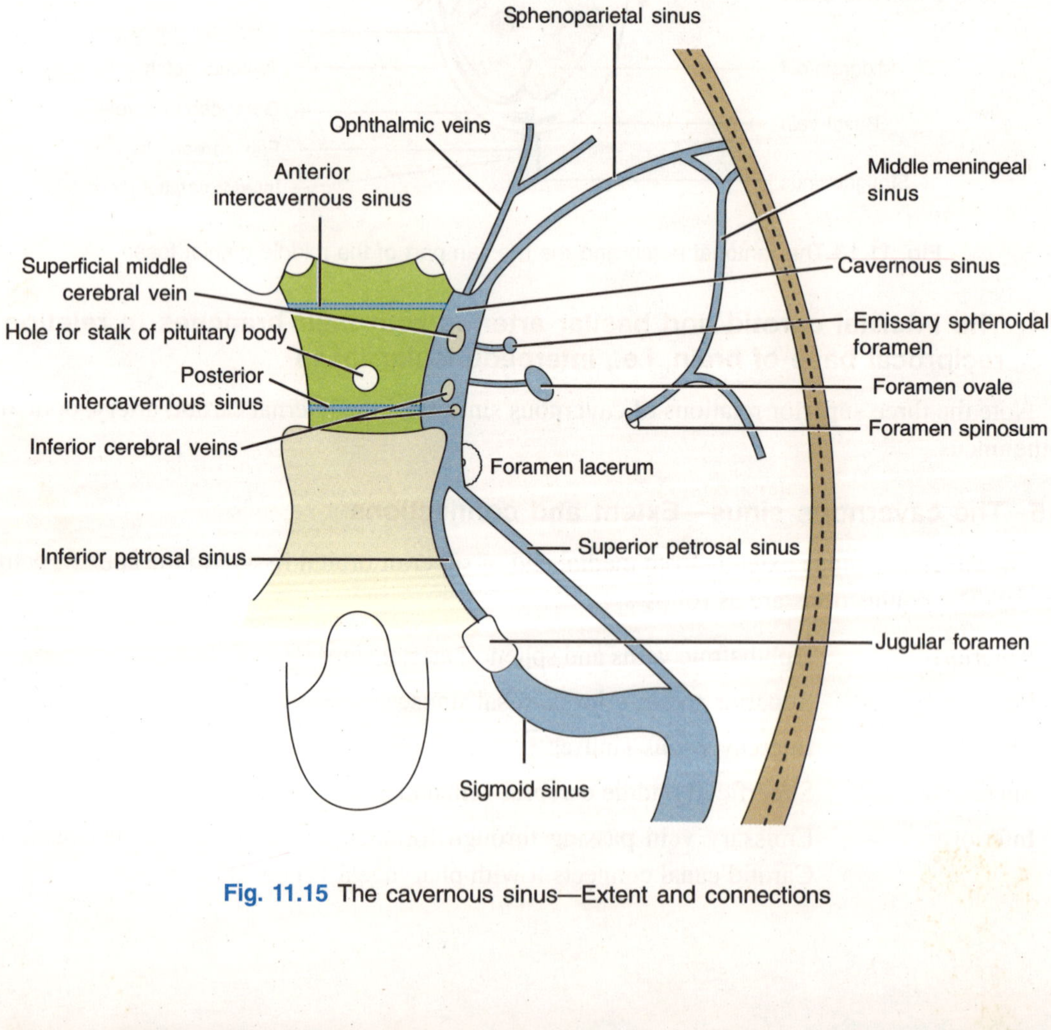

Fig. 11.15 The cavernous sinus—Extent and connections

11.16 The intracranial course of abducent nerve

In the posterior cranial fossa, the abducent nerve passes upwards and forwards and slightly laterally between the pons and the occipital bone. It is crossed Ventrally by the anterior inferior cerebellar artery.

It then pierces the duramater at the back of the basilar portion of occipital bone, crosses the inferior petrosal sinus and runs almost vertically up the back of the petrous temporal near its apex. Arriving at the sharp upper border of the bone, it bends forwards practically at a right angle under the petro-sphenoidal ligament of Gruber and under the superior petrosal sinus to enter the cavernous sinus by an opening which is known as Dorello's canal.

The trigeminal ganglion lies in a bony fossa at the front of the apex of the petrous temporal, and below this covers that part of the foramen lacerum which overlies the internal carotid artery and greater petrosal nerve. To its medial side is the cavernous sinus with its contents.

The ophthalmic division of the trigeminal comes off from the medial and upper part of the convex anterior border of the ganglion and runs forwards in the lateral wall of the cavernous sinus.

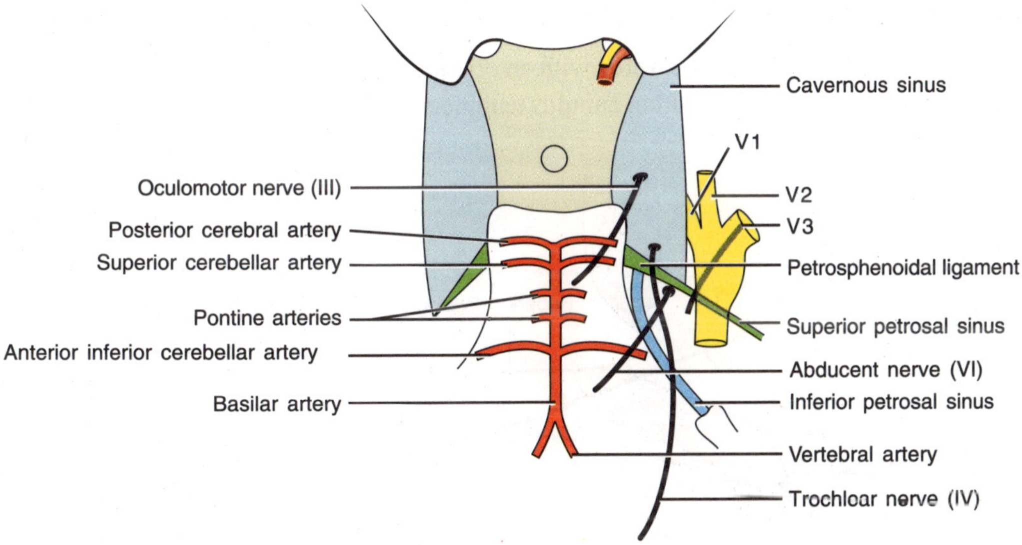

Fig. 11.16 The intracranial course of abducent nerve

BUILDING UP THE LATERAL RELATIONS OF INTERNAL CAROTID ARTERY IN CAVERNOUS SINUS

11.17 Contents of cavernous sinus—Internal carotid artery and abducent nerve (VI)

After entering cavernous sinus, the abducent nerve curves around the ascending part of internal carotid artery and then runs a straight course to enter into the orbit through the superior orbital fissure within the common tendinous ring (annulus tendineus communis). No nerve lies medial to it. The internal carotid artery with its sympathetic plexus is the medial most structure.

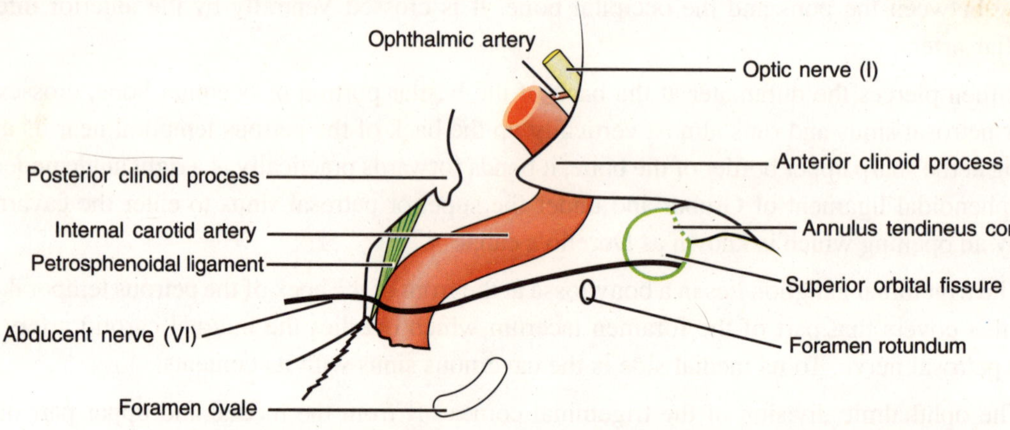

Fig. 11.17 Contents of cavernous sinus—Internal carotid artery and abducent nerve (VI)

11.18 Contents of cavernous sinus *(Contd.)*—III and VI nerve interrelationship

The oculomotor nerve slopes downwards with an oblique course and divides into superior and inferior divisions to pass into the orbit within annulus tendineus communis.

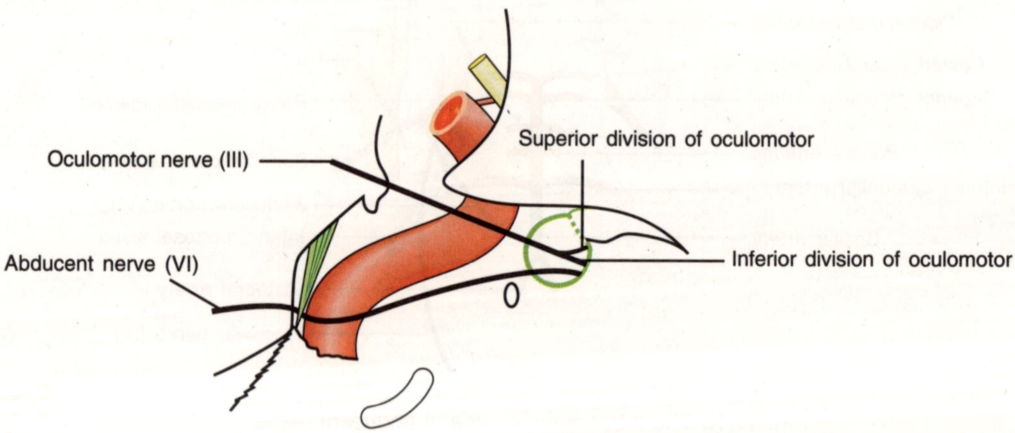

Fig. 11.18 Contents of cavernous sinus—oculomotor (III) and abducent (VI) nerve interrelationship

11.19 Contents of cavernous sinus *(Contd.)*—III, IV and VI nerve interrelationship

The trochlear nerve crosses the oculomotor and is placed lateral to it in the anterior part of cavernous sinus. It passes into the orbit through superior orbital fissure outside annulus tendineus communis.

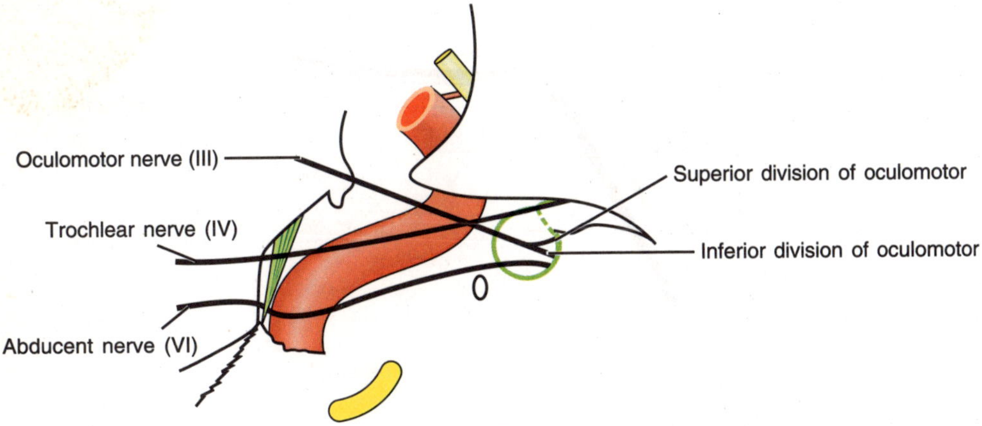

Fig. 11.19 Contents of cavernous sinus—oculomotor (III), trochlear (IV) and abducent (VI) nerve interrelationship

11.20 Contents of cavernous sinus *(Contd.)*—III, IV, V and VI nerve interrelationship

No nerve lies lateral to the ophthalmic division of the trigeminal in its course through cavernous sinus. It crosses the abducent and oculomotor nerves in the anterior part of the sinus. The trochlear nerve runs at a higher level and is therefore not crossed by the ophthalmic nerve. The nasociliary branch is the first to be given off, it goes into orbit within annulus tendineus. The lacrimal and frontal branches given later pass into orbit outside annulus tendineus.

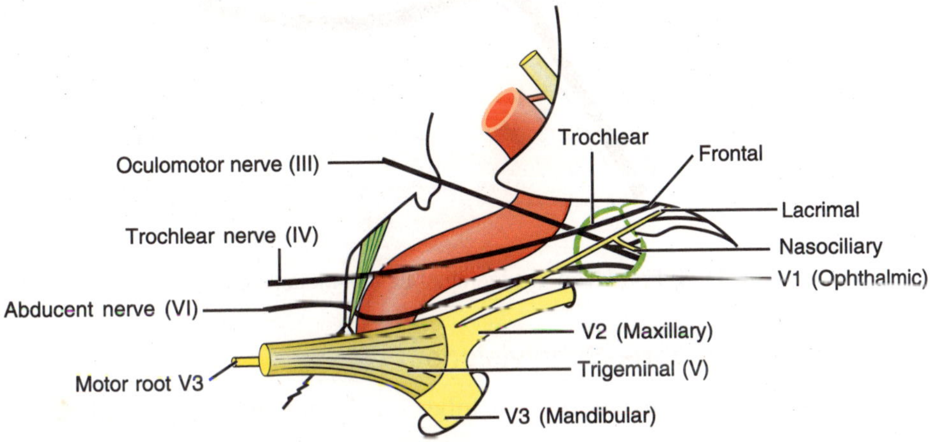

Fig. 11.20 Contents of cavernous sinus—oculomotor (III), trochlear (IV), ophthalmic divisions of trigeminal (V1) and abducent (VI) nerve interrelationship

11.21 Formation of tentorium cerebelli

The arrangement of duramater in middle and posterior cranial fossa in a sagittal section through tentorial attachment lateral to Mekel's cave is shown.

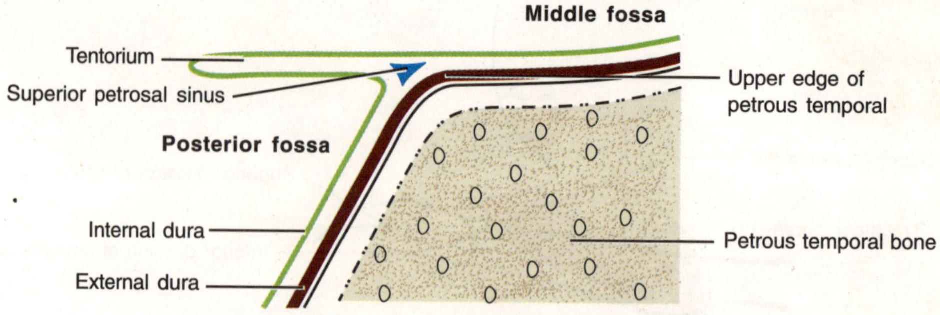

Fig. 11.21 Fromation of tentorium cerebelli

11.22 Formation of the trigeminal cave—Mekel's cave

The two roots of the trigeminal nerve pass frowards and laterally within the posterior cranial fossa and beneath the tentorium cerebelli to cross the superior border of the petrous temporal bone, beneath the superior petrosal sinus. They enter a recess (the trigeminal cave) formed by an evagination of the internal layer of duramater of posterior cranial fossa. This dural recess contains most of the trigeminal ganglion which is homologus with the dorsal root ganglion of a spinal nerve.

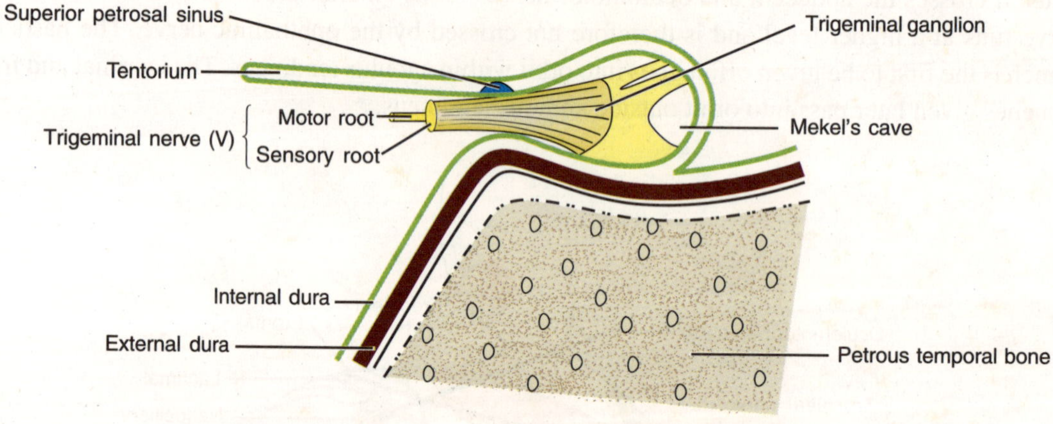

Fig. 11.22 Formation of trigeminal cave—Mekel's cave

11.23 The hypophysis cerebri—Subdivisions

The hypophysis ceretri consists of two lobes—a larger anterior lobe and a smaller posterior lobe.

The posterior lobe is connected with the stalk or infundibulum, a prolongation downwards and forwards from the tuber cinereum.

The anterior lobe is adherent to the posterior lobe by a narrow zone of gland substance that is often divided by a cleft from the main mass of the anterior lobe—this narrow zone is named the pars intermedia. Pars tuberalis, a narrow upward projection of the anterior lobe, partly encircles the infundibulum and may reach the tuber cinereum of the brain.

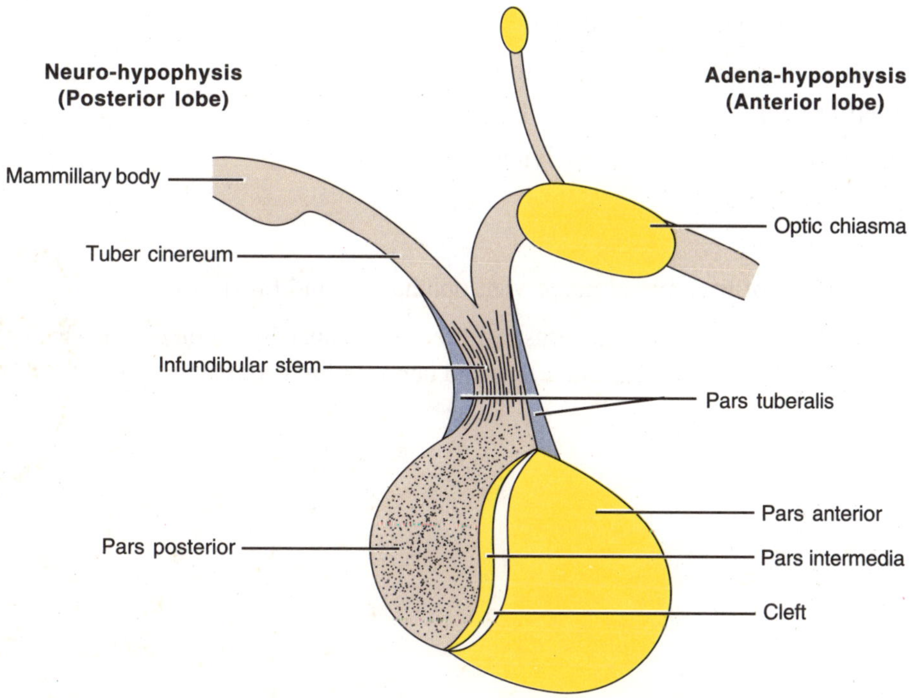

Fig. 11.23 The hypophysis cerebri—Subdivisions

11.24 Coronal section through the sella turcica and cavernous sinus

Note the arrangement of the contents of cavernous sinus. Study the relations of the pituitary gland. Lateral to cavernous sinus is temporal lobe, superiorly it is related to internal carotid artery,

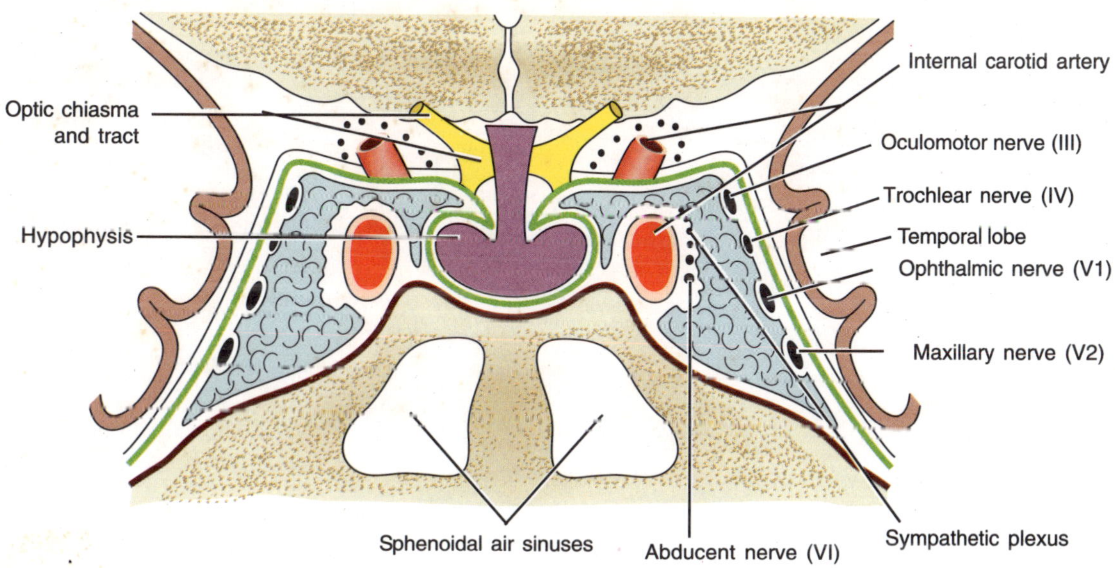

Fig. 11.24 Coronal section through the sella turcica and cavernous sinus

optic tract and uncus, medial is the hypophysis cerebri.

The contents of cavernous sinus are as follows:

- Internal carotid artery surrounded by sympathetic plexus
- Abducent nerve is medial most lying close to the artery
- Oculomotor nerve
- Trochlear nerve
- Two divisions of trigeminial nerve viz., ophthalmic and maxillary

Cavernous sinus is divided into caverns by fibrous septa lined by endothelium, which separates the venous blood from the internal carotid artery and nerves which course through the substance of the trabeculae.

The Orbit

Chapter 12

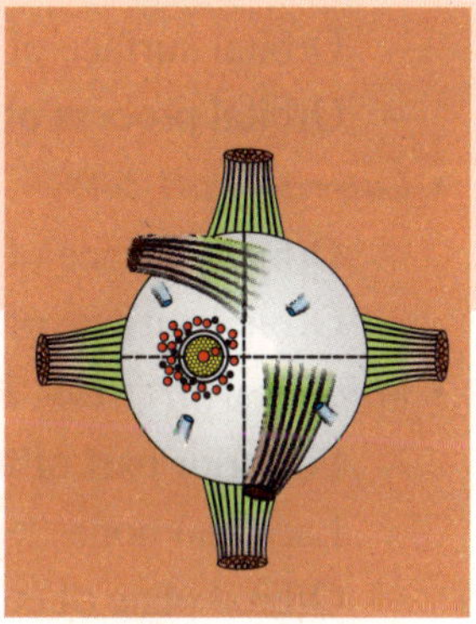

12.1 The orbit—Bony features

The orbit is a pyramidal space with its apex placed deeply and the base open anteriorly. It possesses lateral and medial walls, a roof and a floor. Study their composition. It communicates with the middle cranial fossa through the optic canal and superior orbital fissure, while communication

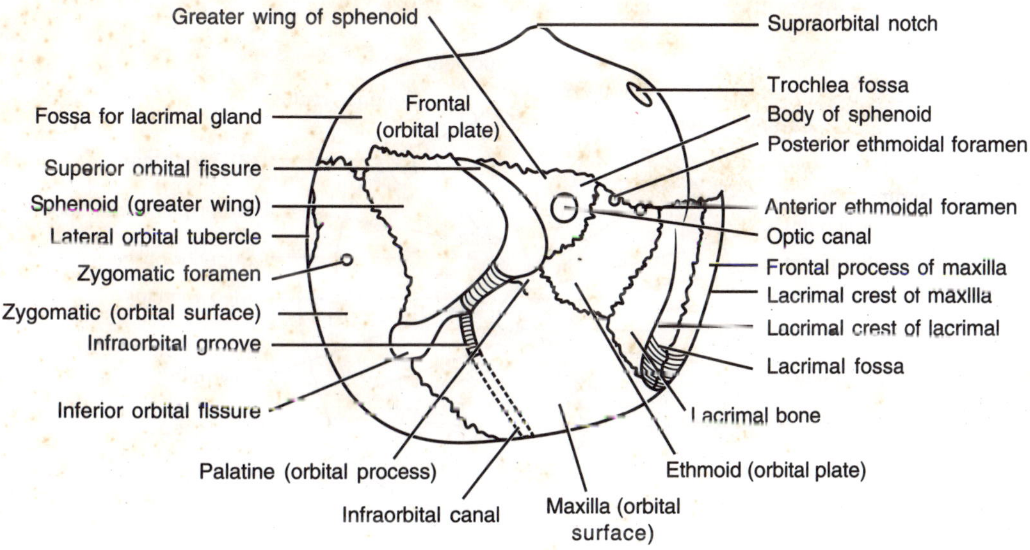

Fig. 12.1 The orbit—Bony features

with the infra-temporal region and pterygo-palatine fossa is through the inferior orbital fissure. Seen from the front the two fissures appear as a continuous L-shaped aperture.

- *Roof*
  - Orbital plate of frontal anteriorly.
  - Lower surface of the lesser wing of sphenoid posteriorly.
- *Floor*
  - Orbital surface of maxilla medially.
  - Orbital surface of zygomatic laterally.
  - Orbital process of palatine posteriorly at the junction of the floor and medial wall.
- *Lateral wall*
  - Orbital surface of the frontal process of zygomatic anteriorly.
  - Orbital surface of greater wing of sphenoid posteriorly.
- *Medial wall from before backwards*
  - Posterior part of the frontal process of maxilla
  - Lacrimal bone
  - Orbital plate of ethmoid
  - Body of sphenoid.

12.2 Ocular muscles—Origin

The four recti originate from the appropriate sides of a common tendinous ring which surrounds the optic canal and medial part of superior orbital fissure. Three additional muscles originate from the bone. Levator palpebrae superior is at the apex of the orbit above the common tendinous ring, the superior oblique at the apex of the orbit and the inferior oblique from the medial side of the floor of the orbit just behind the orbital margin.

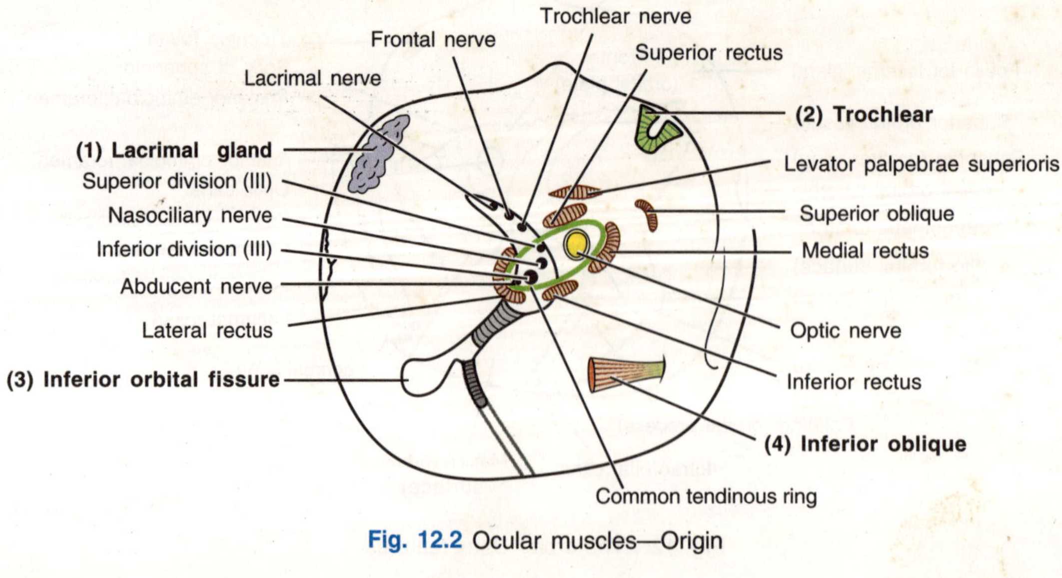

Fig. 12.2 Ocular muscles—Origin

Note the nerves in relation to the common tendinous ring. Note one feature each at the four corners of the orbit (I to IV).

12.3 The routes of entry of nerves into orbit

The ocular muscles form a cone within the bony orbit.

A useful generalisation about the innervation of the ocular muscles is that the lateral rectus (L.R.) is supplied by the abducent (6), the superior oblique (S.O.) is supplied by the trochlear (4) and all other (A.O) are supplied by the oculomotor (3). A convenient formula therefore is LR6SO4AO3.

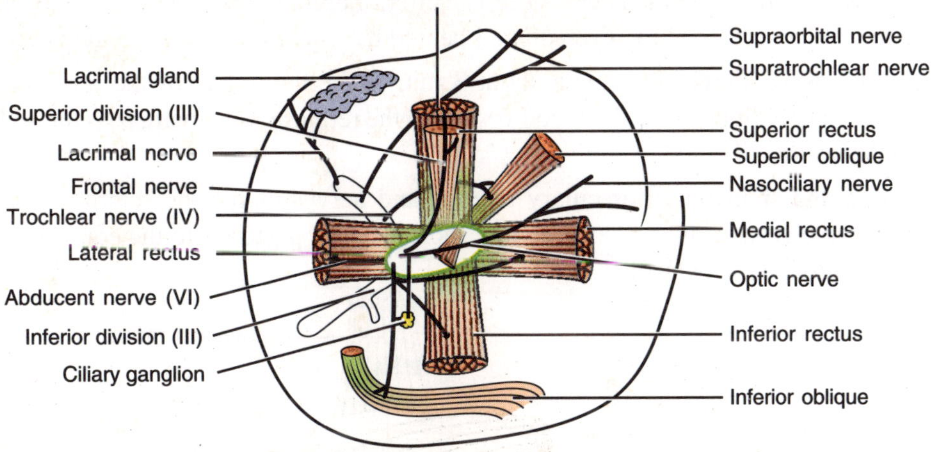

Fig. 12.3 The routes of entry of nerves into orbit

12.4 Ocular muscles—Insertion

The four recti are inserted into the eyeball well in front of its equator (line of maximum circumference) while the obliques are inserted behind this equator.

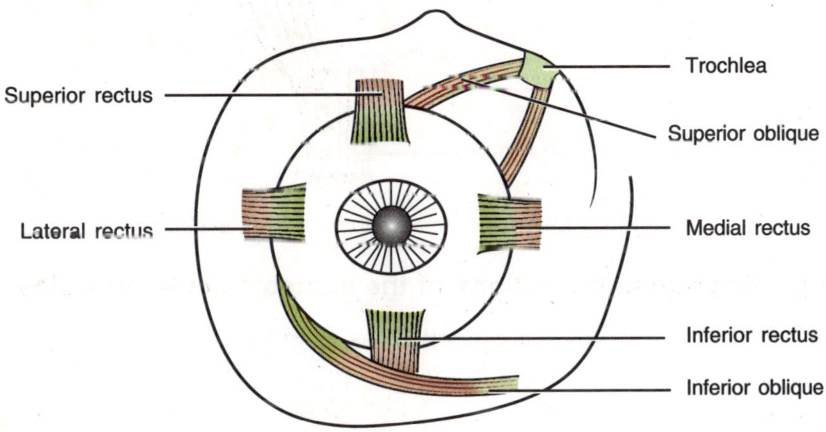

Fig. 12.4 Ocular muscles—Insertion

The superior oblique passes forwards along the medial wall of the orbit above the medial rectus to a fibrous pulley, the trochlea. The tendon passes through this trochlea and then bending sharply, passes laterally and backwards below the superior rectus.

The inferior oblique passes laterally and backwards from its origin. It corresponds to the part of superior oblique beyond the trochlea. Just as superior oblique runs below the superior rectus, so the inferior oblique passes below the inferior rectus.

12.5 The posterior aspect of right eyeball

The superior oblique is inserted as a flat tendon into the upper surface of the eyeball well behind the equator and well to the lateral side. The inferior oblique passes laterally and backwards to insert into the under surface of the eyeball well behind the equator and well to the lateral side.

The optic nerve pierces the sclera about 3 mm to the nasal side of the posterior pole. The bundles of optic nerve fibres, with the blood vessels to the retina among them, pass through a number of holes in the sclera.

The long and short posterior ciliary arteries and nerves pierce the sclera around the optic nerve. Four to five vena vorticosae emerge at a short distance posterior to the equator, more or less equally spaced around the eyeball.

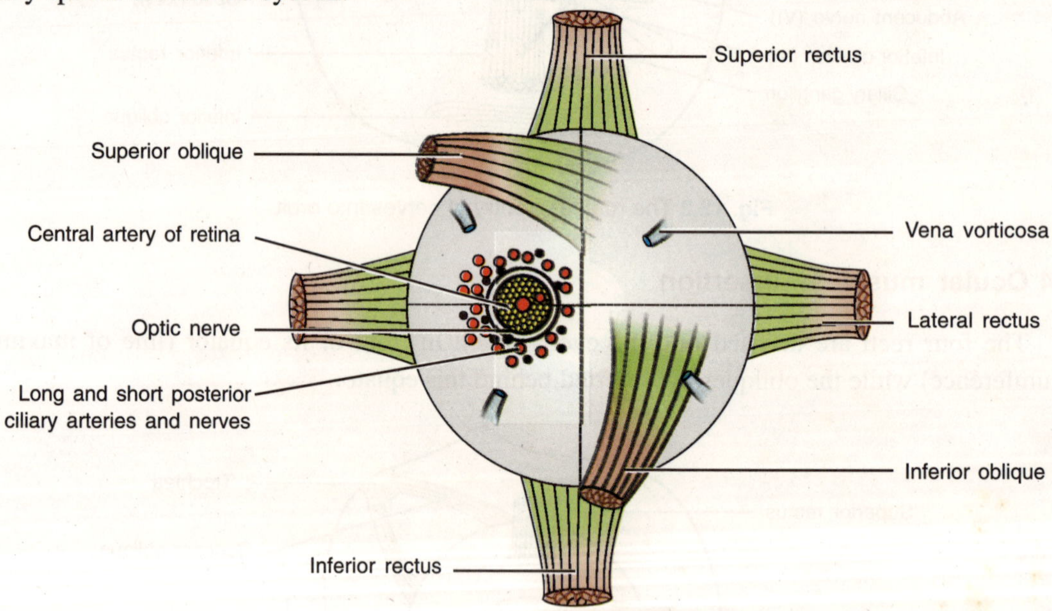

Fig. 12.5 The posterior aspect of right eyeball

12.6 Starling's diagram of the actions of the extrinsic ocular muscles

Superior rectus (S.R.) – rotates the eyeball so as to elevate the cornea and draw it nasally.

Medial rectus (M.R.) – rotates the eye to make the cornea deviate horizontally towards the nasal side.

Inferior rectus (I.R.) – depresses the cornea and deviates it towards the nasal side.

Lateral rectus (L.R.) – deviates the cornea horizontally towards the temporal side.

Superior oblique (S.O.) – depresses the cornea and turns it out towards the temporal side.

Inferior oblique (I.O.) – elevates the cornea and deviates it towards the temporal side.

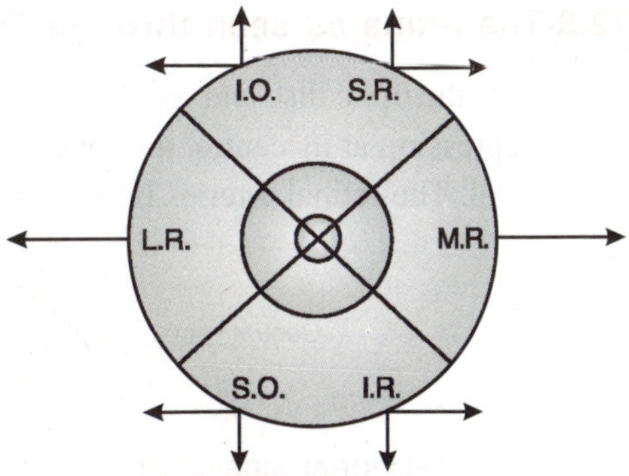

Fig. 12.6 Starling's diagram of the actions of the extrinsic ocular muscles—I.O., Inferior oblique; S.R., Superior rectus; L.R., Lateral rectus; M.R., Medial rectus; S.O., Superior oblique; I.R., Inferior rectus

12.7 The arteries and veins of the orbit

The ophthalmic artery enters the orbit lying below the optic nerve in the optic canal, like the nerve it passes through the tendinous ring into the muscular cone. Begining from a position below the nerve, the artery spirals first to the lateral side and then across the top of the nerve to the medial wall of the orbit. Of its numerous branches, central artery of retina is of particular importance. It arises while the parent trunk is still below the optic nerve itself, and is carried in this position into the eyeball where it is the entire and sole supply of the retina.

The ophthalmic veins are not shown here. They are numerous and lie both within and without the muscular cone and coalesce to form a superior and an inferior ophthalmic vein.

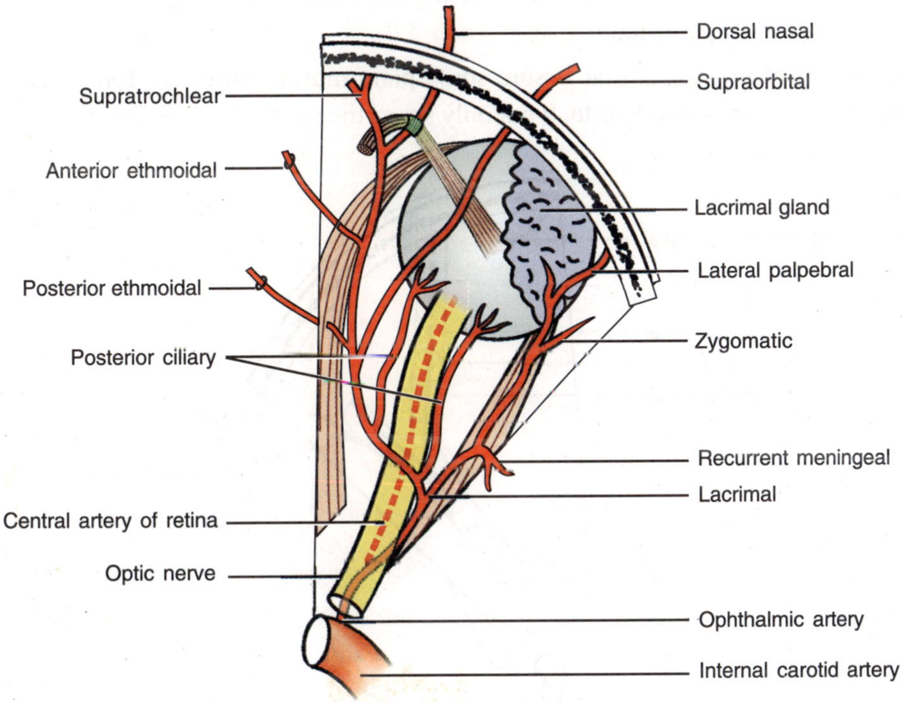

Fig. 12.7 The arteries and veins of the orbit

12.8 The retina as seen through the ophthalmoscope

Note the optic disc and retinal vessels in Figure 12.8. The yellow spot, the macula lutea, with a slight depression at its centre, the fovea centralis, lies in the centre of the retina in the visual axis of the eyeball. The retinal arteries lie superficial to retinal veins.

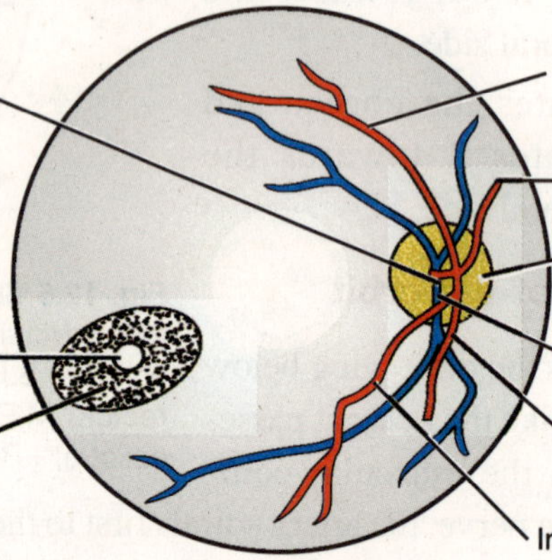

Fig. 12.8 The retina as seen through the ophthalmoscope

BUILDING UP THE CONTENTS OF ORBIT FROM FLOOR TO ROOF

12.9 The nerves outside orbital periosteum

The zygomatic and infraorbital nerves coursing through inferior orbital fissure and infraorbital groove are outside orbital periosteum.

In the region of inferior orbital fissure some plain muscle fibres are found with the orbital periosteum. This is the orbitalis muscle. It not only spans the inferior orbital fissure, but also extends

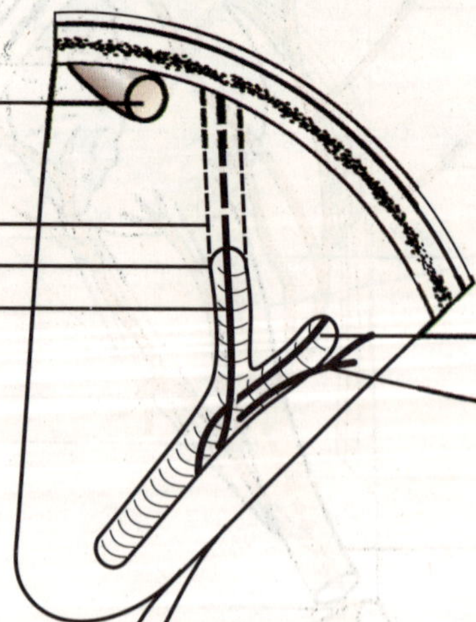

Fig. 12.9 The nerves outside orbital periosteum

backwards, deep to the common tendinous ring, to the front of the cavernous sinus, while anteriorly it gets lost in the orbital periosteum. Its action in man is very doubtful. It has sympathetic supply from pterygo-palatine gangalion.

12.10 The nerves within the muscular cone

The inferior division of the oculomotor is the larger of the two divisions. It supplies three muscles. The medial rectus and inferior rectus are supplied one-third of the way along the orbit on their ocular surface. The branch to the inferior oblique runs along the lateral edge of the inferior rectus and then enters the ocular surface of inferior oblique. It gives the motor root to the ciliary ganglion.

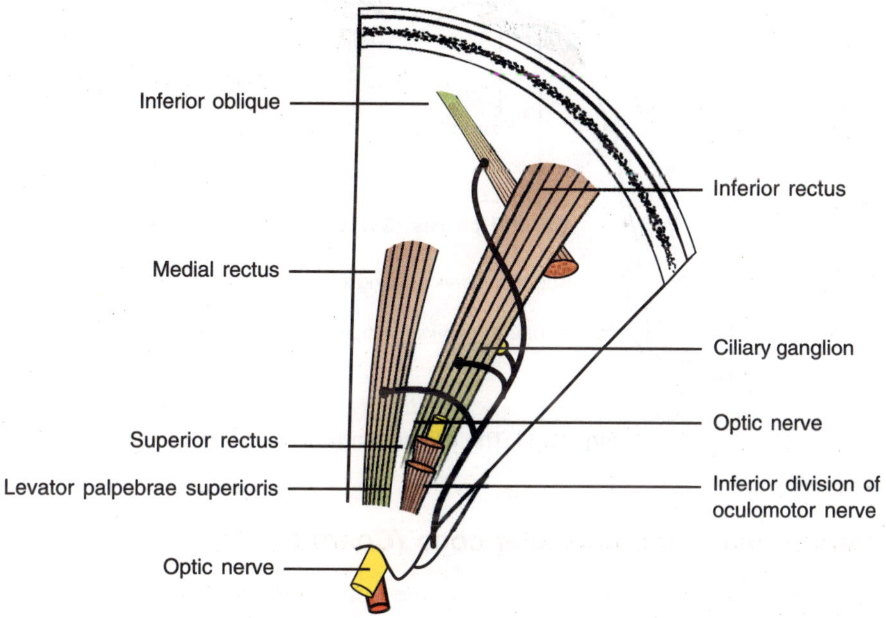

Fig. 12.10 The nerves within the muscular cone

12.11 The ciliary ganglion

It is a minute ganglion about 2 mm in diameter lying on the lateral side of the optic nerve. Three roots enter its posterior end.

Sensory root from nasociliary passes through the ganglion without relay to supply the sensory fibres to the whole eyeball except conjunctiva. Division of this root abolishes corneal reflex but not the conjunctival reflex.

Sympathetic root from cavernous plexus (post-ganglionic fibres) with cell bodies in superior cervical ganglion carries vasoconstrictor fibres to the vessels of the eyeball. The sympathetic supply of the dilator pulpillae enters the eyeball without passing through the ganglion via long ciliary nerves.

Parasympathetic root comes from the inferior division of oculomotor via nerve to inferior oblique. This consists of preganglionic fibres which arise from the Edinger Westphal nucleus. These are the only fibres to relay in the ganglion. They supply constrictor pupillae and ciliary muscle.

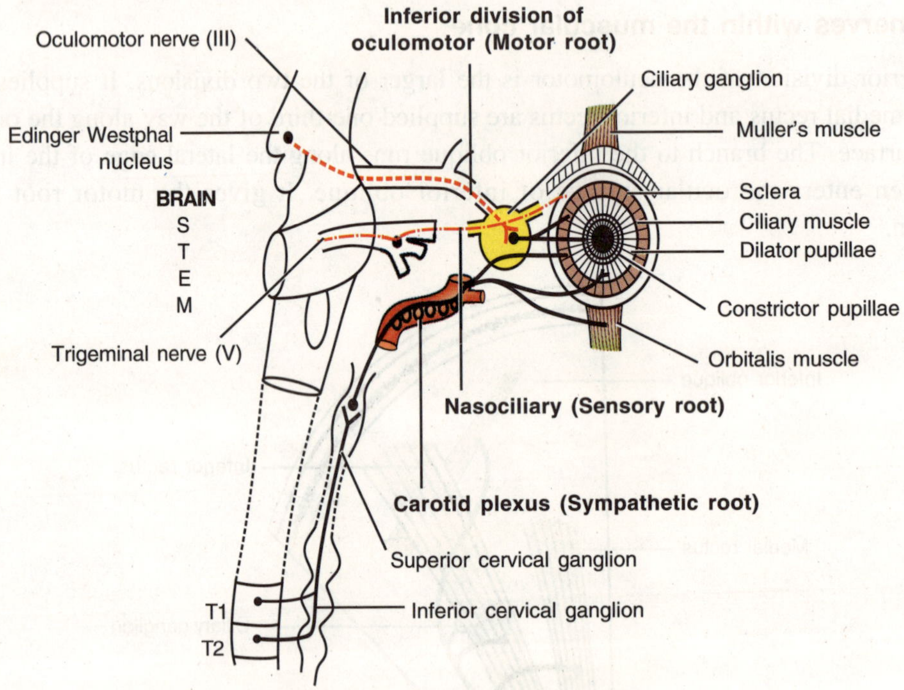

Fig. 12.11 The ciliary ganglion

12.12 The nerves within the muscular cone *(Contd.)*

The nasociliary nerve passes medially across the optic nerve to the medial wall of the orbit where it divides into the anterior ethmoidal and infratrochlear nerves. Before dividing, it gives off a sensory root to the ciliary ganglion and two or three long ciliary nerves directly to the eyeball.

The ciliary ganglion is a minute oval body lying close to the lateral side of the optic nerve. It gives short ciliary nerves to the eyeball.

The abducent nerve lies laterally and passes directly into the lateral rectus.

12.13 The nerves within the muscular cone *(Contd.)*

The superior division of the oculomotor nerve runs forwards above the optic nerve and supplies the overlying superior rectus and levator palpebrae muscle (shown cut) one-third of the way along the orbit. It carries sympathetic fibres from the cavernous plexus to the smooth muscle part of the levator palpebrae superioris (Muller's muscle).

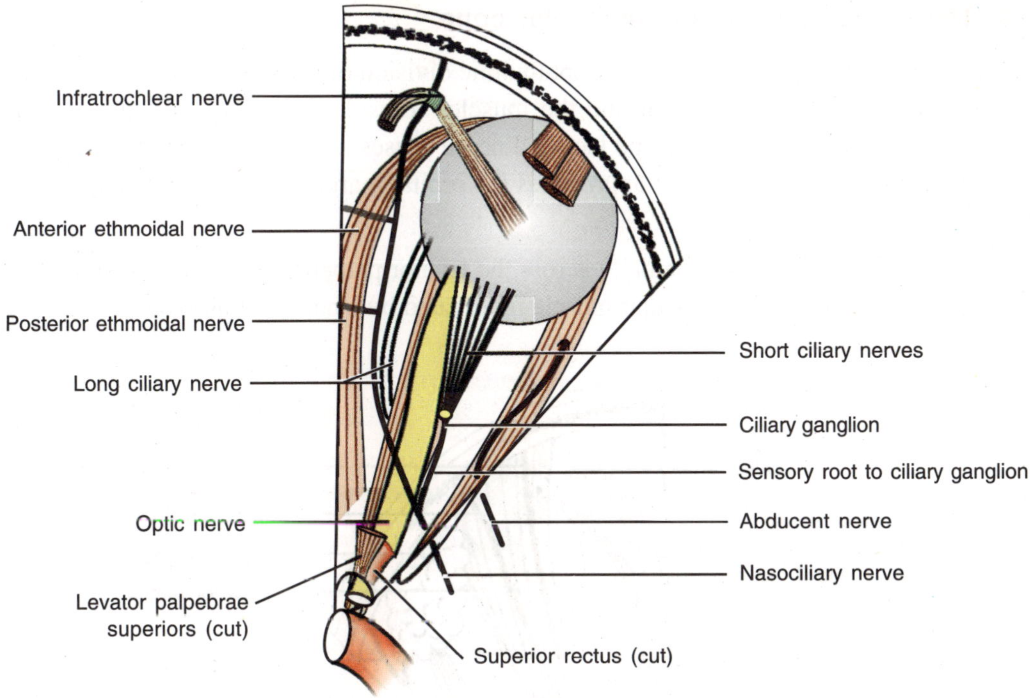

Fig. 12.12 The nerves within the muscular cone (Contd.)

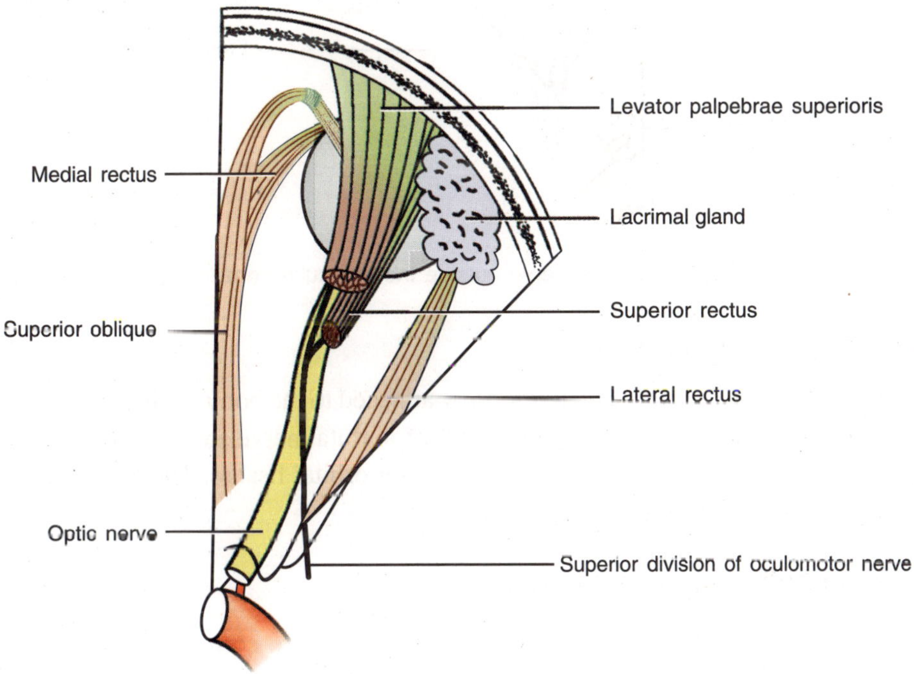

Fig. 12.13 The nerves within the muscular cone (Contd.)

12.14 The nerves outside the muscular cone

The lacrimal and frontal branches of ophthalmic division of trigeminal and the trochlear nerve remain between the roof of the orbit and the muscles (outside the muscular cone) after passing through the superior orbital fissure. The lacrimal nerve passes laterally towards the lacrimal gland. The frontal passes forwards and as it approaches the orbital margin, it divides into supraorbital and supratrochlear nerves.

The trochlear nerve passes medially across the levator palpebrae superioris to supply superior oblique muscle which is the only ocular muscle innervated by a nerve running outside the muscular cone.

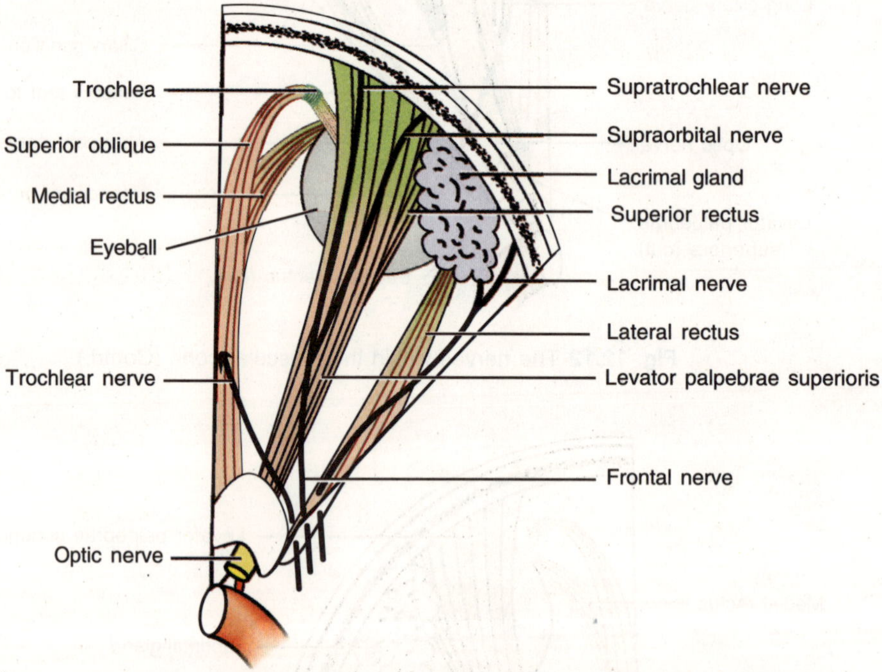

Fig. 12.14 The nerve outside the muscular cone

12.15 The orbital periosteum

It forms a funnel shaped sheath which is loosely attached to the bony walls, and encloses all the contents of the orbit except the zygomatic nerve and infraorbital nerve and vessels. It is continuous with endocranium through the optic canal and the superior orbital fissure. The orbital periosteum is covered over by the bony floor of anterior cranial fossa.

12.16 The facia bulbi (Tenon's capsule)

It is applied like a bursa to the back of the eyeball from sclero-corneal junction to the back of the eyeball. Its inner layer is thin and blended with sclera. Its outer layer is pierced by the tendons of the four recti and two obliques, and is prolonged as tubular investiture proximally along each tendon

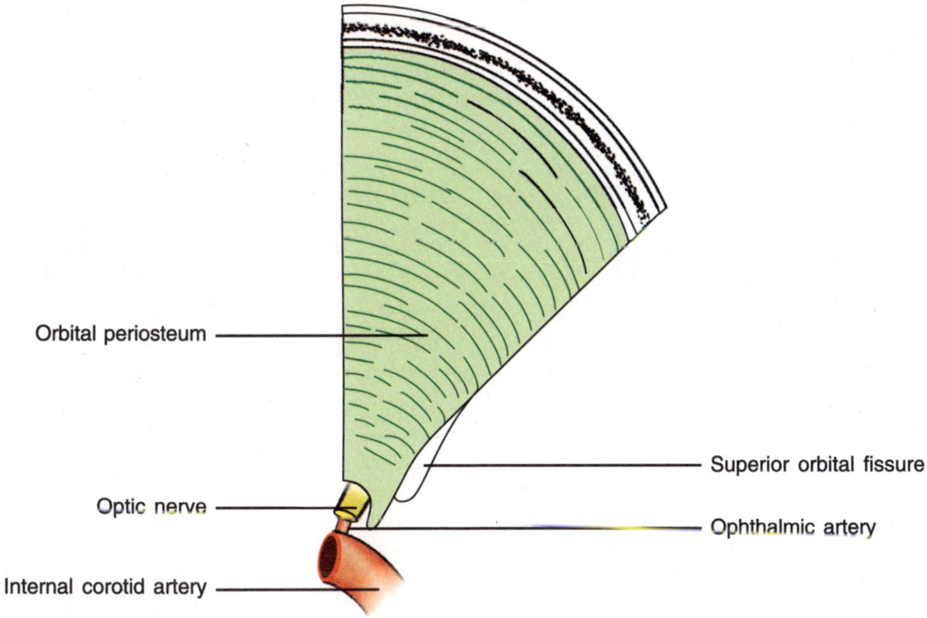

Fig. 12.15 The orbital periosteum

towards the muscle belly. Medial and lateral check ligaments are from the investments on two recti. The suspensory ligament of Lockwood between the check ligaments forms a sling, and is a thickening of fascia bulbi. It supports the eyeball in orbit like a hammock.

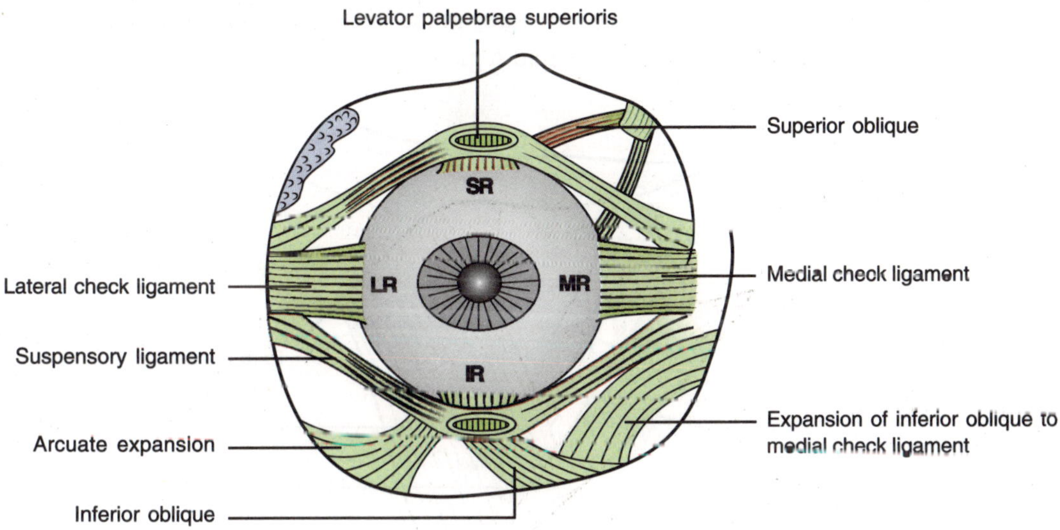

Fig. 12.16 The facia bulbi (Tenon's capsule)

The Parotid Region

Chapter 13

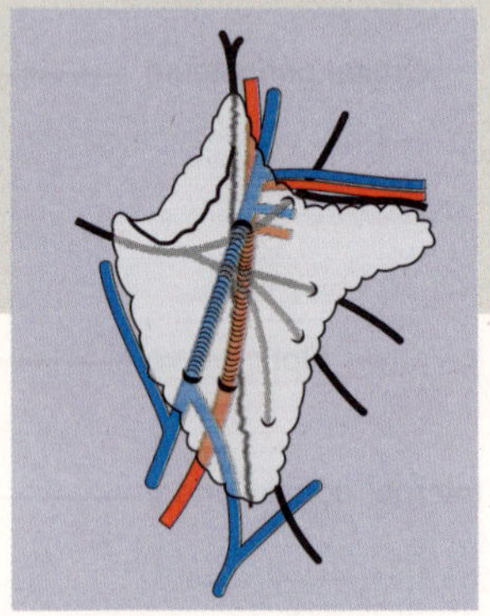

13.1 The parotid bed

The parotid bed is the space in which the parotid gland lies. The space is also known as the retro-mandibular fossa and is the boundary region between the neck and the head, and from the surgical view point is allied closely with the structures in the infra-temporal fossa. It is also in vital connection with the structures in the sternomastoid region.

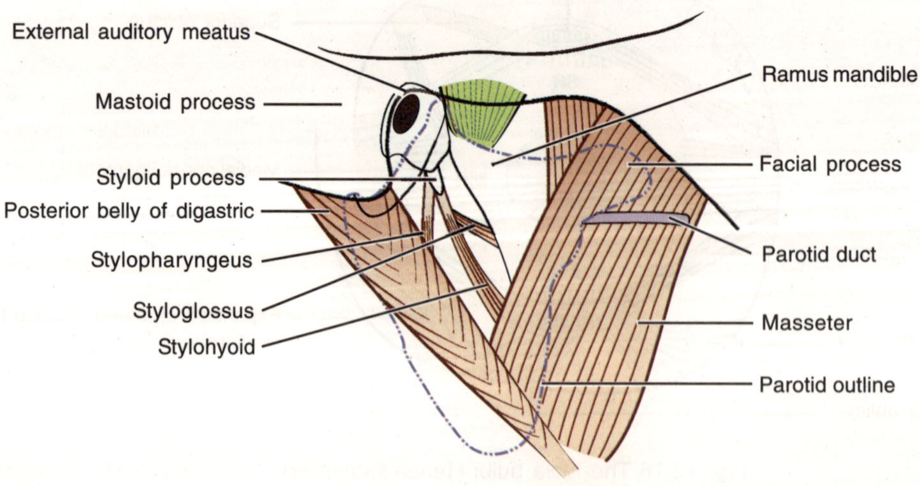

Fig. 13.1 The parotid bed

The anterior boundary is the ramus of mandible sandwiched between the masseter and medial pterygoid muscles. Posterior is the mastoid process between the sternomastoid and the posterior belly of digastric. Superior is the external auditary meatus. Medially is the styloid process with the stylohyoid, styloglossus and stylopharyngeus muscle. Laterally it is limited by the superficial layer of parotid facia attached above to the zygomatic arch.

13.2 The retromandibular fossa

It contains much of the posterior belly of digastric and stylohyoid muscles, trunk of external carotid artery, retromandibular vein, facial nerve and portion of the parotid gland.

The retromandibular vein is formed opposite the temporo-mandibular joint by the union of superficial temporal vein with the maxillary vein.

The superficial situation of facial nerve makes incision into the gland very hazardous.

Immediately deep to the nerve is the retromandibular vein, deepest of all is the external carotid artery.

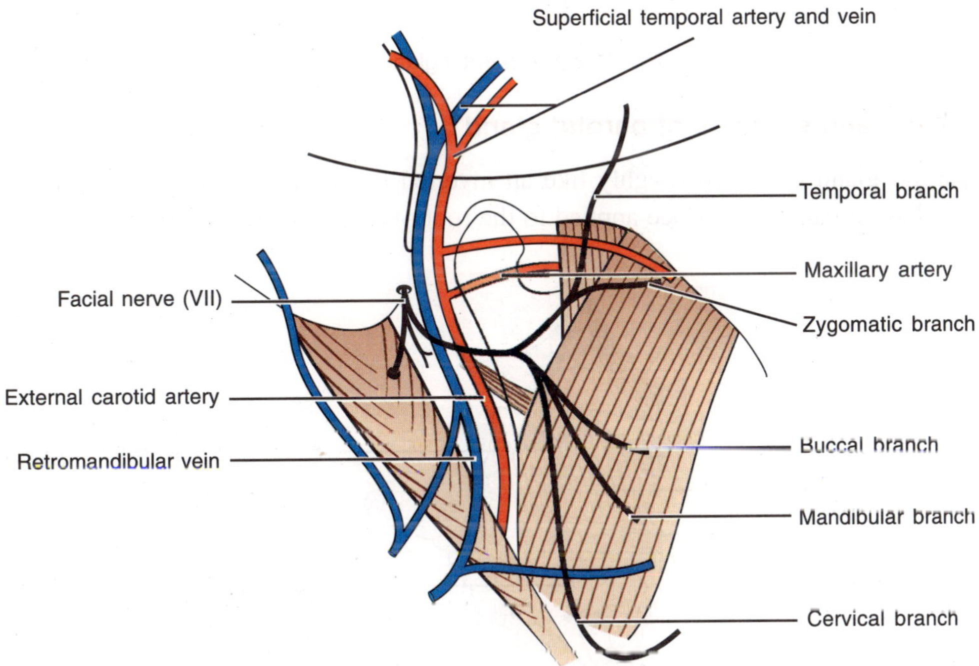

Fig. 13.2 The retromandibular fossa

13.3 The parotid gland

It fills the retromandibular fossa and overflows it to lie on the masseter muscle.

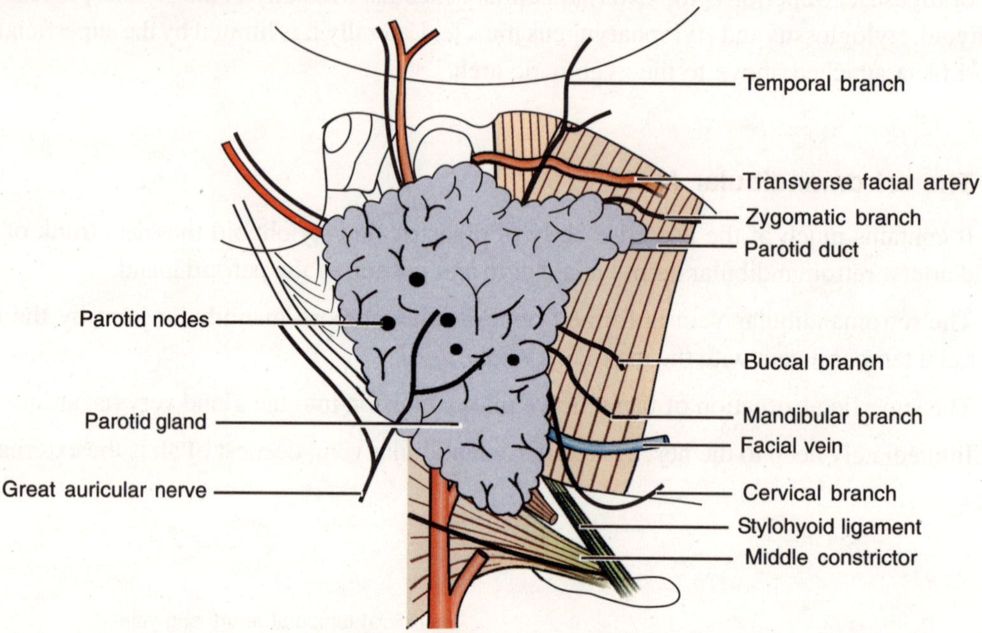

Fig. 13.3 The parotid gland

13.4 The shape and surfaces of parotid gland

The parotid gland is shaped roughly like an inverted pyramid. It presents an apex pointed downwards, a base or superior surface applied to the root of zygoma and the neck of mandible. It

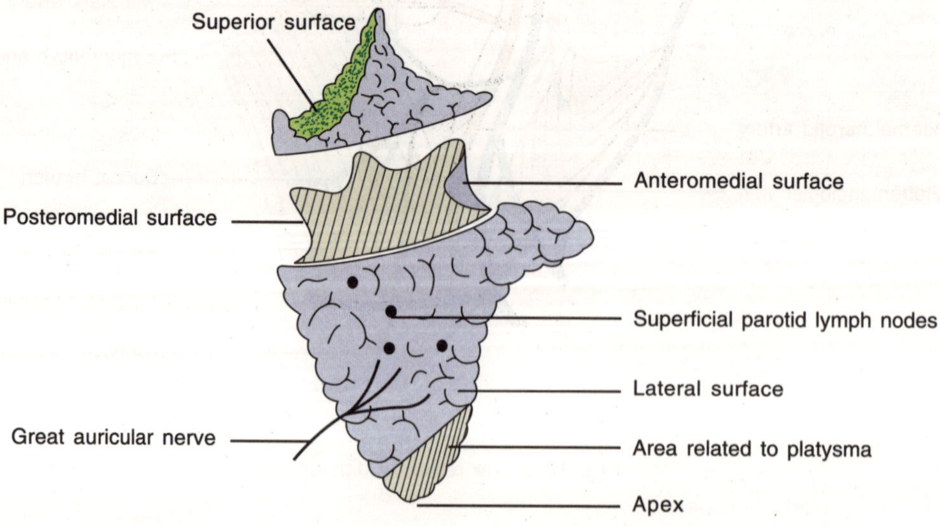

Fig. 13.4 The shape and surfaces of parotid gland

presents lateral, anteromedial and posteromedial surfaces. The gland is shown cut to explain the shape and surfaces.

The superficial surface is related to facial branches of great auricular nerve, superficial parotid lymph nodes, posterior fibres of platysma apart from skin, superficial fascia and parotideo-messetric fascia.

13.5 A transverse section through the parotid gland

The transverse section shows the structures within it which are

- the facial nerve and its terminal branches
- small communicating branches to the facial nerve from the great auricular nerve and larger ones from the auriculotemporal nerve
- the retromandibular vein
- the external carotid artery
- small lymph nodes.

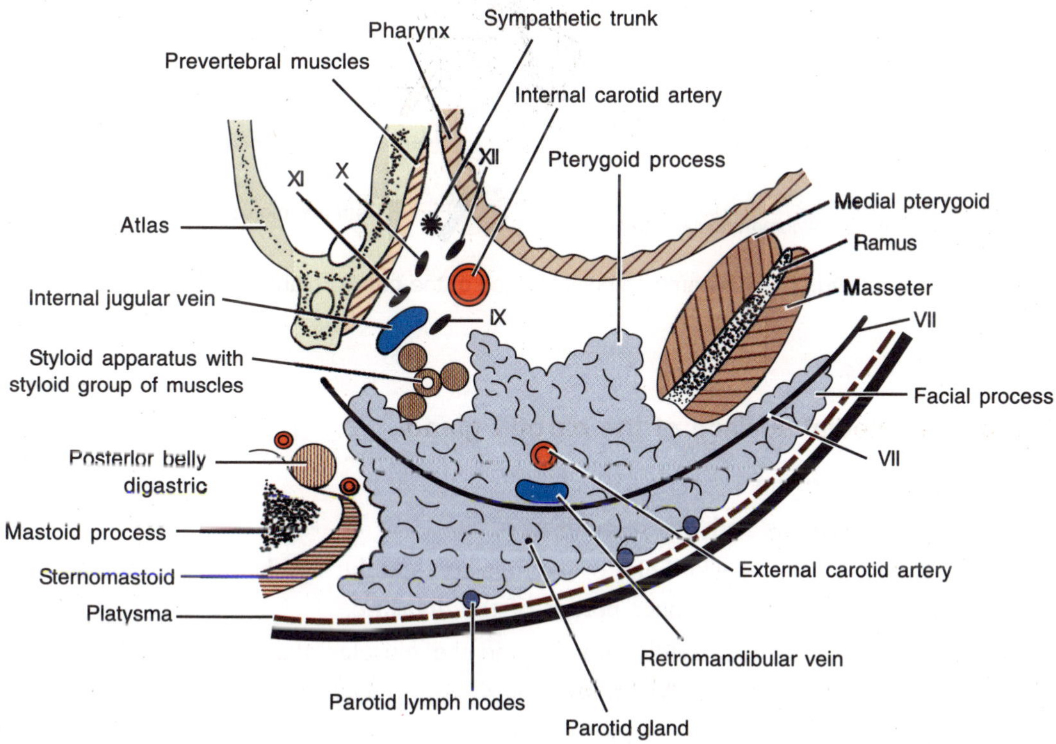

Fig. 13.5 A transverse section through the parotid gland

Note that deep to the styloid group of muscles, the posteromedial surface is related to the carotid sheath and the last four cranial nerves.

13.6 The anteromedial surface of the parotid gland

The surface is grooved by the posterior border of the ramus of mandible. It covers the posteroinferior part of the masseter muscle, the lateral aspect of temporomandibular joint and the adjoining part of the mandibular ramus. It passes forwards on the deep aspect of the ramus to reach the medial pterygoid muscle and this is called the pterygoid process. The maxillary artery comes out of this process to enter the infratemporal fossa. The lower part of the surface is separated from the submandibular salivary gland by the stylomandibular ligament.

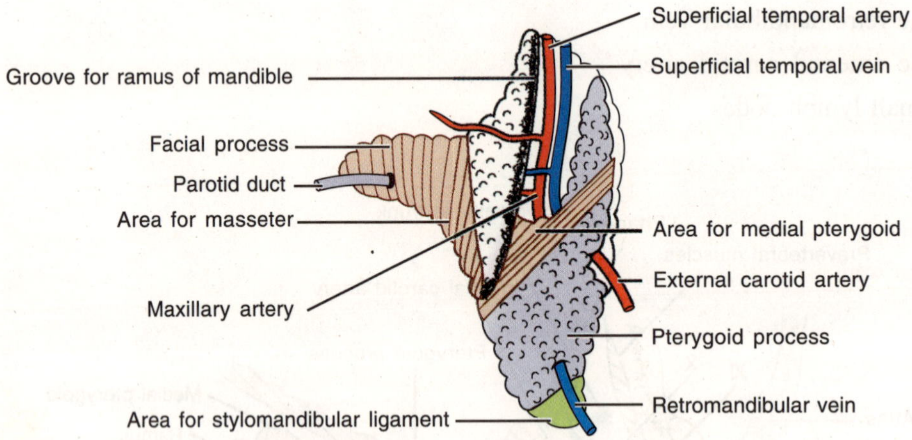

Fig. 13.6 The anteromedial surface of the parotid gland

13.7 The posteromedial surface of the parotid gland

It is related to the following:

- The mastoid process and the sternomastoid.
- More deeply to the posterior belly of the digastric and the stylohyoid, with the posterior auricular artery along the upper border of the digastric.
- More deeply still to the styloid process and the muscles attached to it. The external carotid artery enters this surface above the digastric. The cervical branch of the facial nerve and the branches of the posterior facial vein emerge below the digastric. The facial nerve enters between the digastric and the styloid process.

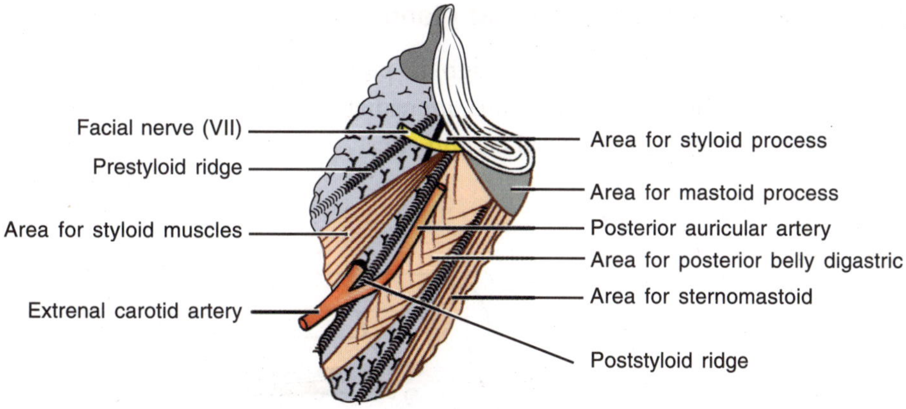

Fig. 13.7 The posteromedial surface of the parotid gland

13.8 Patey's faclo-venous plane within the parotid gland

The gland is shaped like a collar stud (inset) with the large part of the stud superficial and forming the superficial lobe. The deep part or the deep lobe is joined to the superficial lobe by the neck or isthmus. The facial nerve with its branches passes forwards on either side of the neck of the stud. The stippled area represents the deep lobe of the gland. The plane between the superficial and deep lobe in which the nerve and the vein lie has been designated by Patey as the facio-venous plane.

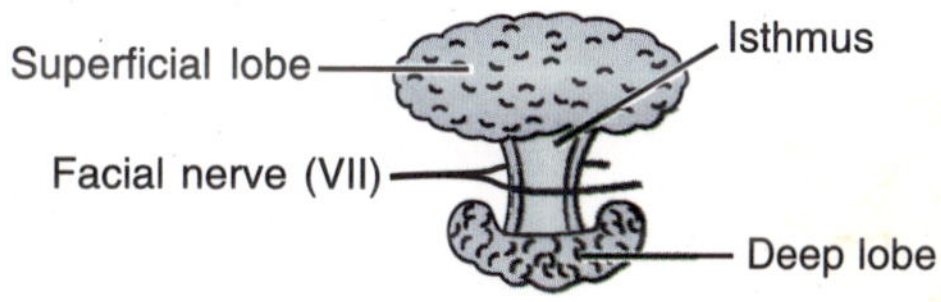

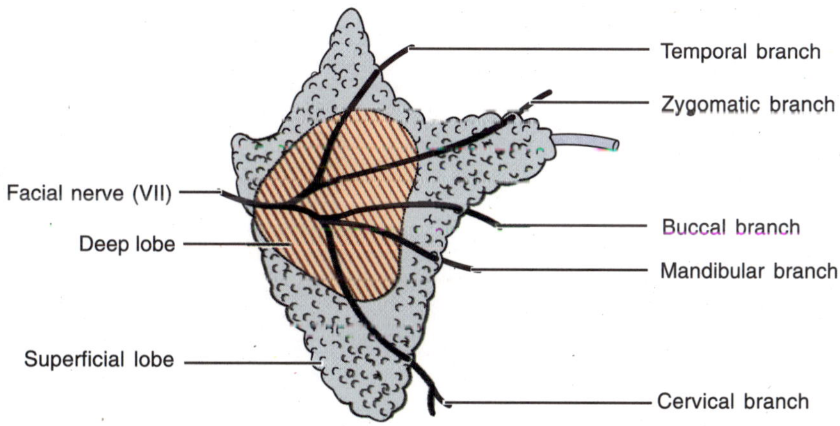

Fig. 13.8 Patey's facio-venous plane within the parotid gland

13.9 The structures within the parotid gland

There are three structures passing through the parotid gland. The most superficial is the facial nerve with its branches forming pes anserinus, immediately deep to the nerve is the retromandibular vein and the deepest of all is the external carotid artery.

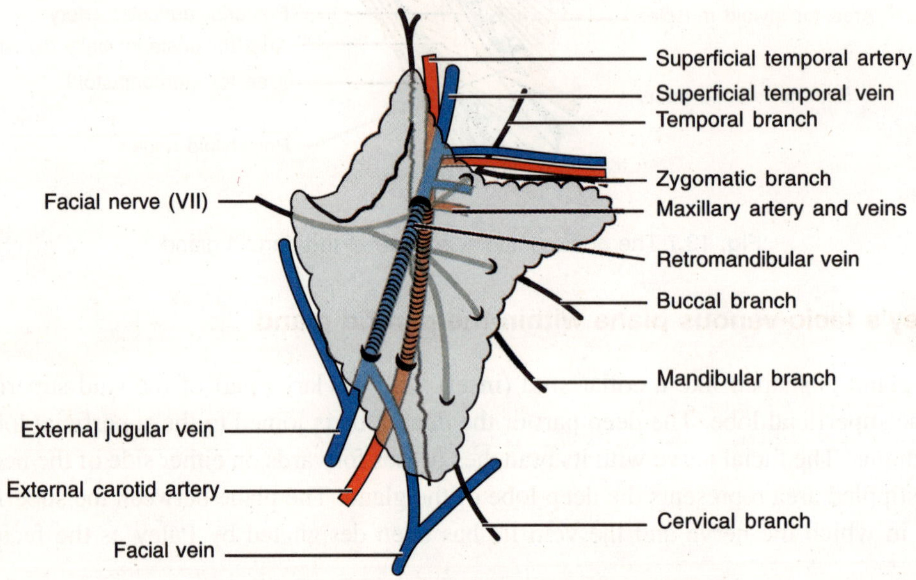

Fig. 13.9 The structures within the parotid gland

The Infratemporal Region

Chapter **14**

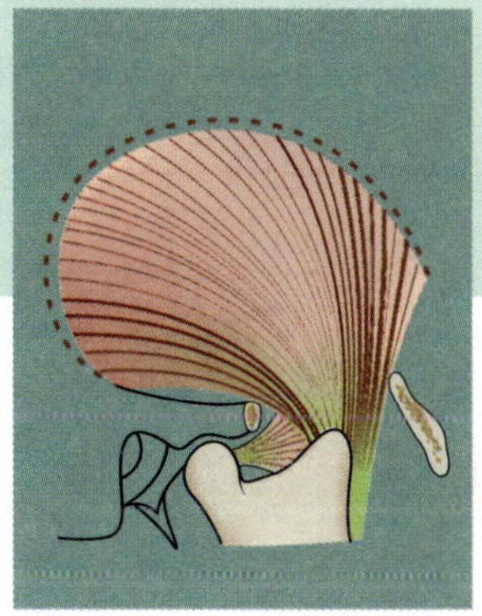

14.1 The scheme of infratemporal fossa represented as a cube

The fossa lying below the back of the skull is best visualised as a cube with no floor. The roof is pierced by two foramina. The anterior wall is separated by fissures from the roof and the medial wall.

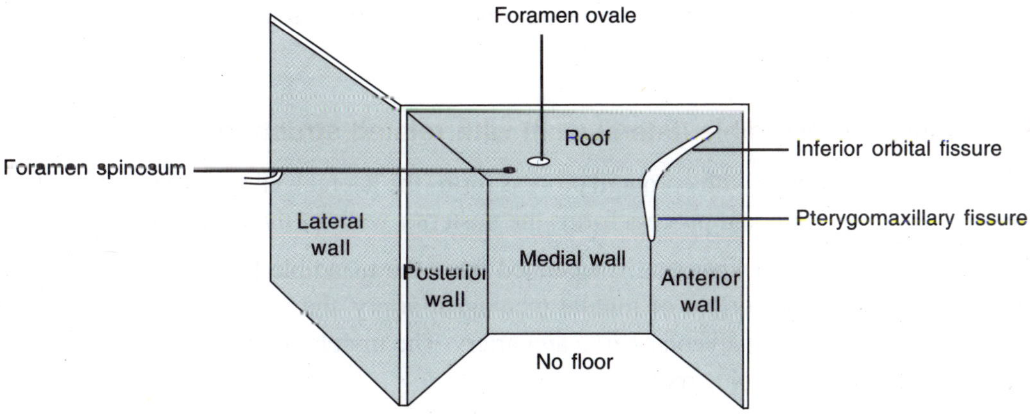

Fig. 14.1 The scheme of infratemporal fossa represented as a cube

14.2 The bony walls of infratemporal fossa

Lateral wall	–	Ramus of mandible with coronoid process (seen rotated laterally).
Medial wall	–	Lateral pterygoid plate.
Anterior wall	–	Lateral part of the posterior surface of maxilla.
Posterior wall	–	Anterior surface of the condyloid process of the mandible.
Roof	–	Inferior surface of greater wing of sphenoid and part of squamous temporal bone.
Floor	–	No anatomical floor as the fossa is continuous downwards into the tissue spaces of the neck, lateral to the pharynx.

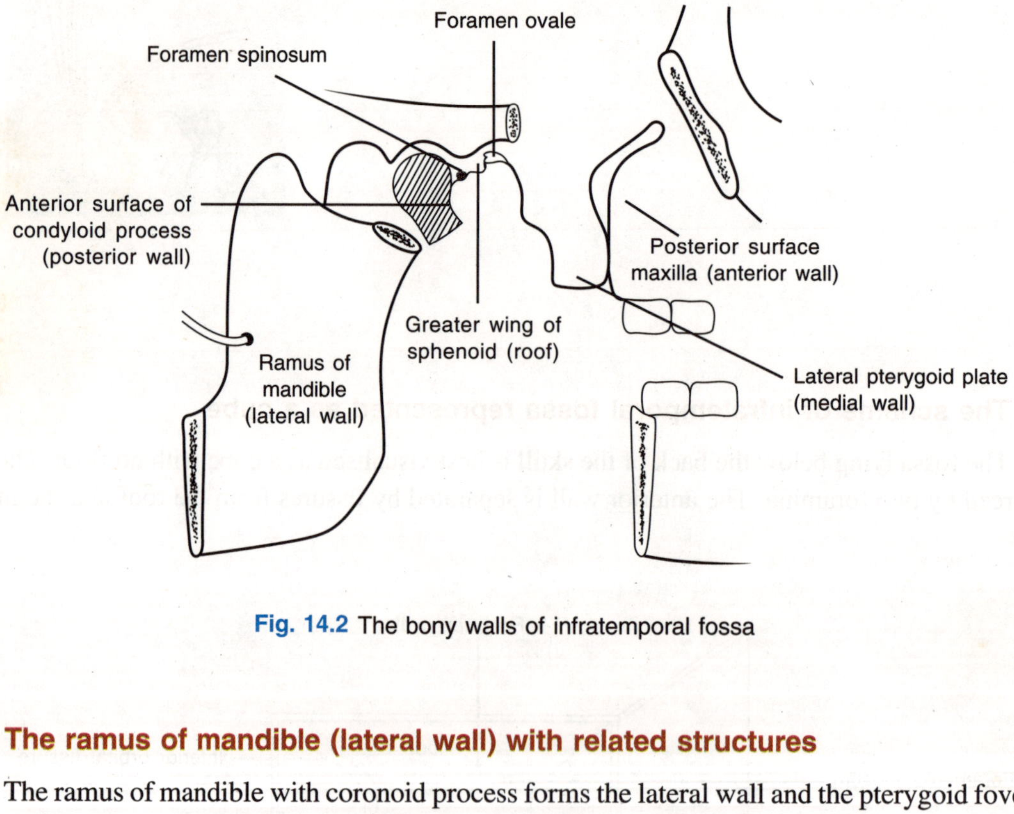

Fig. 14.2 The bony walls of infratemporal fossa

14.3 The ramus of mandible (lateral wall) with related structures

The ramus of mandible with coronoid process forms the lateral wall and the pterygoid fovea on the anterior aspect of condyloid process forms the posterior wall of the infratemporal fossa.

The sphenomandibular ligament is separated from the mandible from above downwards by auriculotemporal nerve, the origin of middle meningeal artery, the maxillary artery, a porcess of parotid gland and the inferior alveolar nerve and artery. The mylohyoid nerve and artery pierce the ligament to reach the mylohyoid groove.

Note that the lingual nerve lies behind the last molar tooth where it may be injured during extraction of this tooth.

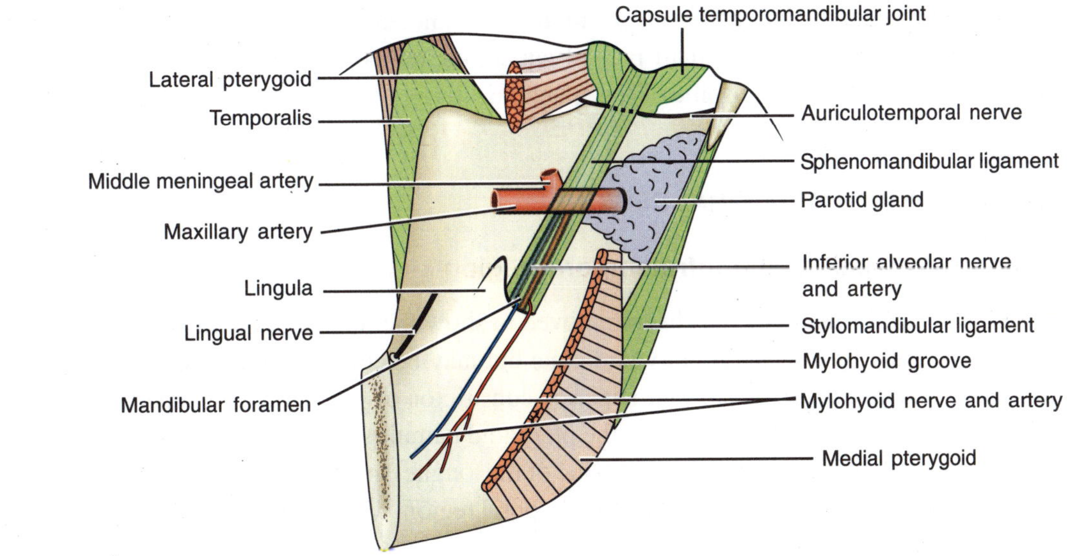

Fig. 14.3 The ramus of mandible (lateral wall) with related structures

14.4 The infratemporal region of base of the skull (roof)

The basal aspect of the greater wing of sphenoid between infratemporal crest and lateral pterygoid plate should be noted. It narrows to the posterior angle where it bears the spine of sphenoid.

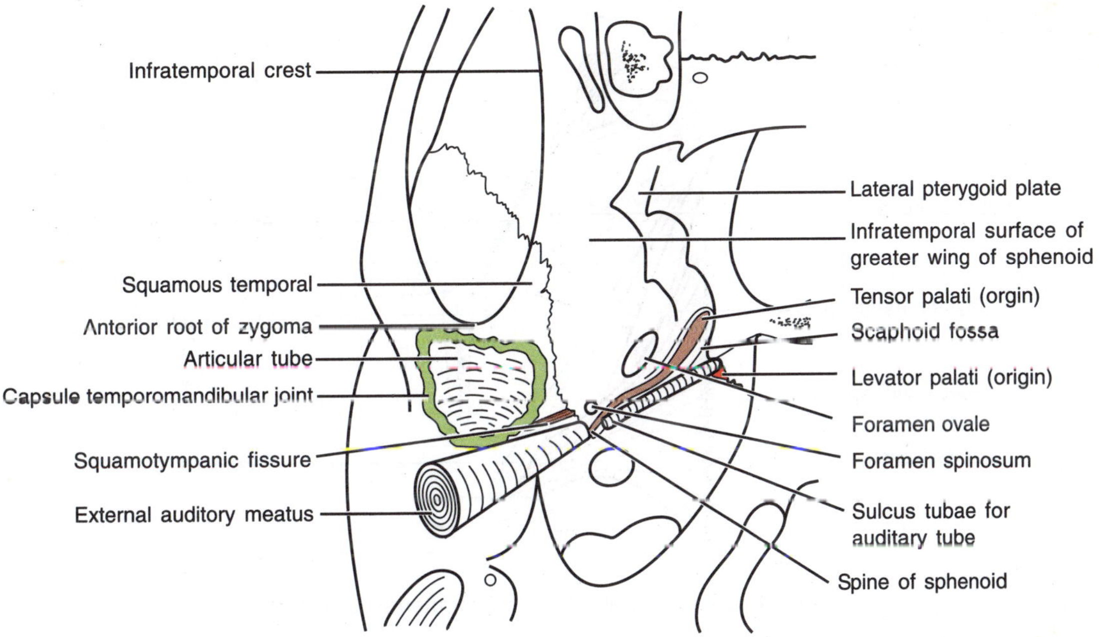

Fig. 14.4 The infratemporal region of base of the skull (roof)

Along the posteromedial edge the tensor palati arises, immediately lateral to which is the foramen ovale and foramen spinosum. A small part of squamous temporal forms the roof. The squamo-tympanic fissure is lateral to the spine of the sphenoid.

BUILDING UP OF INFRATEMPORAL REGION

14.5 The medial limit of the infratemporal region

The ramus of the mandible has been removed to show the medial boundary of this area which is formed principally by the lateral pterygoid plate but may be considered to extend further back to include tensor palati, levator palati and superior constrictor of pharynx. The superior constrictor slopes steeply inward from its origin (from the pterygoid hamulus, the pterygomandibular raphe, the posterior end of mylohyoid line and from the side of the tongue) towards the midline raphe behind the pharynx. This accounts for the fact that the infratemporal region, which it helps to bind, is considerably deepened posteriorly.

Note that the Eustachian tube lies at the skull base between tensor palati laterally and levator palati medially.

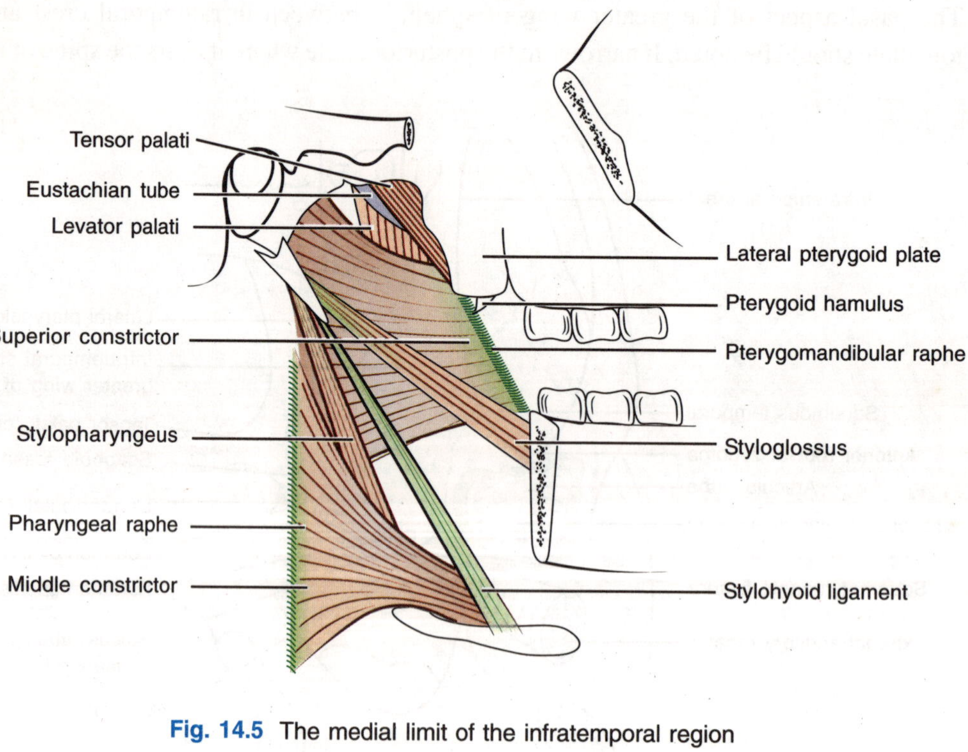

Fig. 14.5 The medial limit of the infratemporal region

14.6 The superficial relations of the superior constrictor of pharynx

The styloglossus, the stylopharyngeus and upper fibres of middle constrictor of pharynx muscles and stylohoid ligament lie superficial to the superior constrictor of pharynx.

Study the course of the facial artery and its two branches viz., ascending palatine and tonsillar artery over the muscle. The styloglossus muscle intervenes between these branches.

- The glossopharyngeal nerve runs forwards on the lateral side of stylopharyngeus muscle to enter the pharynx in the interval between the middle and superior constrictors of pharynx where it usually lies deep to stylohyoid ligament. It then reaches the base of the tongue. The maxillary artery commences its course on the superior constrictor of the pharynx.

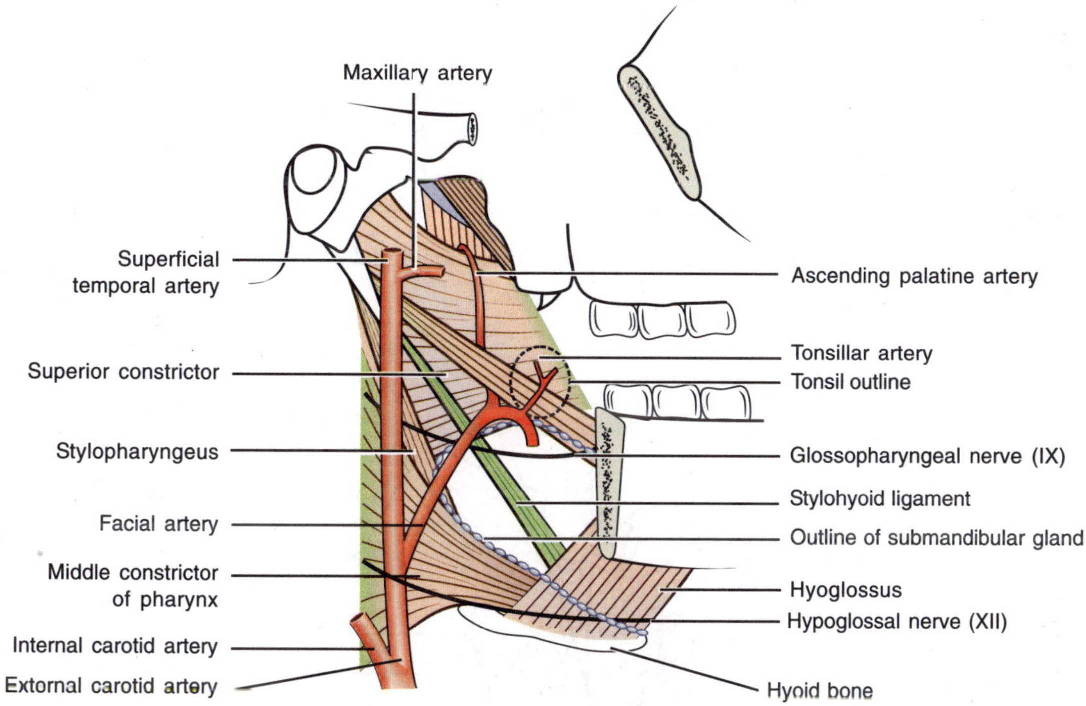

Fig. 14.6 The superficial relations of the superior constrictor of pharynx

14.7 The medial pterygoid muscle and the deeper contents of infratemporal fossa

The medial pterygoid muscle is bicipital in origin. The superficial head is small and arises from the maxillary tuberosity and pyramidal process of palatine while the bigger deep head arises from the medial aspect of lateral pterygoid plate. The two heads unite and get inserted into the rough area between the mandibular foramen and angle of mandible.

The mandibular nerve descends into the infratemporal fossa through foramen ovale. It soon divides into an anterior and posterior division.

Branches

- From the main trunk
  - Nervous spinosus for duramater of middle cranial fossa by passing through foramen spinosum
  - Nerve to medial pterygoid which also supplies the tensor tympani and tensor palati muscles
- From anterior division
  - Masseteric nerve for masseter
  - Anterior and posterior deep temporal nerves for temporalis
  - Buccal nerve (sensory) for mucous membrane of cheek and gums
  - Nerve to lateral pterygoid
- From posterior division
  - Auriculotemporal (sensory) for tragus, upper part of pinna, external auditory meatus, outer surface of tympanic membrane and temporomandibular joint
  - Inferior alveolar nerve gives mylohyoid branch for mylohyoid muscle. Rest is sensory for teeth of lower jaw
  - Lingual nerve (sensory) for tongue

The chorda tympani, a branch of facial nerve, joins the lingual nerve. Note the middle meningeal artery arising from the first part of the maxillary artery.

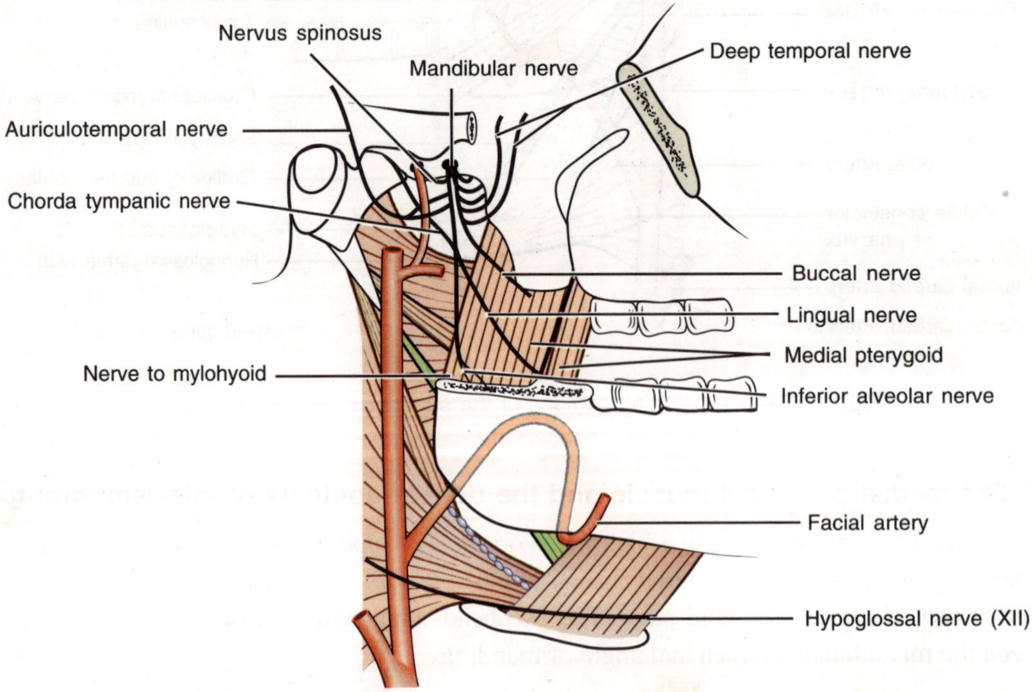

Fig. 14.7 The medial pterygoid muscle and the deeper contents of infratemporal fossa

14.8 The otic ganglion

It is situated medial to the mandibular nerve trunk and lateral to the tensor palati muscle.

Sympathetic root – from plexus around middle meningeal artery for blood vessels of the parotid gland

Somatic motor root – from nerve to medial pterygoid for tensor palati and tensor tympani muscles

Parasympathetic root – from glossopharyngeal nerve via tympanic and lesser petrosal nerves for parotid gland. These are the only fibres which synapse in the ganglion. After a relay in the ganglion, the fibres of the nerve join the auriculotemporal nerve to reach the parotid gland.

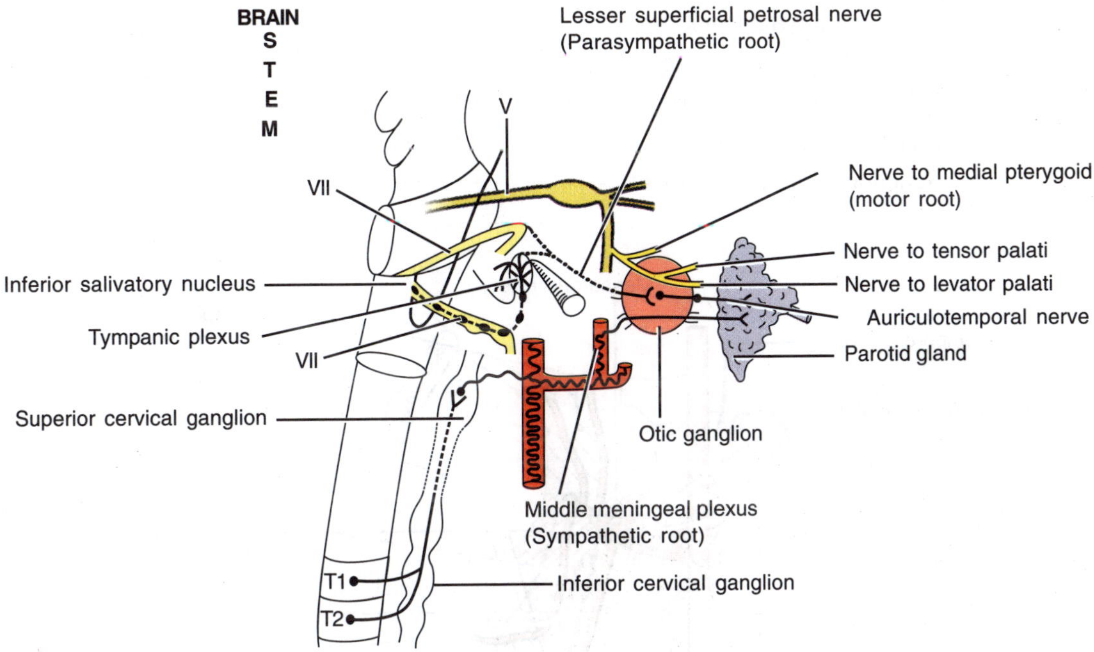

Fig. 14.8 The otic ganglion

14.9 The lateral pterygoid muscle and the superficial contents

The lateral pterygoid arises by two heads. The smaller upper head springs from the infratemporal crest and infratemporal surface of the greater wing of the sphenoid. The lower head arises from the lateral surface of the lateral pterygoid plate. It is inserted into the pterygoid fovea on the front of the neck of the mandible, the capsule and the articular disc of the temporo-mandibular joint. It is the key muscle of the region. The nerve of the region viz., mandibular nerve lies deep to it while the artery of the region viz., the maxillary artery lies superficial to it. As this artery enters the region postero-inferiorly, so all its branches lie posterior to the branches of the mandibular nerve which enters the region in an anterior plane.

The branches of anterior division of mandibular nerve, with the exception of buccal, are motor and are distributed to the muscles of mastication, as well as tensor palati and tensor tympani through the otic ganglion. All the branches of posterior division are sensory except the nerve to mylohyoid whose component fibres travel in the inferior alveolar nerve but leave it before it enters the mandibular foramen.

Relations of this key muscle are as follows:

- Deep (Fig. 14.7 *Refer* page 102)
  - Lingual nerve
  - Inferior alveolar nerve
  - Main mandibular trunk
  - Medial pterygoid muscle
  - Middle meningeal artery
  - Pterygoid venous plexus
  - Sphenomandibular ligament

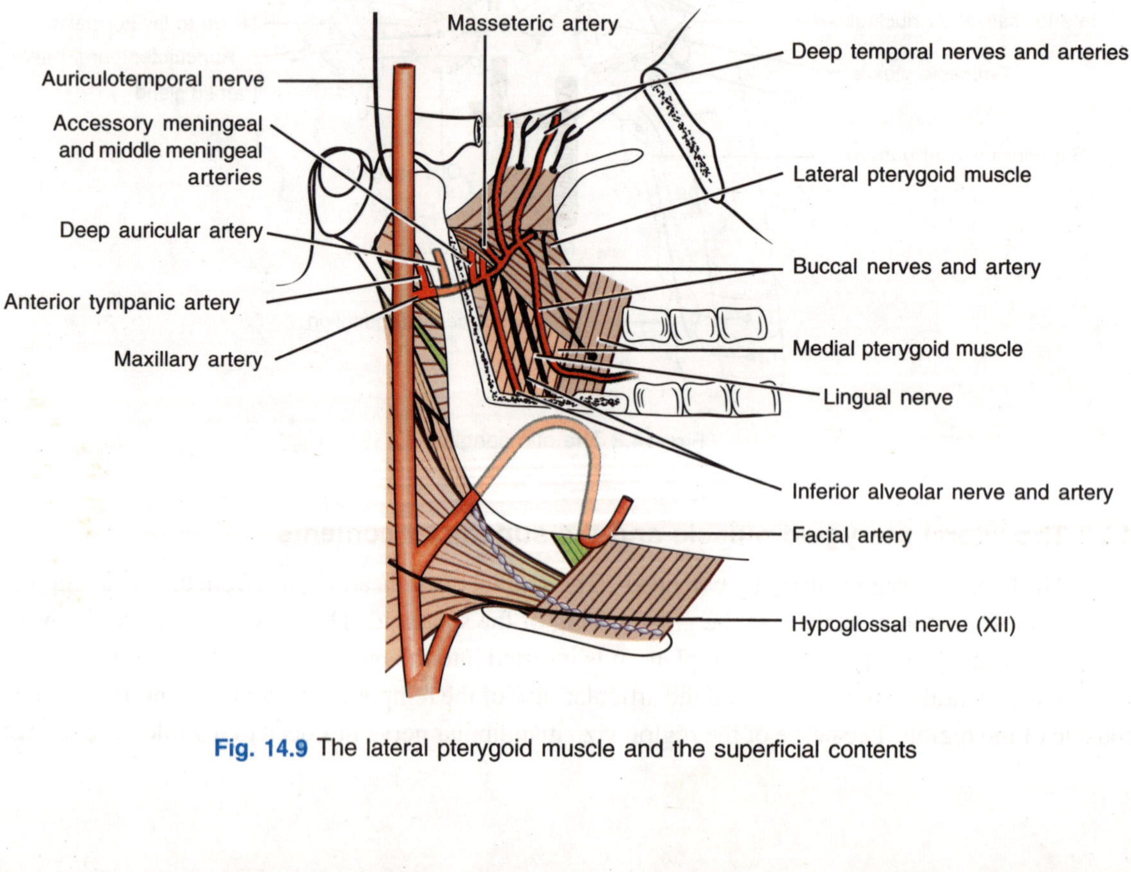

Fig. 14.9 The lateral pterygoid muscle and the superficial contents

- Superficial
  - Ramus of mandible
  - Masseter muscle
  - Temporalis muscle
  - Second part of maxillary artery
  - Deep temporal arteries
- Emerging along the upper border
  - Deep temporal nerves
  - Masseteric nerve
- Emerging at the lower border
  - First part of maxillary artery
  - Lingual nerve
  - Inferior alveolar nerve
- Disappearing under the lower border
  - Middle meningeal artery
  - Accessory meningeal artery

14.10 The temporalis muscle

The third muscle of mastication, the large and powerful, temporalis is shown here. It arises from the skull over the whole temporal fossa as well as from the temporal facia which is superficial to it. The muscle forms a flat tendon which inserts into the margins and deep surface of the coronoid process of the mandible and is lateral to the lateral pterygoid muscle. Its anterior fibres are vertical, posterior fibres horizontal and in between run with different degrees of obliquity.

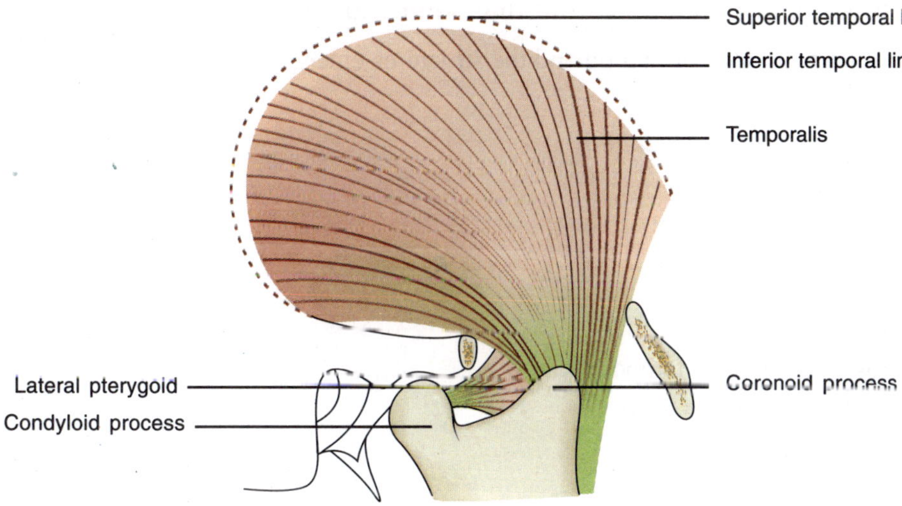

Fig. 14.10 The temporalis muscle

14.11 The masseter muscle

It is the most superficial of the four muscles of mastication. It arises from the lower border and deep surface of the whole zygomatic arch. The anterior two-third of the muscle runs down and back to insert into the ramus of mandible, close to its lower border. The posterior third of the muscle runs down with a slight anterior inclination to insert deep to the anterior part into the upper part of the ramus.

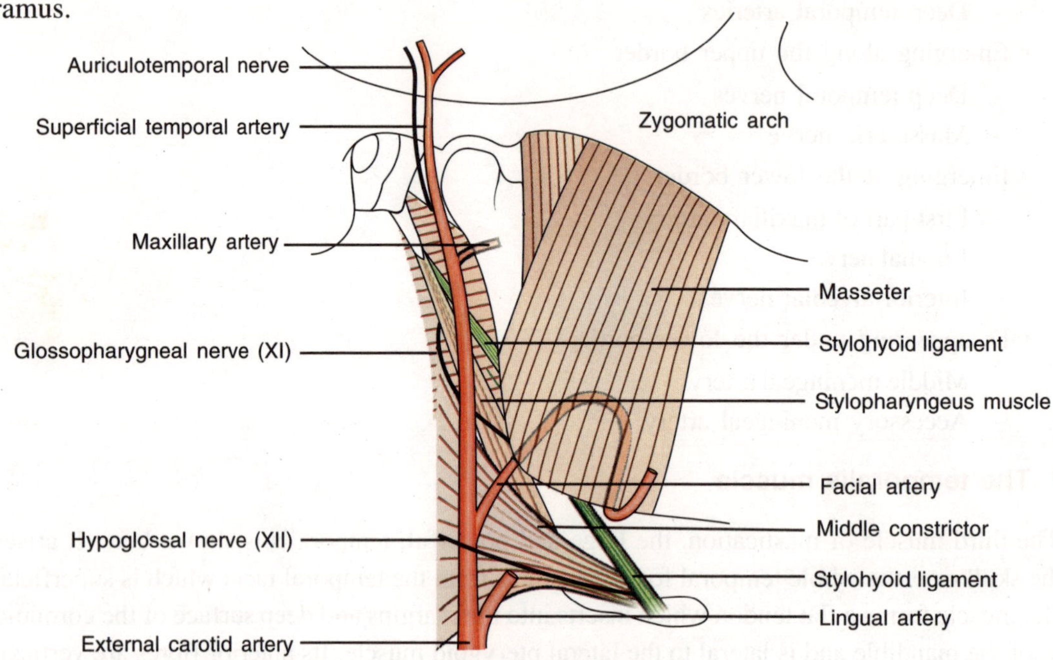

Fig. 14.11 The masseter muscle

14.12 The superficial relations of the masseter muscle

Note the superficial lobe of parotid and the structures emerging from underneath it and lying superficial to the masseter muscle.

Action of muscles of mastication:

- Protraction
  - Lateral pterygoid
  - Medial pterygoid
  - Masseter
- Retraction
  - Posterior fibres of temporalis
  - Deep fibres of masseter
- Elevation
  - Medial pterygoid
  - Masseter
  - Vertical fibres of temporalis

- Depression
  - Lateral pterygoid assisted by gravity
- Side to side movements of chewing
  - Lateral pterygoid
  - Medial pterygoid

Protraction at one joint is accompanied by retraction at the other.

Nerve supply:

All the muscles of mastication are supplied by the mandibular nerve.

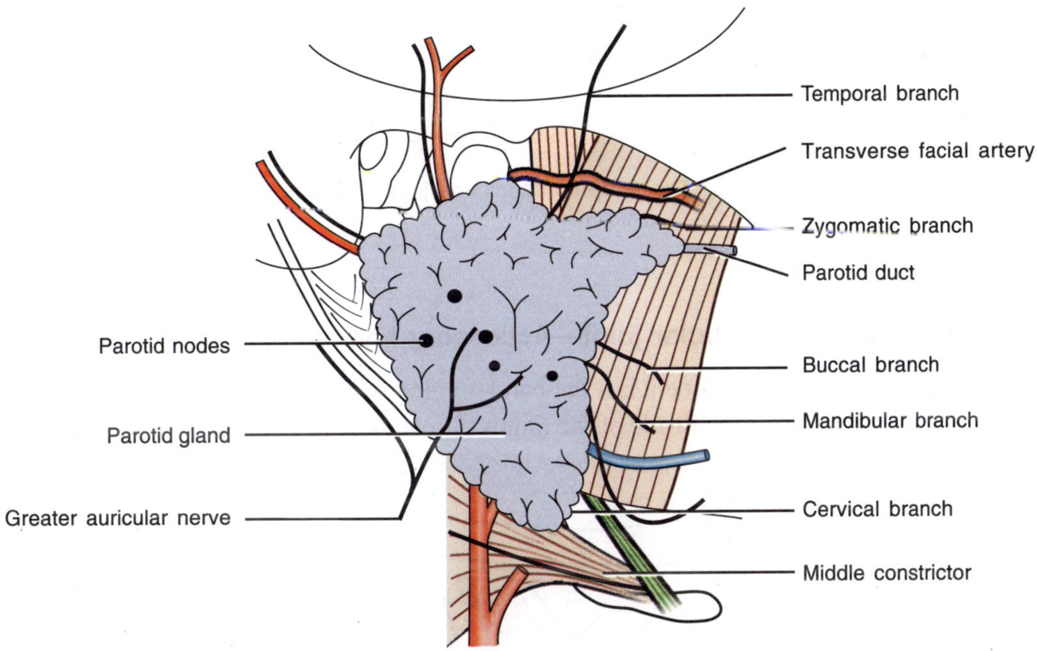

Fig. 14.12 The superficial relations of the masseter muscle

14.13 The temporomandibular joint—Fibrous capsule

It is attached above to the margins of the articular area on the temporal bone and below to the neck of the mandible.

The temporomandibular ligament is a thickened part of the capsule and is triangular in shape. Its base is attached to the zygomatic process of the temporal bone and the tubercle at its roots and its apex is attached to the lateral side of the neck of the mandible.

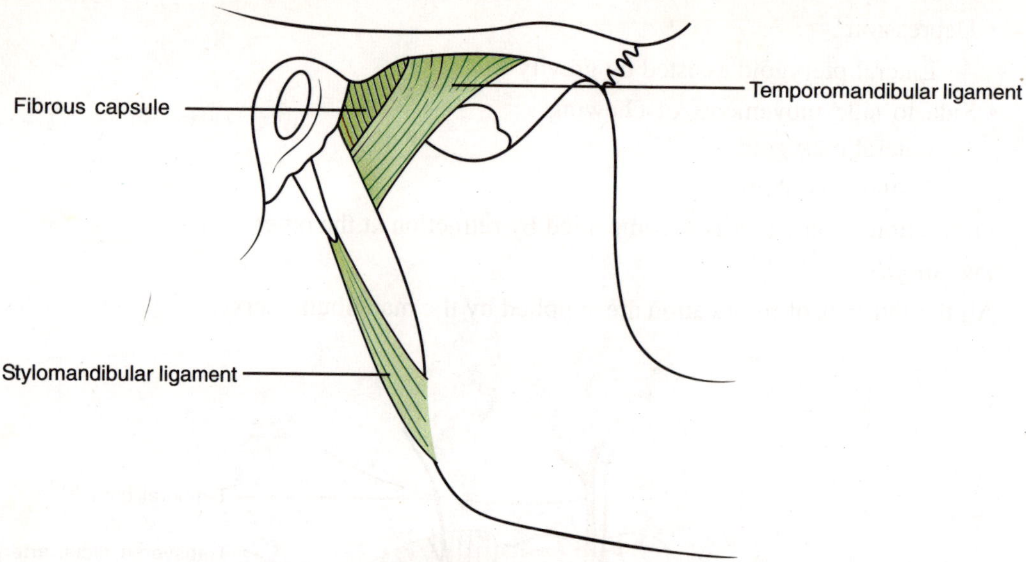

Fig. 14.13 The temporomandibular joint—Fibrous capsule

14.14 The temporomandibular joint—Accessory ligaments

The sphenomandibular ligament is a flat band running from the spine of the sphenoid above to the lingula at the midpoint of the inside of the ramus of mandible below.

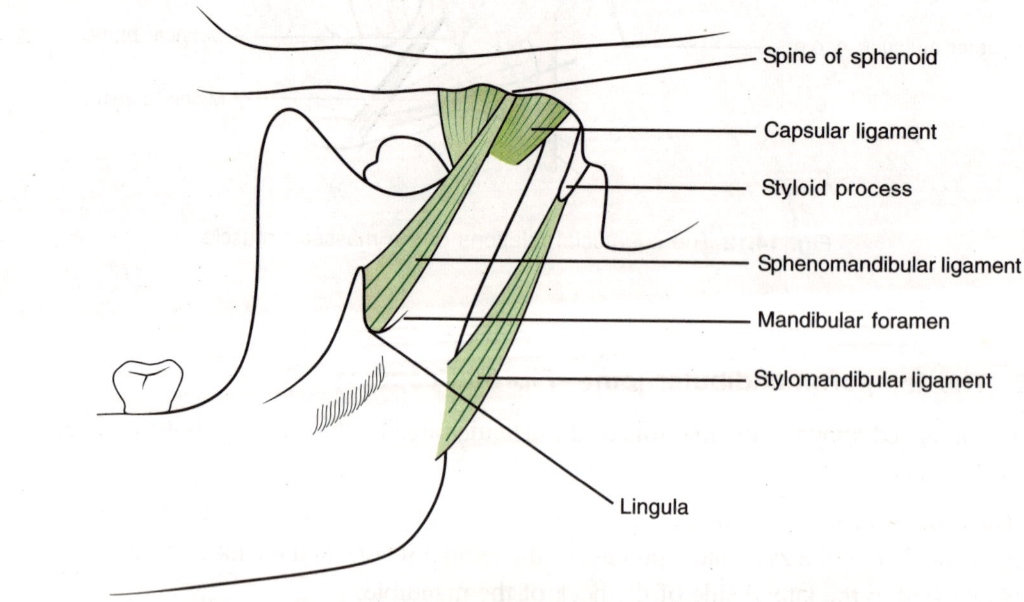

Fig. 14.14 The temporomandibular joint—Accessory ligaments

The stylomandibular ligament joins the styloid process to the angle of the mandible. This ligament, which is superficial to all the muscles originating from the styloid process, separates the parotid gland above from the submandibular gland below.

14.15 The temporomandibular joint—Articular disc and synovial membrane—Mouth closed

The articular disc is an oval plate of dense fibrous tissue which is fused with the fibrous capsule around its periphery. The upper surface of the disc is concavo—convex to fit the articular tubercle and the mandibular fossa. The concave inferior surface fits the head of the mandible. The joint thus has upper and lower compartments lined by synovial membrane.

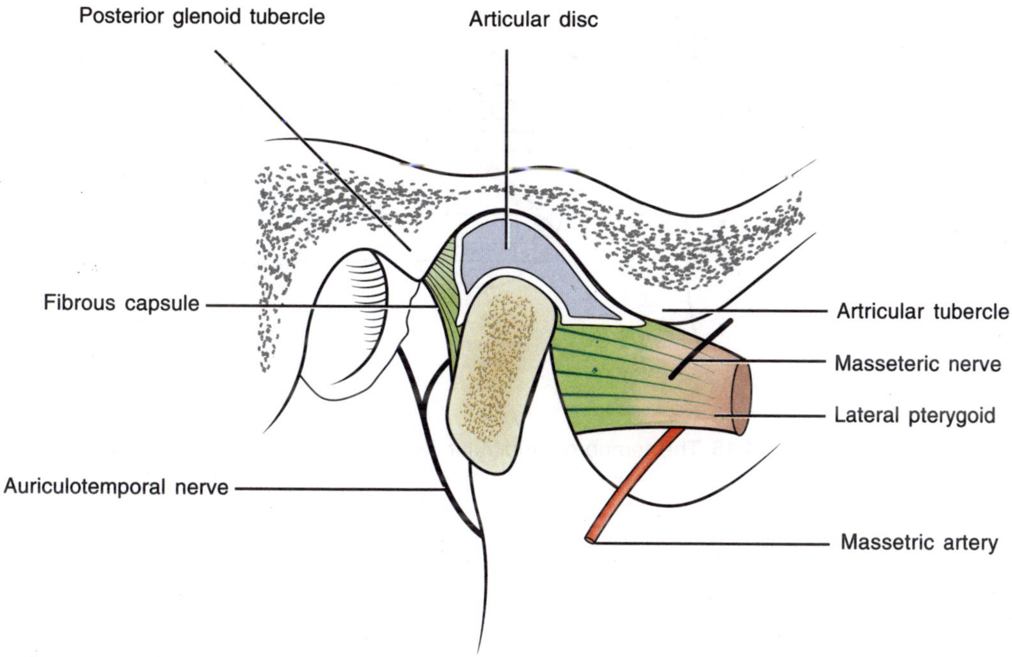

Fig. 14.15 The temporomandibular joint—Articular disc and synovial membrane—Mouth closed

14.16 The temporomandibular joint—Mouth opened

The relationship between the articular disc, head of mandible and articular tubercle with the mouth opened is shown.

Compare the diagram with Figure 14.15 which shows the structures with mouth closed.

The joint is supplied by masseteric nerve which enters from the anterior aspect and the auriculotemporal nerve which enters from the posterior aspect.

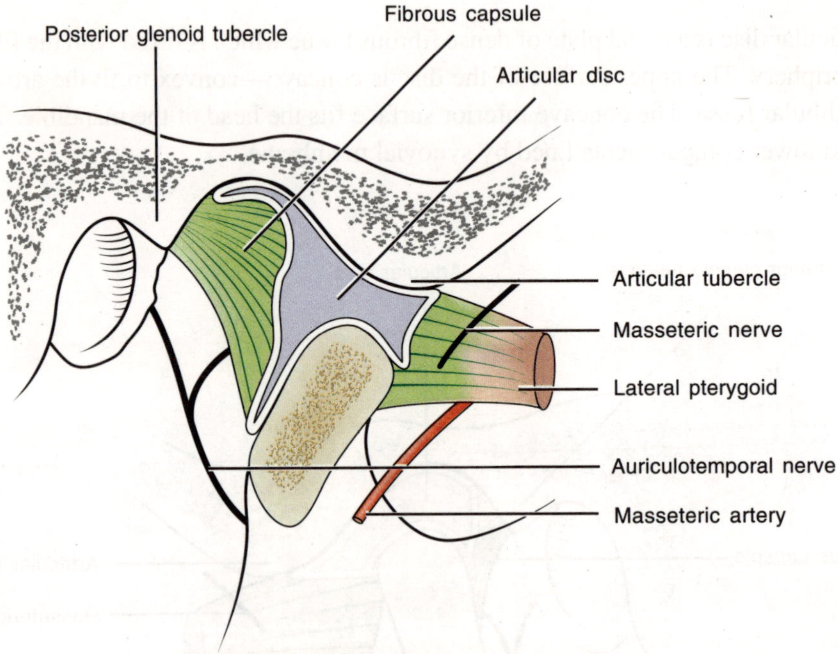

Fig. 14.16 The temporomandibular joint—Mouth opened

The Pterygo-palatine Fossa

Chapter **15**

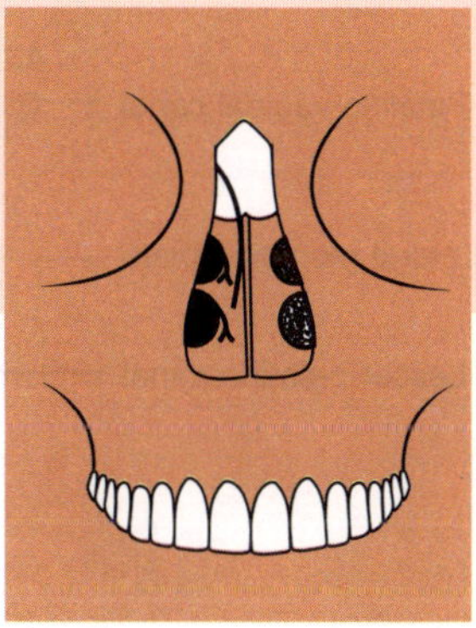

15.1 The pterygo-palatine fossa—Bony features and extent

A deep fissure, the pterygo-maxillary fissure, separates the pterygoid plates from the back of the maxilla. This fissure deepens considerably at its upper end, almost extending through into the nasal cavity. This upper portion is termed the pterygo-palatine fossa and is concerned with the blood supply and nerve supply to the upper jaw.

It is bounded as mentioned below:

Anteriorly – the extreme medial part of posterior surface of maxilla below the apex of the floor of the orbit. Inferior orbital fissure connects it with the orbit.

Posteriorly – the lateral pterygoid plate and a part of the medial plate. The pterygoid and palatino-vaginal canals connect it with the region of naso-pharynx.

Medially – the perpendicular plate of palatine. The spheno palatine foramen connects it with nasal fossa.

Laterally – there is pterygo-maxillary fissure so there is no wall. The fissure connects it with infratemporal fossa.

Roof – the undersurface of greater wing of sphenoid. The foramen rotundum connects it with the middle cranial fossa.

Floor – this is absent as the posterior wall (pterygoid plates) meets with the anterior wall (posterior surface of maxilla). Between the two lies the greater palatine canal which opens below at a foramen on the hard palate connecting the fossa with the oral cavity.

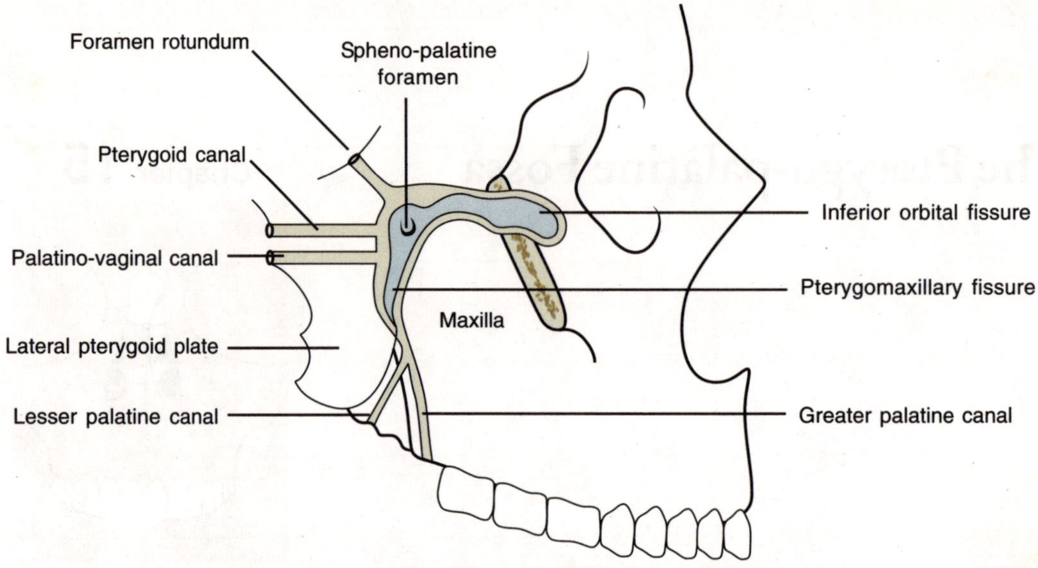

Fig. 15.1 The pterygo-palatine fossa—Bony features and extent

15.2 The medial wall of the pterygo-palatine fossa

The position of spheno-palatine foramen has been shown as it is related to the lateral wall of nose. It normally closed in life by the muco-periosteum of the nose. The shaded area indicates the extent of the fossa.

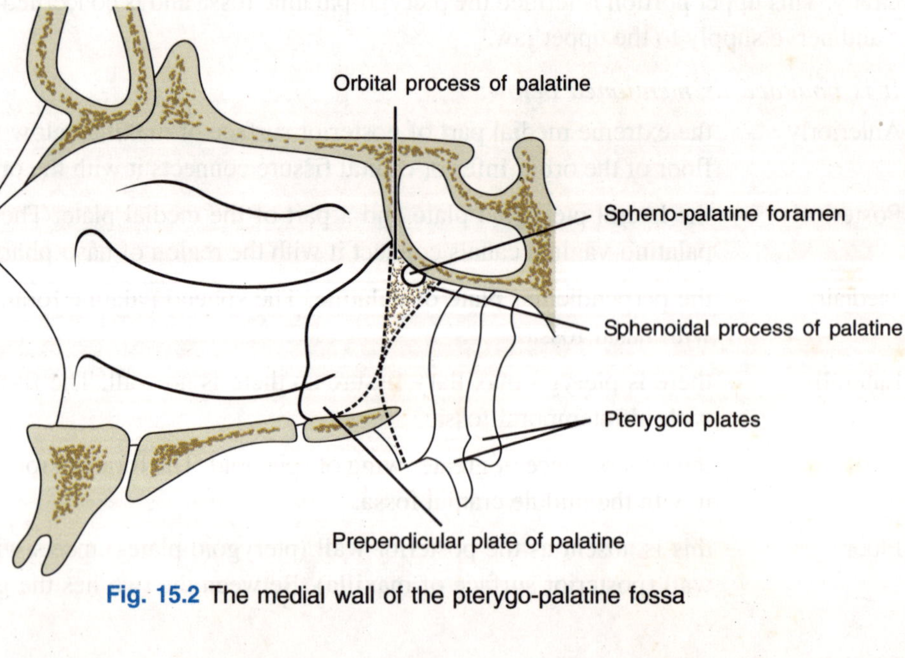

Fig. 15.2 The medial wall of the pterygo-palatine fossa

15.3 The maxillary nerve—Course and branches

The maxillary nerve and vessels and the pterygo-palatine ganglion occupy the fossa. The maxillary nerve courses from the middle cranial fossa through foramen rotundum into the pterygo-palatine fossa, then passes into the orbit through the inferior orbital fissure and then lies in infra orbital groove. In the fossa the pterygo-palatine ganglion is suspended by two short thick pterygo-palatine branches from the maxillary nerve. Study the other branches of maxillary nerve which have been labelled.

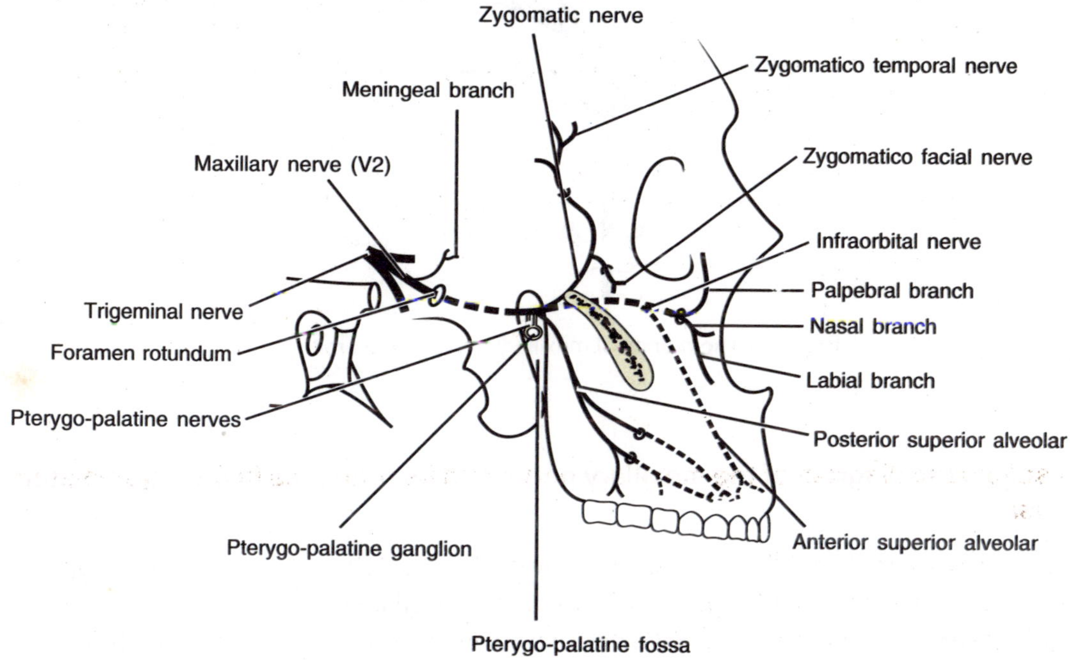

Fig. 15.3 The maxillary nerve—Coruse and branches

15.4 The branch of maxillary nerve in the orbit

The maxillary nerve deviating laterally in the fossa divides at the inferior orbital fissure into two branches, the infraorbital and the zygomatic, both of which enter the orbit and are distributed to the skin of the face.

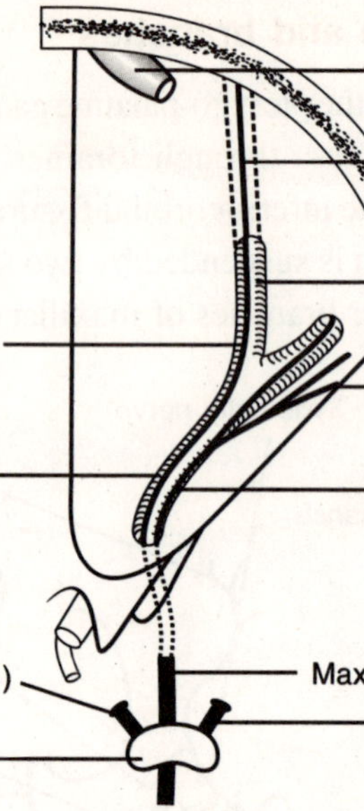

Fig. 15.4 The branch of maxillary nerve in the orbit

15.5 A schematic diagram of the maxillary nerve and its branches in pterygo-palatine fossa

Note the two pterygo-palatine nerves, which suspend the ganglion, and the posterior superior alveolar nerves, which run down the posterior aspect of the maxilla to enter the bone above the last molar tooth. At the inferior orbital fissure it divides into zygomatic and infra-orbital branches.

15.6 The Pterygo-palatine ganglion and its roots and branches in a schematic representation of the pterygo-palatine fossa

The ganglion lies just below the maxillary nerve in the pterygo-palatine fossa. The sensory fibres are received through the pterygo-palatine branches of maxillary nerve. Sympathetic and parasympathetic nerve fibres enter the ganglion in the nerve of the pterygoid canal fromed by the greater petrosal (geniculate ganglion) and deep petrosal (internal carotid plexus) nerves.

The branches given off by the ganglion are the orbital (ascending), the greater and lesser palatine (descending), the nasopalatine and posterior nasal (passing inwards) and the pharyngeal (passing backwards).

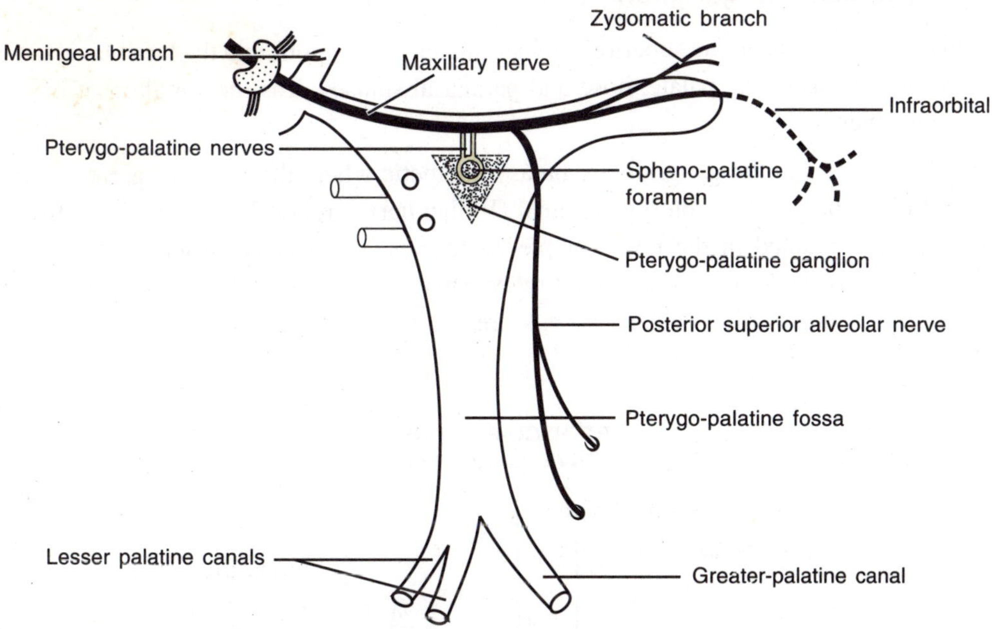

Fig. 15.5 A schematic diagram of the maxillary nerve and its branches in pterygo-palatine fossa

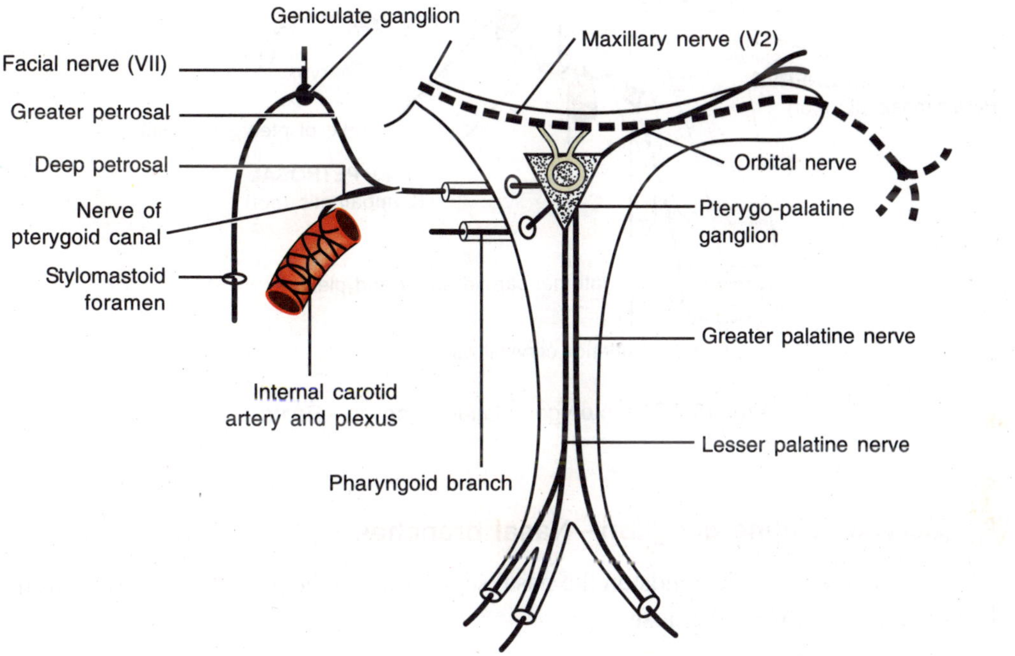

Fig. 15.6 The pterygo-palatine ganglion and its roots and branches in a schematic representation of the pterygo-palatine fossa

15.7 The pterygo-palatine ganglion—Roots

It is a relay station between the superior salivary nucleus in the pons and the lacrimal gland and mucous and serous glands of the palate, nose and paranasal sinuses. It is the ganglion of hayfever (running nose and eyes).

The only cell bodies in the ganglion are parasympathetic where the fibres of greater petrosal nerve contained in the nerve of the pterygoid canal (Vidian nerve) relay. The sympathetic fibres of deep petrosal nerve contained in the nerve of pterygoid canal are vasoconstrictors. The sensory fibres of maxillary nerve are sensory and do not relay. There are five branches, each branch carries a mixture of all three kinds of fibres viz, sensory, secretomotor and sympathetic.

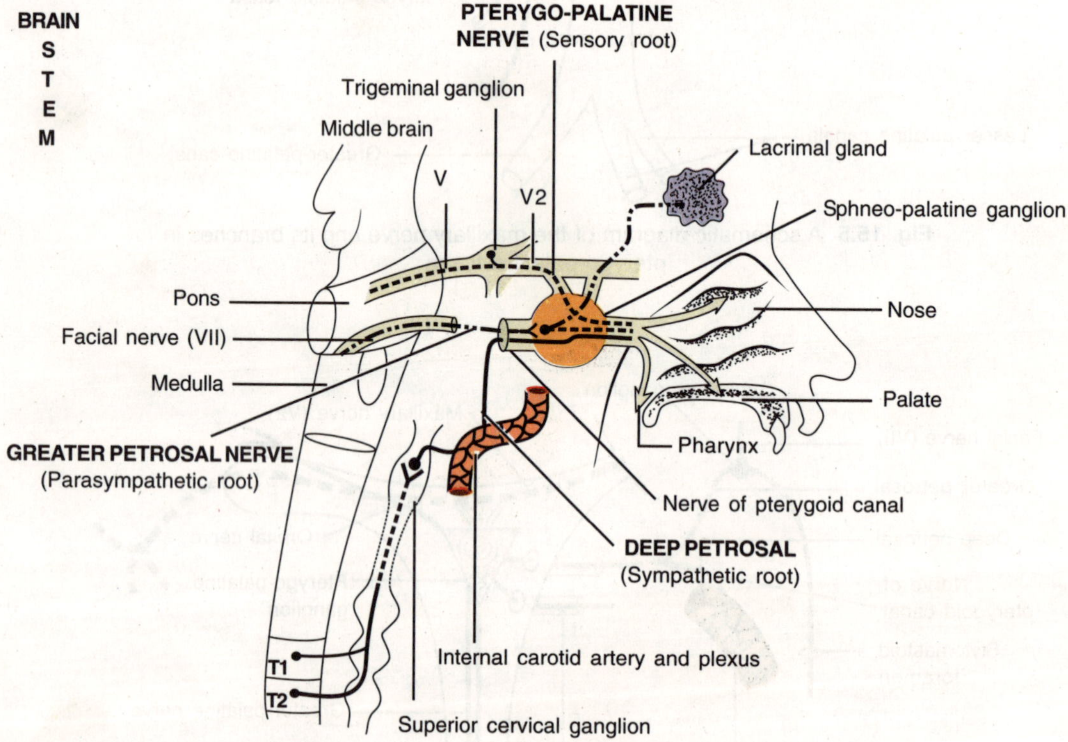

Fig. 15.7 The pterygo-palatine ganglion—Roots

15.8 The pterygo-palatine ganglion—Nasal branches

The naso palatine nerve descends on the nasal septum while the posterior superior nasal nerve descends on the lateral wall of the nose.

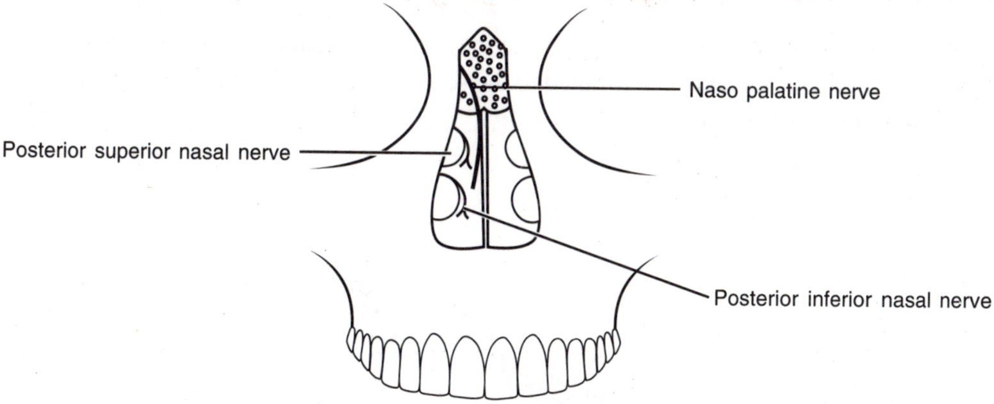

Fig. 15.8 The pterygo-palatine ganglion—Nasal branches

15.9 The branches of pterygo-palatine ganglion on the lateral wall of nose

The posterior superior lateral nasal nerves (short spheno-palatine) pass through the spheno-palatine foramen and turn forwards to supply the postero-superior quadrant of the lateral wall of the nose.

The posterior inferior lateral nasal nerves are given off by greater (anterior) palatine nerve to supply the postero-inferior quadrant of the lateral wall of the nose. The greater and lesser palatine nerves supply the palate and tonsil.

The pharyngeal branch passes back through the palatino-vaginal canal and emerges at the roof of the nose to supply the mucous membrane of the naso-pharynx.

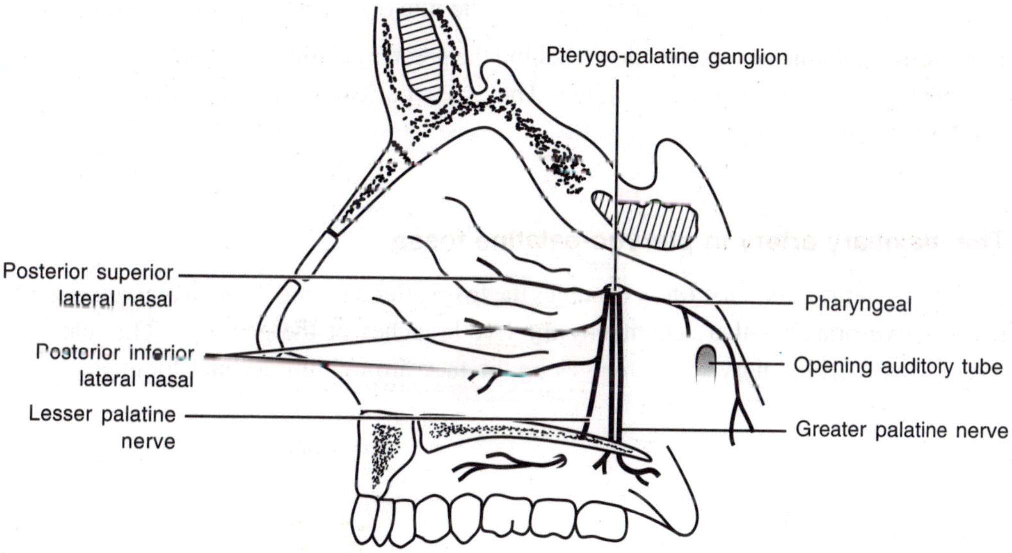

Fig. 15.9 The branches of pterygo-palatine ganglion on the lateral wall of nose

15.10 The branches of pterygo-palatine ganglion on the septum of nose

The naso-palatine nerve (long spheno-palatine) passes through the spheno-palatine foramen, crosses the roof of the nose, and is distributed to the septum and incisive gum of the hard palate after passing through incisive foramina (Fig. 15.11).

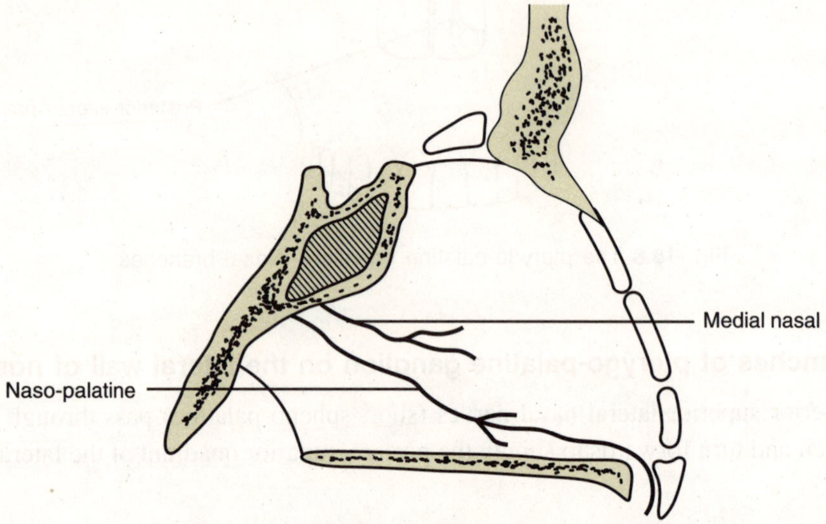

Fig. 15.10 The branches of pterygo-palatine ganglion on the septum of nose

15.11 The branches of pterygo-palatine ganglion on the palate

The greater palatine (anterior palatine) passes down through the greater palatine canal and at the greater palatine foramen turns forwards to supply the mucous membrane of the hard palate.

The two lesser palatine nerves pass down behind the greater palatine nerve and emerge through the medial and lateral lesser palatine foramina. They pass backwards to soft palate and mucous membrane of supratonsilar recess.

15.12 The maxillary artery in pterygo-palatine fossa

The third part of the maxillary artery occupies the fossa after entering through pterygo-maxillary fissure. It gives five branches that accompany the five branches of the ganglion. The main trunk accompanies the infraorbital nerve and emerges on the face through infraorbital foramen.

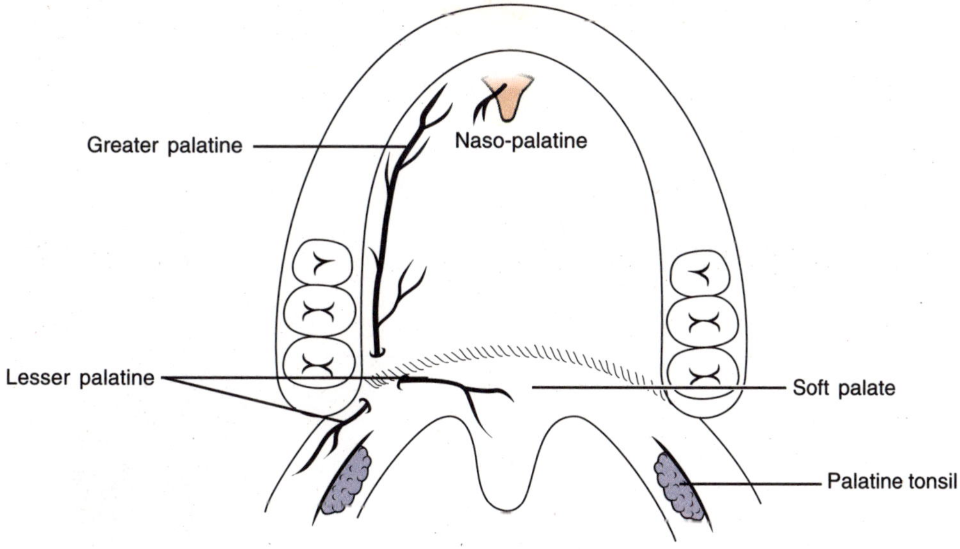

Fig. 15.11 The branches of pterygo-palatine ganglion on the palate

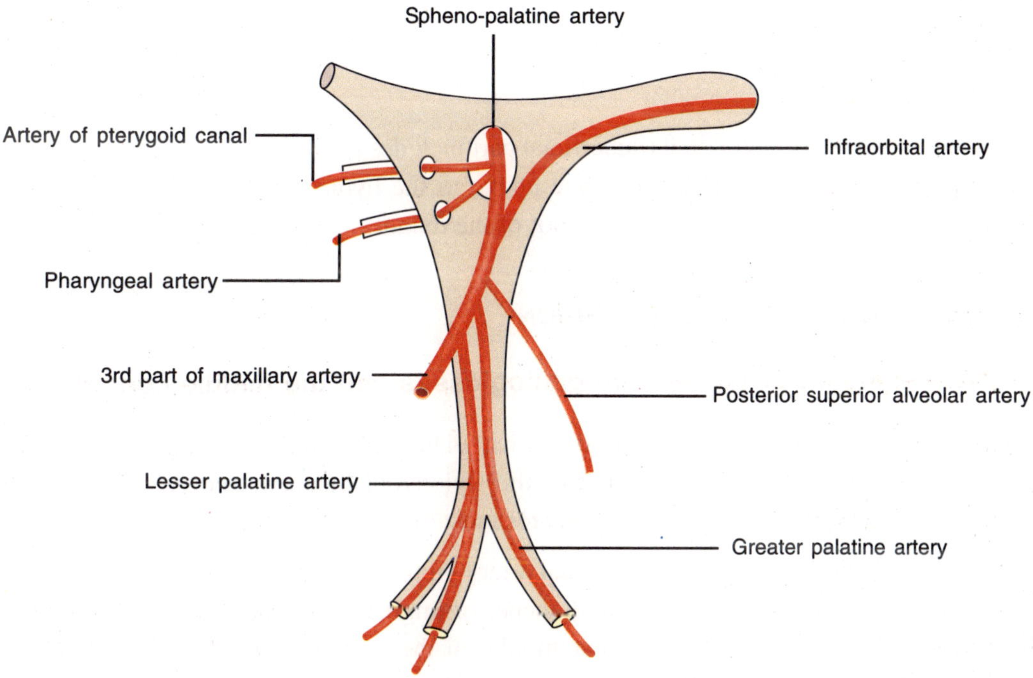

Fig. 15.12 The maxillary artery in pterygo-palatine fossa

The Submandibular Region

Chapter **16**

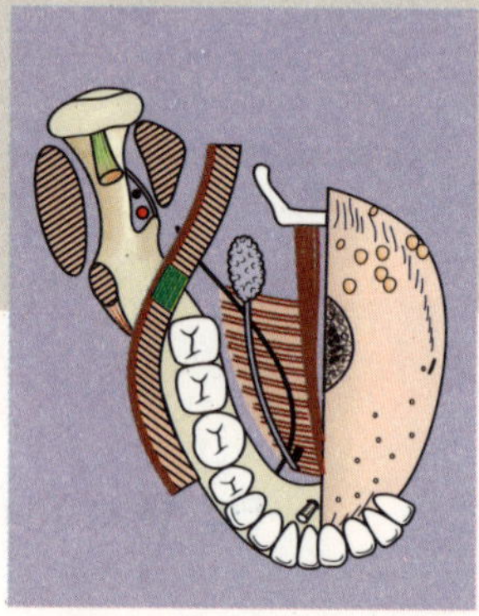

The submandibular region in its superficial part includes the submental and digastric triangles. The region extends from the mylohyoid line above to the hyoid bone below and deals with the structures in the floor of the mouth and the root of the tongue.

BUILDING UP THE SUBMANDIBULAR REGION

16.1 The first muscular plane—The genioglossus and the middle constrictor

These muscles together form a smooth vertical plane between the hyoid bone and the tongue. Three structures, the glossopharyngeal nerve, the stylohyoid ligament and the lingual artery, lie superficial to the genioglossus which accounts for most of the bulk of the tongue.

Note the characteristic loop of the lingual artery on the middle constrictor muscle. The two or more dorsalis linguae arteries are the main branches of lingual artery and run up to supply the body of the tongue and contribute to the vascular supply of the palatine tonsil. The geniohyoid is seen below the genioglossus. These structures are deep relations of the hyoglossus muscle.

The superior constrictor forms the wall of the oral pharynx and the palatine tonsil lies against its medial side.

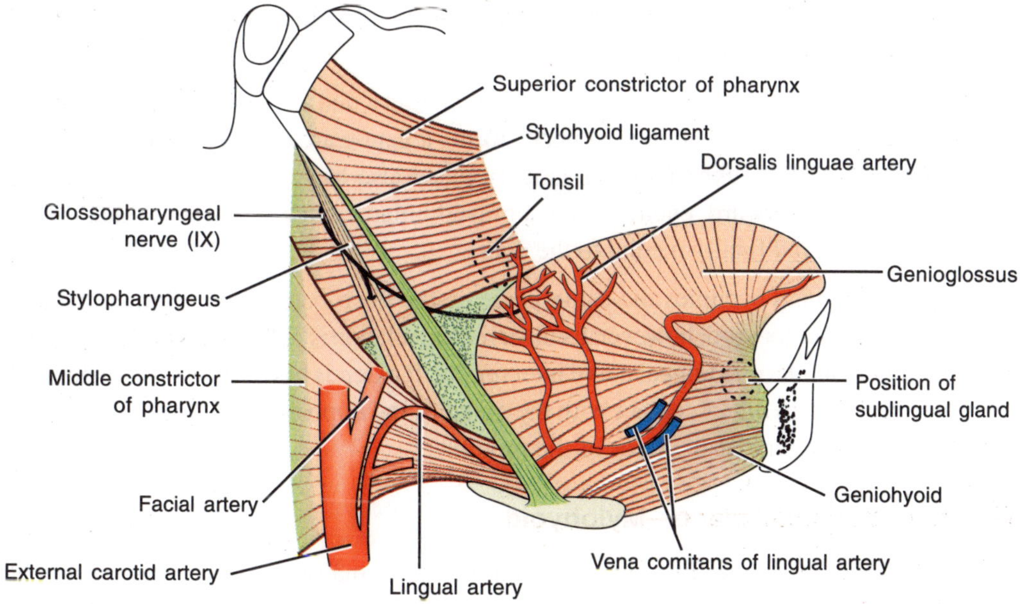

Fig. 16.1 The first muscular plant—The genioglossus and the middle constrictor

16.2 The second muscular plane—Hyoglossus and the styloglossus

These muscles form a second group of tongue muscles. The hyoglossus is the key to the floor of the mouth. It extends as a quadrilateral sheet on the side of the tongue and its upper border

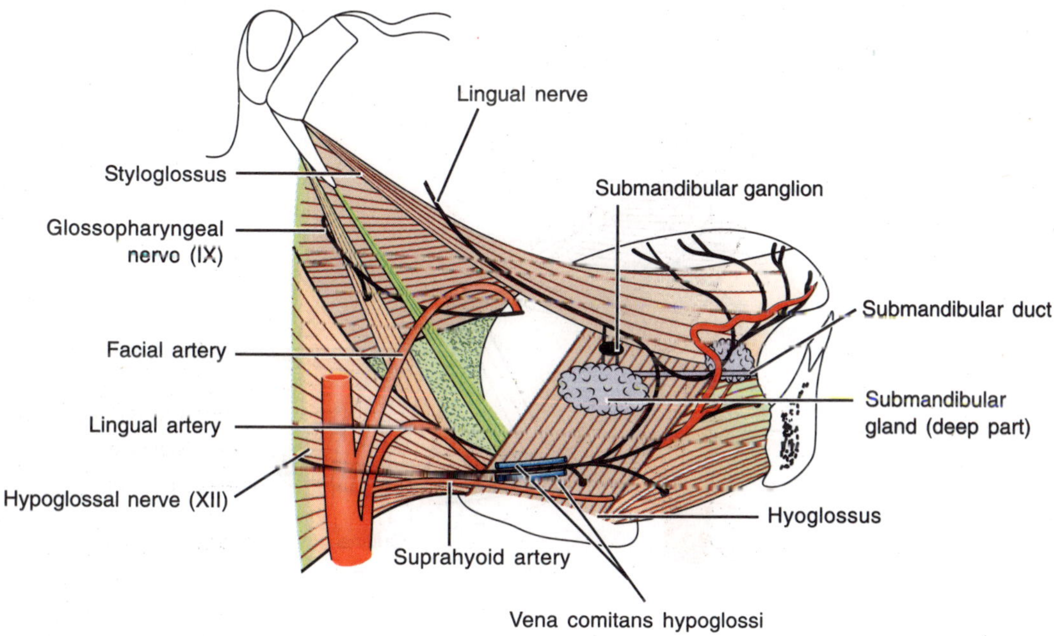

Fig. 16.2 The second muscular plane—Hyoglossus and the styloglossus

interdigitates with the fibres of styloglossus. Three structures, the lingual nerve, deep part of submandibular gland with its duct and hypoglossal nerve, lie superficial to it.

The hypoglossal nerve crosses the loop of lingual artery and then is separated from it by the posterior border of hyoglossus. The lingual nerve forms a gentle arc on hyoglossus before entering the tongue. The deep part of submandibular salivary gland also lies on the hyoglossus muscle. The lingual nerve, in arching forward, encircles the submandibular duct (Wharton's) so that the nerve is first lateral, then below and finally medial to the duct.

The sublingual gland occupies the same plane as the deep part of the submandibular gland, because it is placed further forward; however, its main medial relation is not hyoglossus but genioglossus, with the submandibular duct and lingual nerve intervening. It extends beyond the limit of genioglossus so that its anterior part is in direct contact with the gland of the opposite side. The gland lies directly below the mucous membrane of the floor of the mouth.

16.3 The third muscular plane—Mylohyoid

It is the 'diaphragm of the floor of the mouth' (diaphragma oris). Above this muscle lies the mouth, below it lies the neck. It arises from mylohyoid line, its posterior quarter is inserted into the body of the hyoid bone and the anterior three quarters interdigitate in a midline raphe extending from chin to hyoid bone.

Note the deep relations of the submandibular salivary gland within its transparent outline depicted in the diagram.

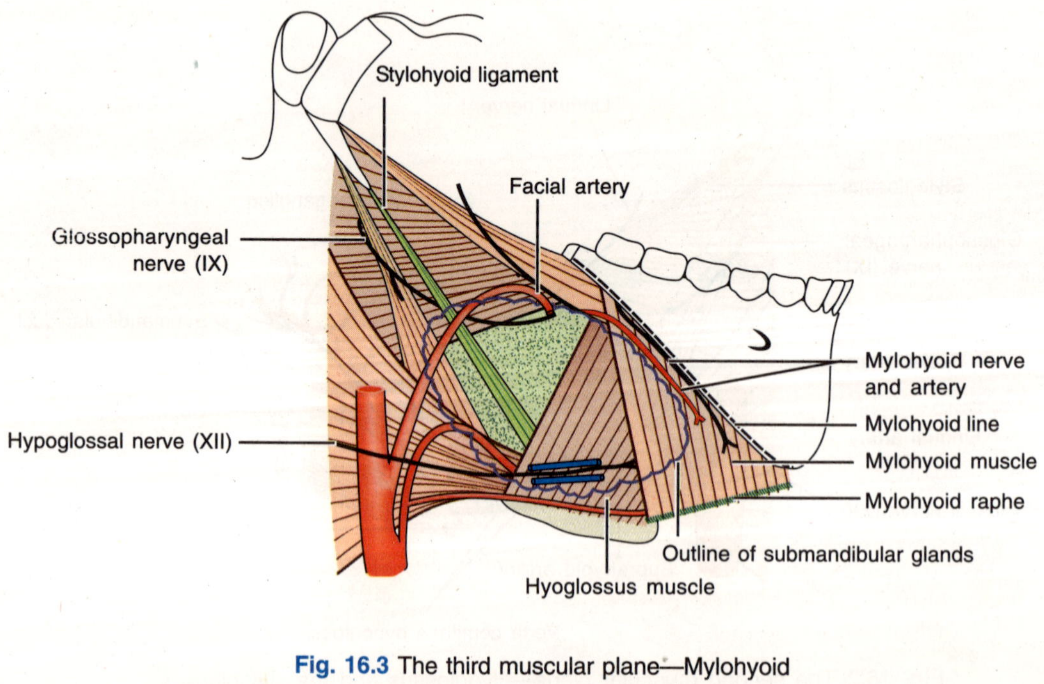

Fig. 16.3 The third muscular plane—Mylohyoid

16.4 The fourth muscular plane—Stylohyoid and digastric

The anterior and posterior bellies insert into an intermediate tendon which passes through the split in the tendon of stylohyoid.

The posterior belly of the digastric crosses the external carotid artery, the origin of the facial artery and the loop of the lingual artery. The glossopharyngeal nerve and the hypoglossal nerve are directly deep to this muscle.

The facial artery runs upwards to form its loop on styloglossus, then runs downwards, forwards, and laterally grooving the postero-superior part of the submandibular salivary gland. It then loops around the lower border of the mandible to enter the face.

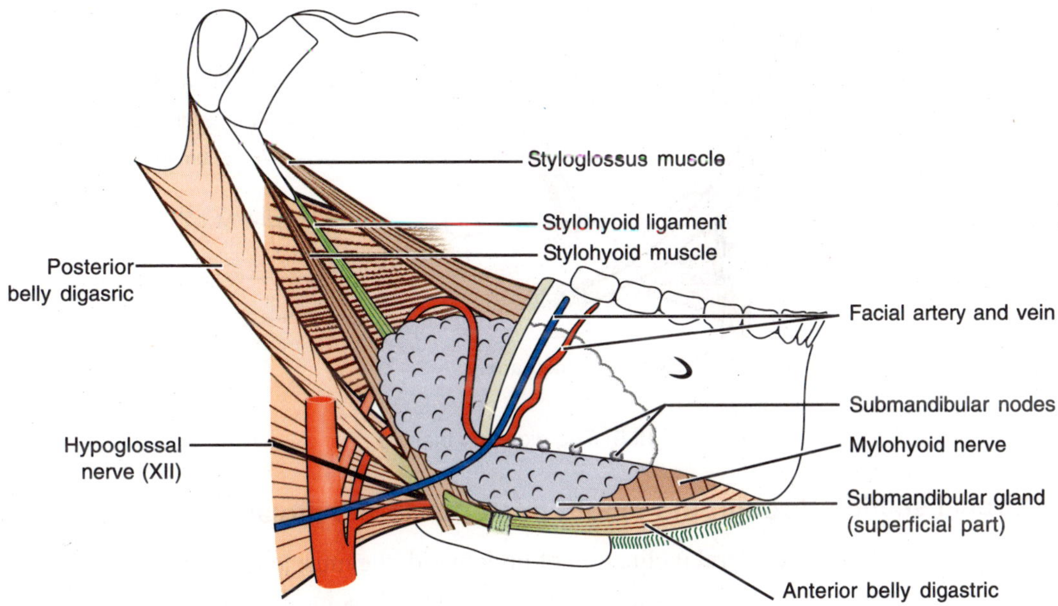

Fig. 16.4 The fourth musclar plane—stylohyoid and digastric

16.5 The digastric triangle

The digastric triangle, a part of the submandibular region, is bounded by the digastric and the stylohyoid muscles and the lower border of the mandible. Its roof is formed by the mylohyoid and hyoglossus muscles.

The lower part of the submandibular gland almost fills the triangle. The submandibular lymph nodes lie on the surface of the gland, specially along the lower border of the mandible.

The facial vein pierces the deep fascia at the lower border of the mandible and crosses the gland. The facial artery curves round the lower border of the mandible to enter the face.

The mylohyoid nerve lies on the anterior surface of the mylohyoid near the mandible and supplies it as well as the anterior belly of digastric.

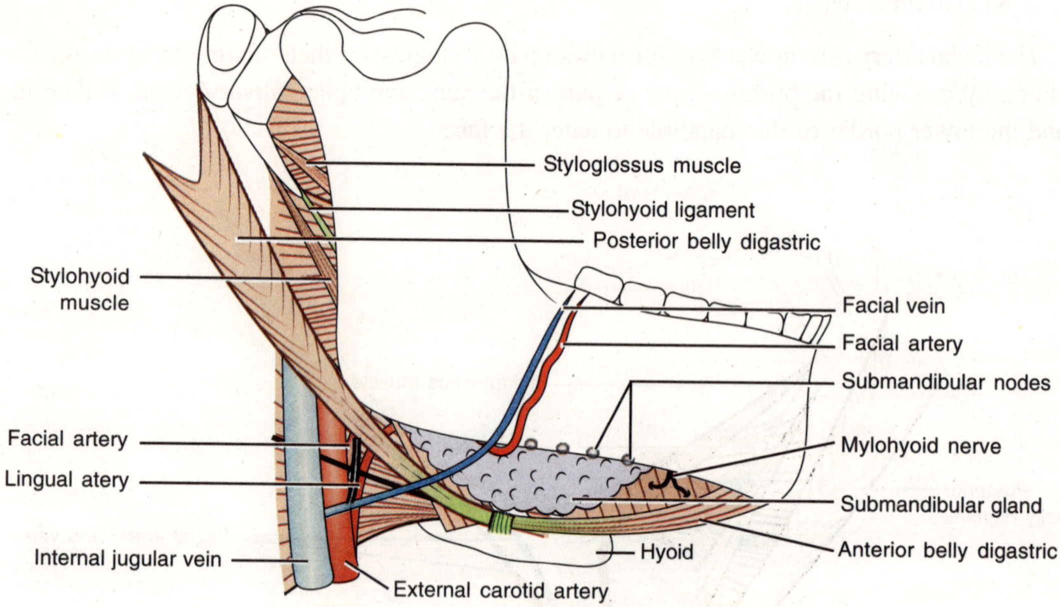

Fig. 16.5 The digastric triangle

16.6 Coronal section through the mouth posterior to the molar teeth

Note that because of the lateral inclination of mylohyoid, the muscle forms an acute angle with the hyoglossus leaving a deep V-shaped trough between them. It is in this trough that the deep part of the submandibular gland lies with its accompanying lingual and hypoglossal nerves. The superficial part of the gland does not lie in the trough but lies subcutaneously under cover of the body of the mandible with both mylohyoid and hyoglossus as its medial relations.

16.7 The submandibular ganglion—Roots and branches

It is a relay station for the parasympathetic secreto-motor fibres in the chorda tympani for submandibular and sublingual salivary glands and some small glands in the floor of the mouth.

Parasympathetic root – Fibres come from superior salivary nucleus in pons through the nervus intermedius of facial nerve. They leave the facial nerve in chorda tympani and join lingual nerve to reach the ganglion where they relay.

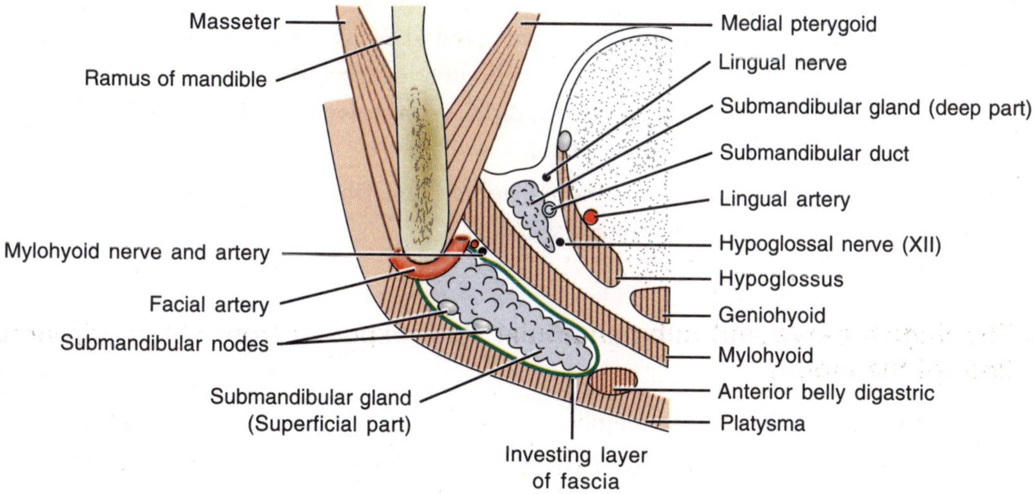

Fig. 16.6 Coronal section through the mouth posterior to the molar teeth

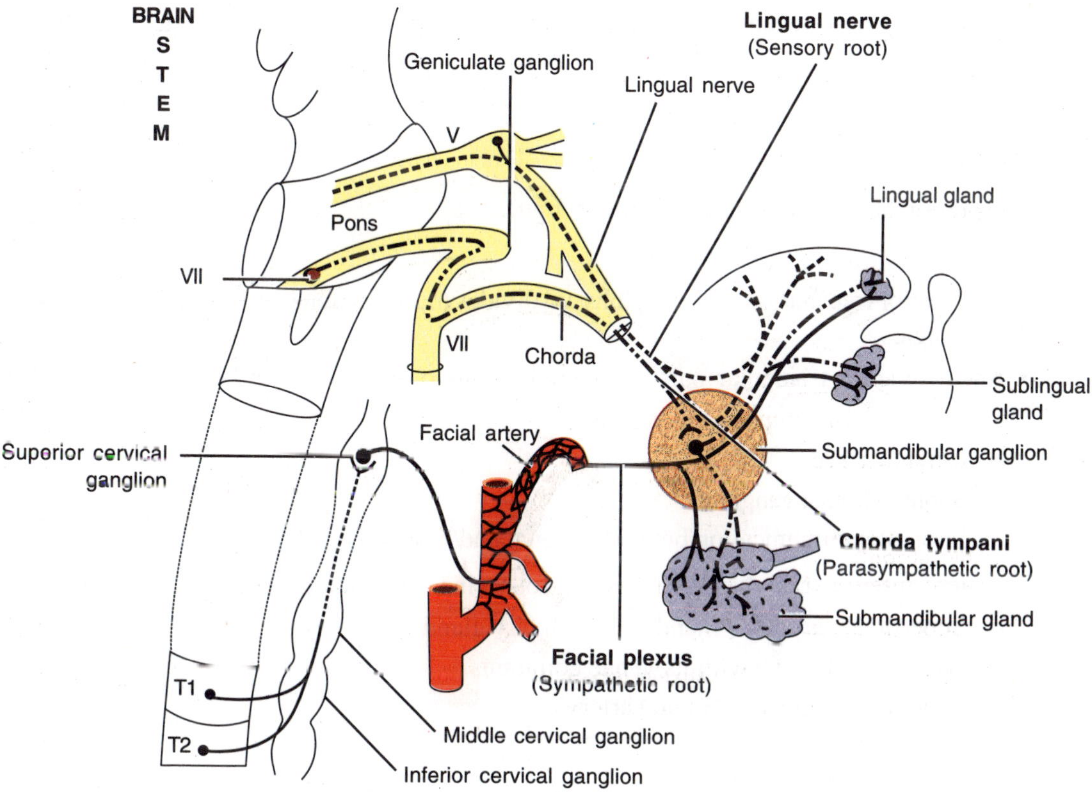

Fig. 16.7 The submandibular ganglion—Roots and branches

Sympathetic root – From the plexus around facial artery. These are postganglionic with cell bodies in superior cervical ganglion and pass through the ganglion to supply blood vessels in the submandibular and sublingual salivary glands.

Sensory root – From lingual nerve. The fibres rejoin lingual nerve and are distributed with it.

16.8 The lingual nerve and submandibular duct exposed from above through the floor of the mouth

An incision through the mucous membrane just lateral to the tongue passes into the area on the lateral side of hyoglossus into the V-shaped trough between it and mylohyoid. It gives a clear view of the sublingual gland, of the lingual nerve and of the deep part of the submandibular gland with its duct. Indeed, by retracting the submandibular gland it is even possible to expose the hypoglossal nerve.

The hyoglossus is important as it is the key muscle of the floor of the mouth.

Origin:

- Upper source of the entire length of the greater cornua of hyoid bone, external to middle constrictor
- Body of hyoid bone

Insertion:

- Posterior half of the margin of the tongue.

Superficial relations:

The posterior free margin of the mylohyoid divides the superficial surface of hyoglossus into two triangles.

- Anterosuperior triangular part is covered by mylohyoid and is related to:
  - Deep part of submandibular gland
  - Lingual nerve
  - Submandibular ganglion
  - Loop of communication between lingual and hypoglossal nerves
- Postero-inferior triangular part has the following superficial relations:
  - Superficial part of submandibular salivary gland
  - Hypoglossal nerve with its venae comitants
  - Suprahyoid branch of lingual artery

Deep relations:

- Posterior part of genioglossus anteriorly
- Middle constrictor posteriorly

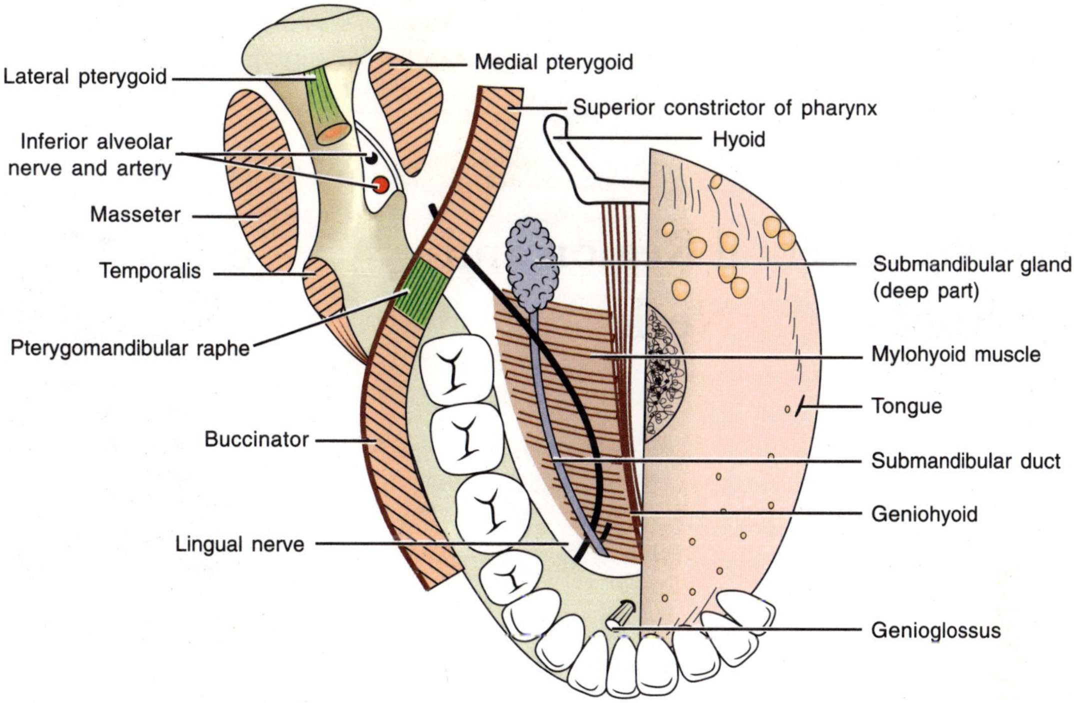

Fig. 16.8 The lingual nerve and submandibular duct exposed from above through the floor of the mouth

- Glossopharyngeal nerve
- Stylohyoid ligament
- Second part of lingual artery

The Prevertebral Region and the Root of the Neck

Chapter 17

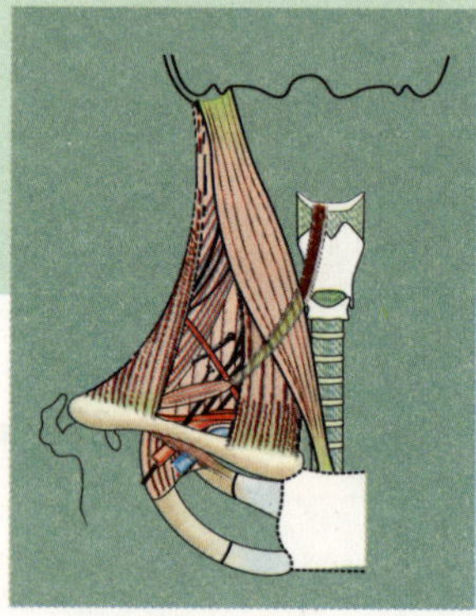

BUILDING UP THE PREVERTEBRAL REGION AND ROOT OF THE NECK

17.1 The bony framework of the neck

The neck consists of the seven cervical vertebrae and may be considered to include the superior surface of the manubrium sterni and the first rib which slopes downwards and forwards.

The levator scapulae is shown attached to transverse processes of C1 and C2 and posterior tubercles of C3 and C4. The scalenus posterior is attached to the posterior tubercles of C4, C5 and C6. The suprapleural membrane is attached to transverse process of C7 above and to the inner border of the first rib below and covers the apex of the lung and cervical pleura which fill the concavity of the first rib.

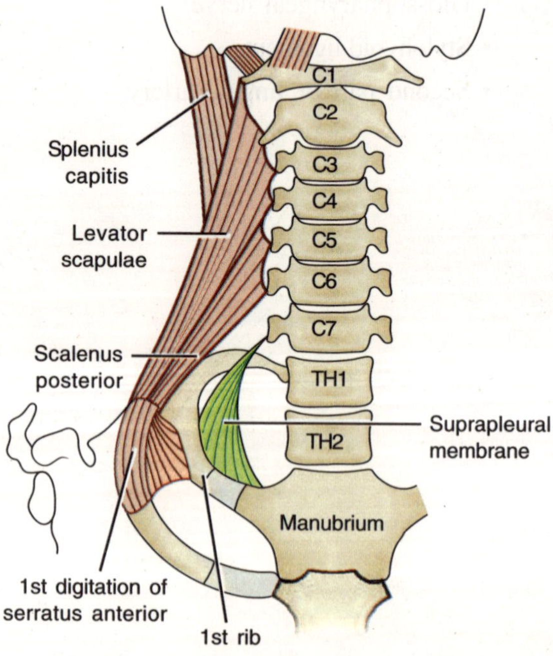

Fig. 17.1 The bony framework of the neck

17.2 The prevertebral muscles

The prevertebral muscles are week flexor muscles lying in front of the vertebral column from the skull to superior mediastinum. They are covered by prevertebral fascia.

The rectus capitis anterior and rectus capitis lateralis lie edge to edge with each other and extend from lateral mass of atlas to the front of foramen magnum and the jugular process of occipital bone, respectively.

The longus cervicis extends from the anterior tubercle of atlas to the lower border of T3 in the superior mediastinum. Laterally it is attached to the anterior tubercles of the typical cervical vertebrae (C3 to C6). It has middle vertical part and upper and lower oblique parts. The infero-lateral edge of the muscle is of importance in connection with its relations as it forms the medial boundary of the triangle of vertebral artery and covers the head of the first rib.

Note the sympathetic trunk, the first posterior intercostal vein, superior intercostal artery and the first thoracic nerve forming anterior relations of neck of the first rib from medial to lateral side. The upper two ribs and intercostal spaces lie posterior to cervical pleura.

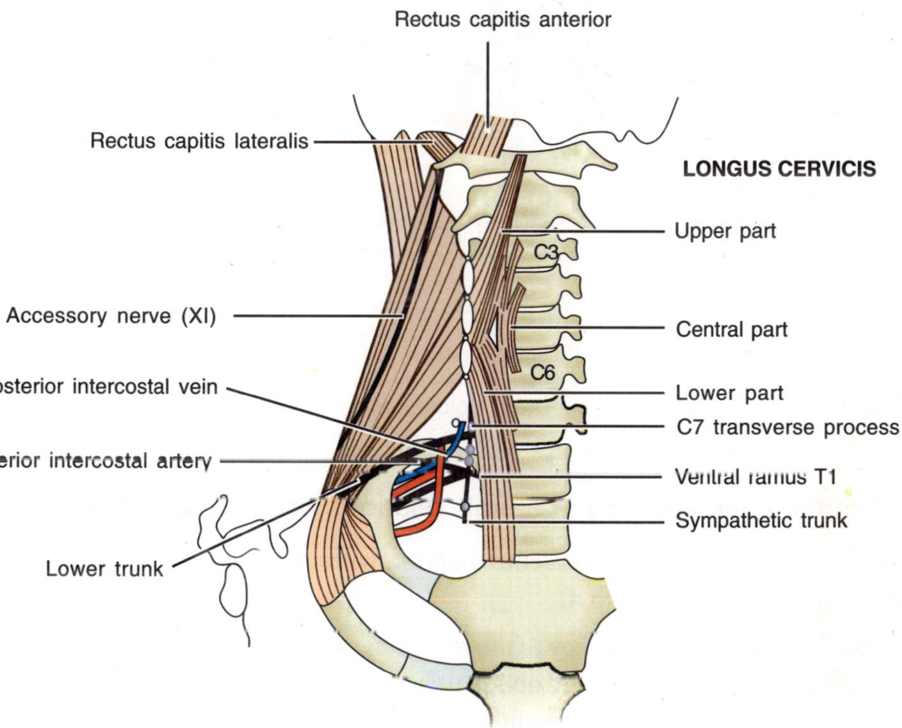

Fig. 17.2 The prevertebral muscles

BUILDING UP THE RELATIONS OF THE APEX OF THE LUNG

17.3 The root of the neck—The structures adjacent to the cervical pleura

The root of the neck lies above the apex of the lung. Relations of the apex of the lung comprise all that needs to be known about the root of the neck. The structures arching over the apex of the lung are the costo-cervical trunk and its highest intercostal branch which arches over the dome of the cervical pleura from the anterior to the posterior surface.

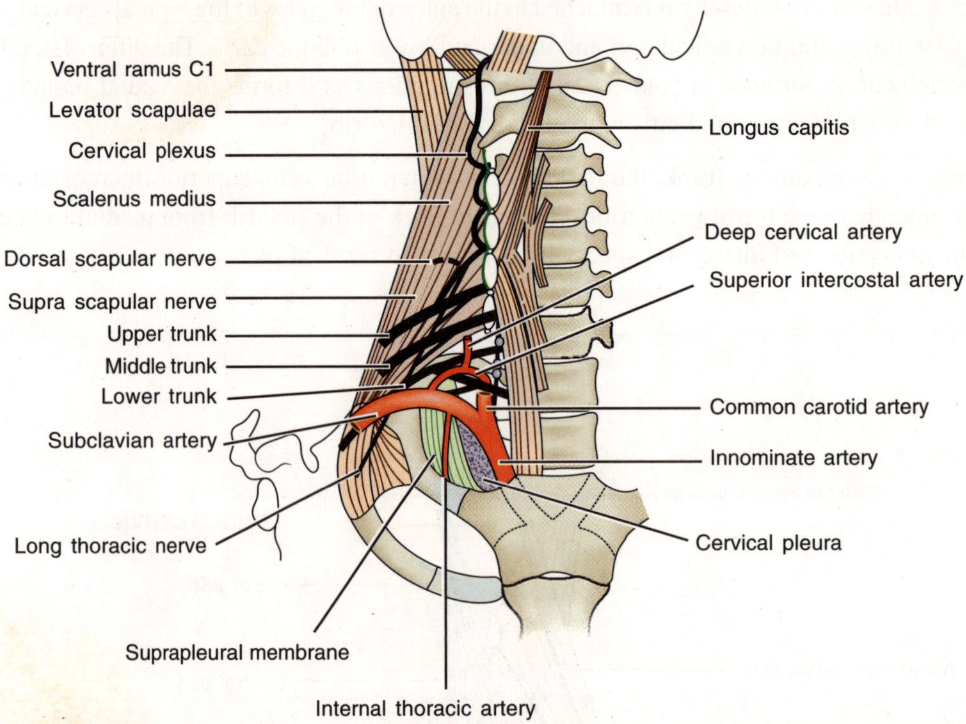

Fig. 17.3 The root of the neck—The structures adjacent to the cervical pleura

17.4 The root of the neck *(Contd.)*—Lateral relations of the apex of the lung

Lateral to the cervical pleura is the scalenus anterior, with the subclavian artery and the lower trunk of the branchial plexus posterior to it.

The scalenus anterior muscle is the key to the root of the neck. The medial edge of the scalenus anterior with the lateral edge of the lower oblique part of longus cervicis forms the triangle of vertebral artery (Grant). The apex of the vertebral artery is the carotid tubercle (transverse process of C6) and the base is formed by the first part of subclavian artery. In its floor lie the ventral rami of C7 and C8, neck of the first rib and the supra pleural membrane covering the apex of the lung.

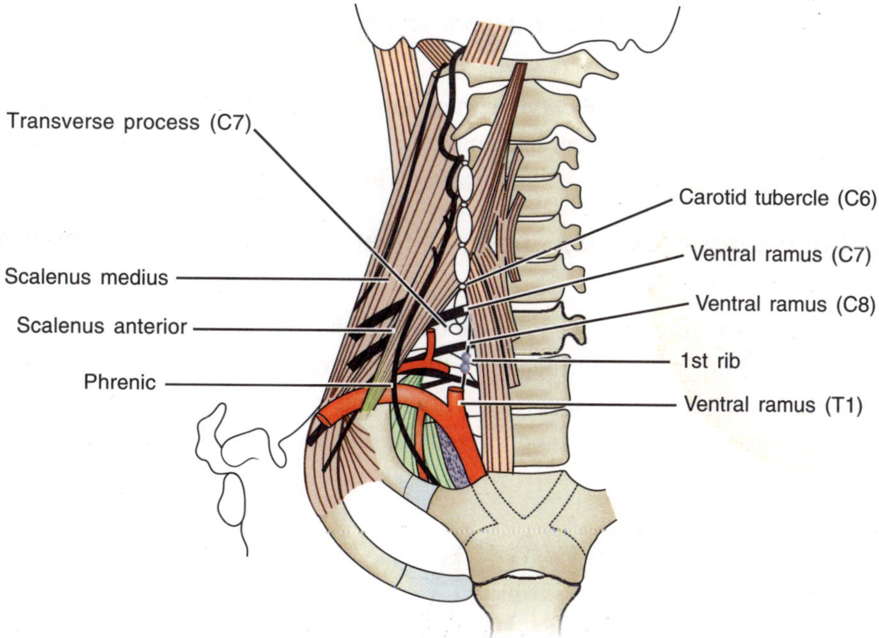

Fig. 17.4 The root of the neck—Lateral relations of the apex of the lung

17.5 The root of the neck *(Contd.)*—Anterior relations of the apex of the lung on right side

Anterior to the apex of the lung are the great vessels of the upper limb and head and neck. Because the subclavian artery lies on the anterior surface of the cervical pleura, its ascending (vertebral

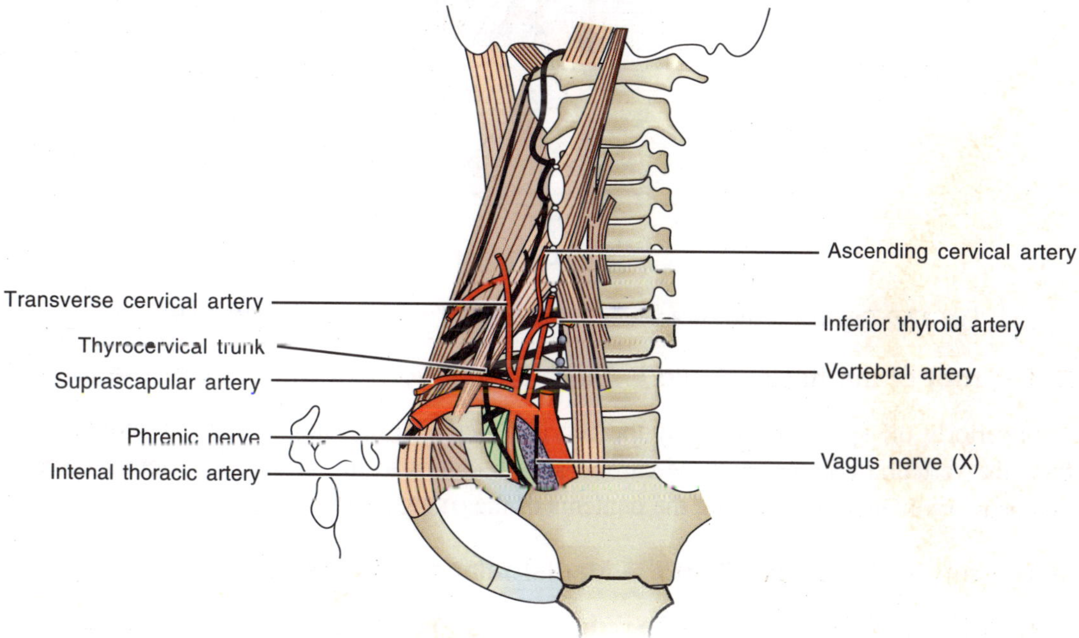

Fig. 17.5 The root of the neck—Anterior relations of the apex of the lung on right side

and inferior thyroid) and descending (internal thoracic) branches also lie in anterior relationship with the apex of the lung.

The phrenic nerve crosses the subclavian artery and its internal thoracic branch and lies behind the subclavian vein. It lies on suprapleural membrane and then passes medially to the apex of the lung, then in fornt of the vagus nerve, to enter the superior mediastinum.

17.6 The root of the neck *(Contd.)*—Anterior relations of the apex of the lung on left side

In addition to the structure on right side, the thoracic duct arches over the apex of the left lung and subclavian artery to enter the confluence of the subclavian and internal jugular veins. In this course it crosses the sympathetic chain, vertebral artery and vein (vertebral system) and lies behind the common carotid artery, vagus nerve and internal jugular vein (carotid system).

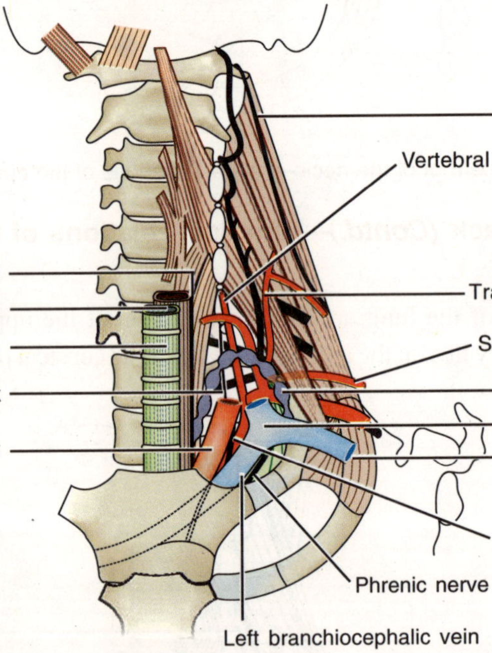

Fig. 17.6 The root of the neck—Anterior relations of the apex of the lung on left side

17.7 The root of the neck *(Contd.)*—Superior relations of the apex of the lung

Superiorly the space occupied by the cervical pleura disappears so that the vertebral artery reaches the vertebral column, and the carotid sheath comes to lie on the prevertebral fascia and sympathetic trunk, thereby covering the contents of the triangle of vertebral artery.

17.8 The root of the neck *(Contd.)*—Medial relations of the apex of the lung

Medial to the cervical pleura are the vertebral bodies, oesophagus and trachea with the thoracic duct and recurrent laryngeal nerve on the left side.

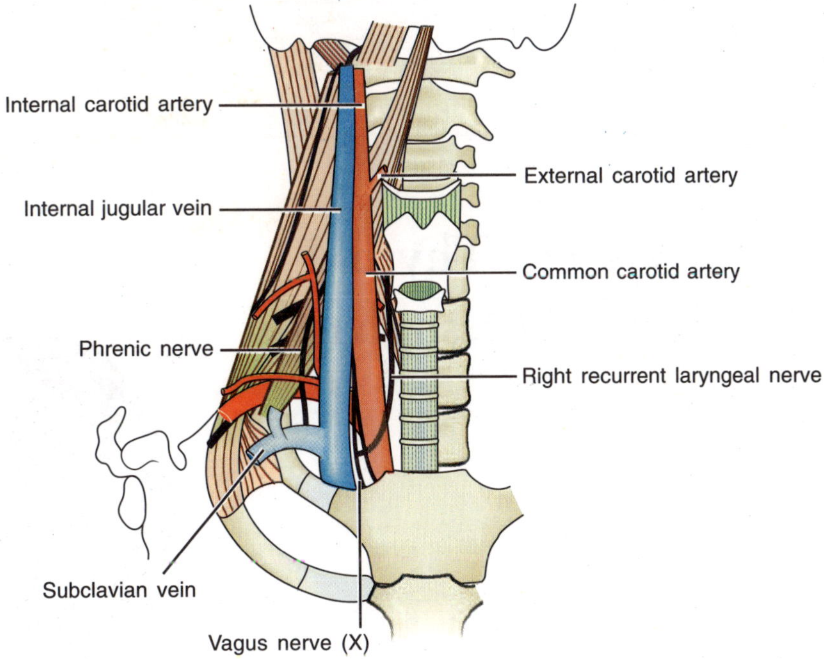

Fig. 17.7 The root of the neck—Superior relations of the apex of the lung

The clavicular head of sternomastoid muscle covers the scalenus anterior muscle and the carotid sheath. The triangular interval between its two heads lies over the termination of internal jugular vein.

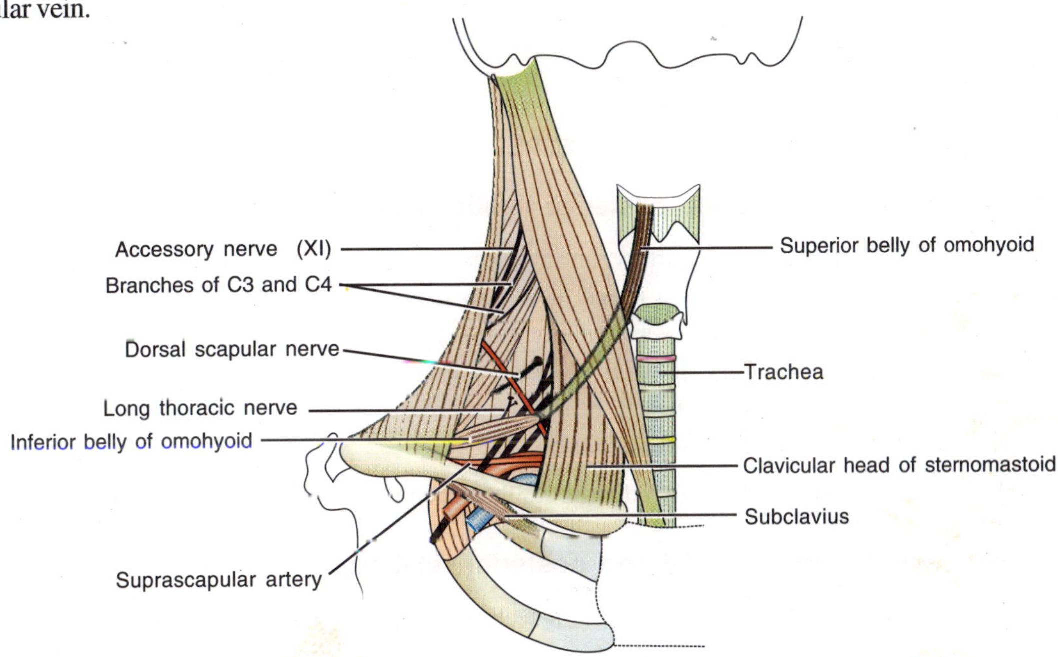

Fig. 17.8 The root of the neck—Medial relations of the apex of the lung

The Cervical Viscera-Thyroid Gland, Trachea and Oesophagus

Chapter **18**

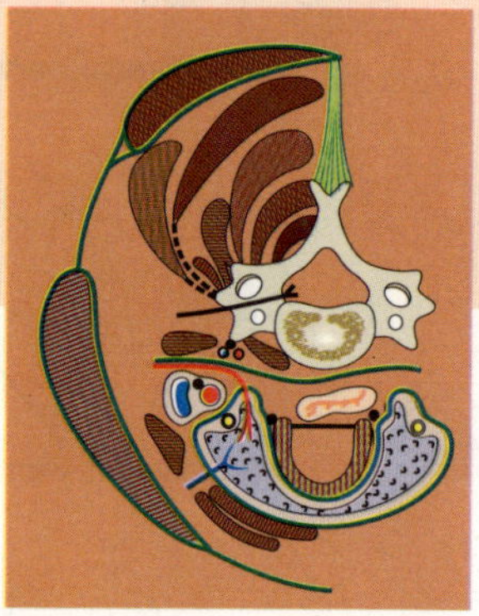

The space bounded by the great vessels on either side and by longus cervicis and capitis behind is primarily occupied by a group of structures aptly termed cervical viscera (Grant), which includes the cervical parts of the alimentary tract (mouth, pharynx and oesophagus), the respiratory tract (pharynx, larynx and trachea) and the thyroid gland.

RELATIONS OF THYROID GLAND FROM DEEPER TO SUPERFICIAL ASPECT

18.1 The thyroid gland—Deep posterior relations of a thyroid lobe

Note that the inferior thyroid artery, an important posterior relation, forms an S-shaped loop with a general medial direction. First it lies medial to scalenus anterior, then crosses between the common carotid and vertebral arteries and finally loops in towards the deep aspect of the lower pole. As it crosses the vertebral artery, it is enveloped by strands of sympathetic trunk. The recurrent laryngeal nerve lies behind the branches of the inferior thyroid artery before they pierce the pretracheal fascia and is therefore always behind this fascia.

The isthmus of thyroid is firmly adherent to the second, third and fourth rings of the trachea.

18.2 The thyroid gland—Medial and posterior relations

Each lateral lobe is roughly triangular on section. The medial surface is related to two tubes viz., oesophagus and trachea; two nerves viz., recurrent and external laryngeal; two muscles viz., inferior constrictor and cricothyroid.

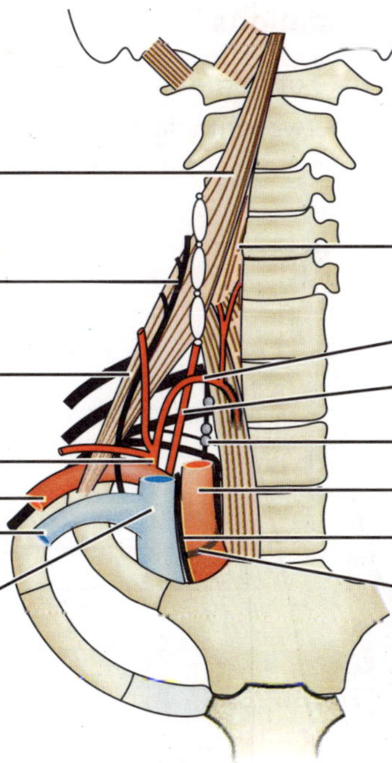

Fig. 18.1 The thyroid gland—Deep posterior relations of a thyroid lobe

The posterior surface overlaps the common carotid artery and covers the terminal part of the inferior thyroid artery, which is a deep posterior relation as already described above.

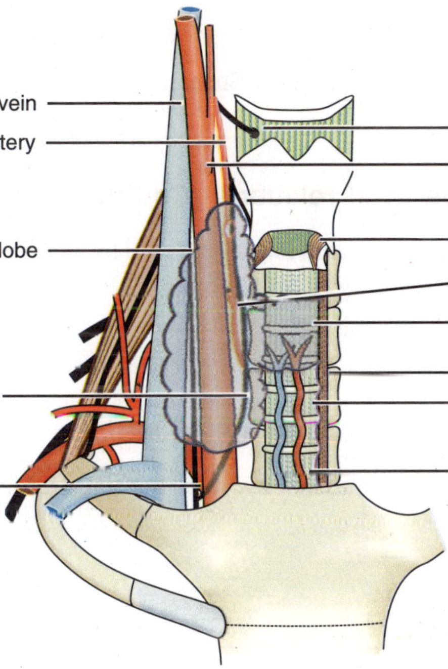

Fig. 18.2 The thyroid gland—Medial and posterior relations

18.3 The thyroid gland—Superficial relations

The thyroid lobe lies directly under cover of sterno-thyroid muscle. The upper pole lies trucked away beneath the upper end of this muscle between it and the ala of the thyroid cartilage.

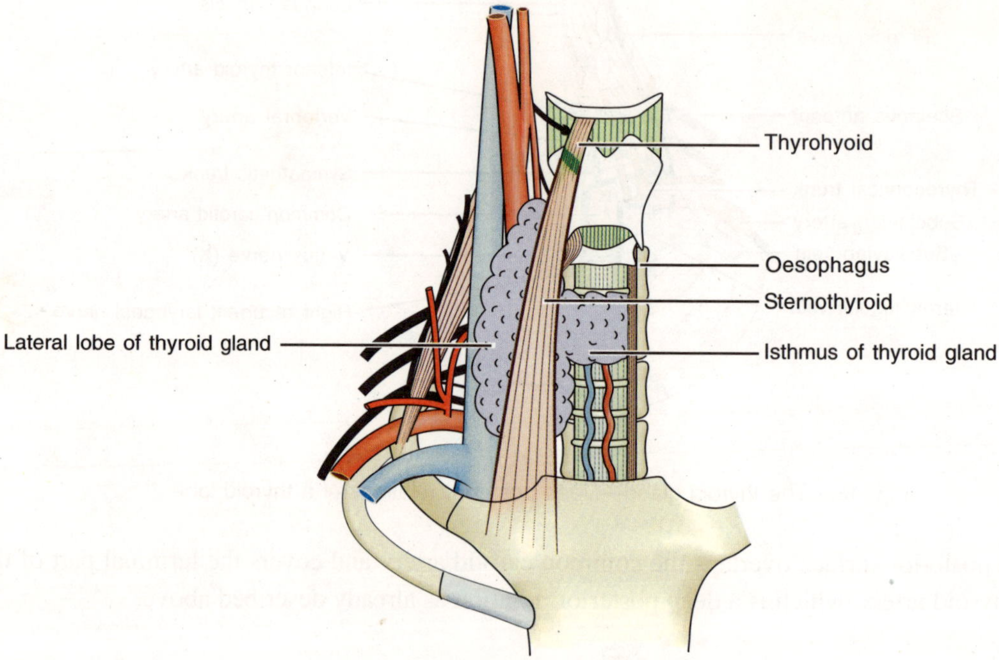

Fig. 18.3 The thyroid—Superficial relations

18.4 The thyroid gland—Superficial relations *(Contd.)*

Over the sternothyroid muscle the thyroid lobe is covered by sternohyoid. Also lying superficial but lateral to these muscles is superior belly of omohyoid.

18.5 The thyroid gland—Superficial relations *(Contd.)*

The anterior border of sternocleidomastoid overlaps the flat strap like infrahyoid muscles.

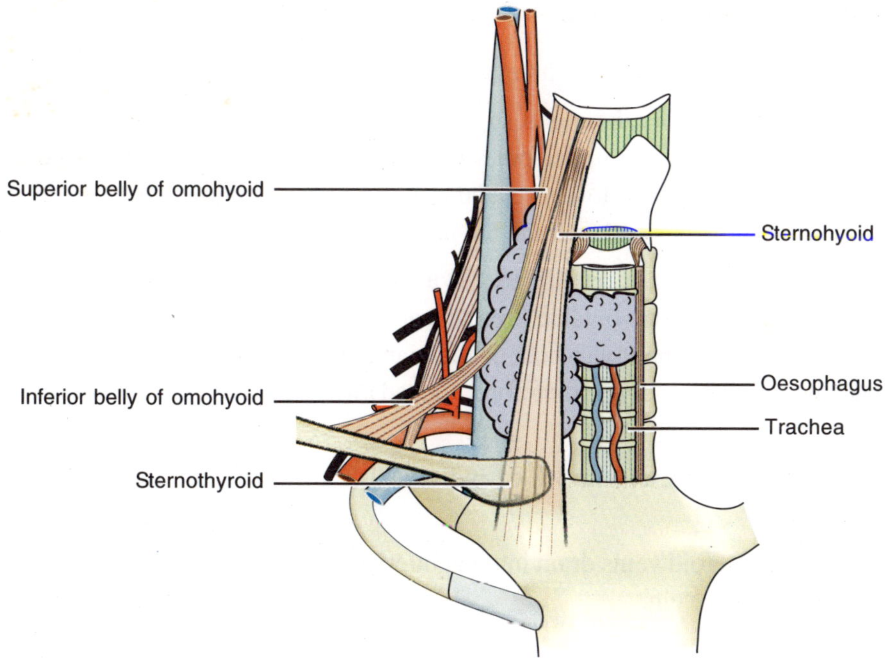

Fig. 18.4 The thyroid gland—Superficial relations *(Contd.)*

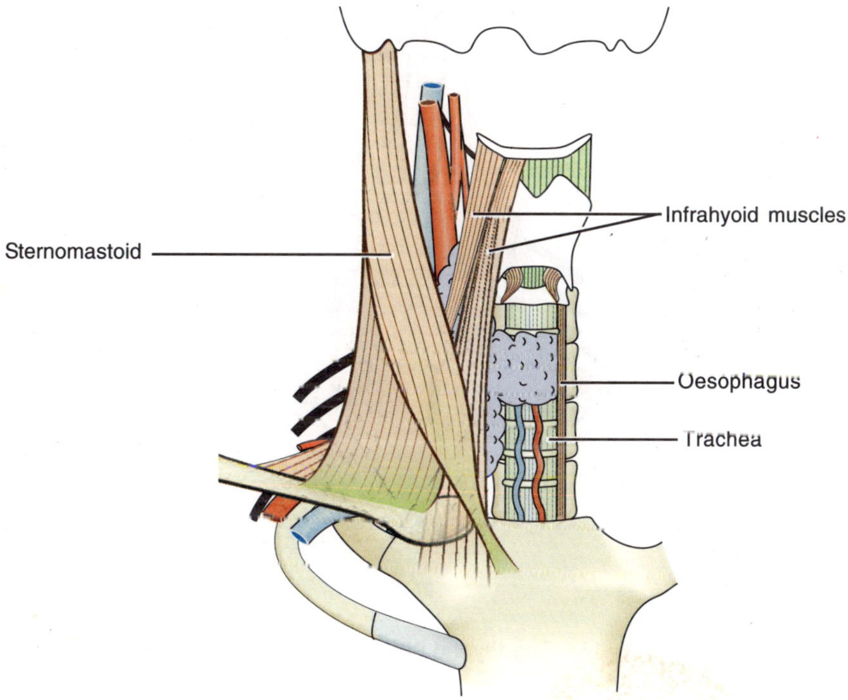

Fig. 18.5 The thyroid gland—Superficial relations *(Contd.)*

18.6 The thyroid gland—Vascular supply

There are on each side two arteries and three veins.

The superior thyroid artery enters the gland superficially, pierces the pretracheal fascia as a single vessel to reach the summit of the upper pole where it divides into anterior and posterior branches. The external laryngeal nerve is closely related to it. A ligature is placed close to the upper pole to include the two set of branches and exclude the nerve in the surgery on thyroid.

The inferior thyroid artery shown in Figure 18.1 is a deep posterior relation of the gland and enters from its deep surface and divides outside pretracheal fascia into four or five branches that pierce the fascia separately to reach the lower pole of the gland. These terminal branches are close to the recurrent laryngeal nerve. The artery is, therefore, ligated away from the gland in its transverse portion.

The thyroidea ima artery is present in 3% of individuals, and enters the lower part of the isthmus.

The superior and middle thyroid veins drain into the internal jugular. The inferior thyroid veins drain into the left-brachio-cephalic vein.

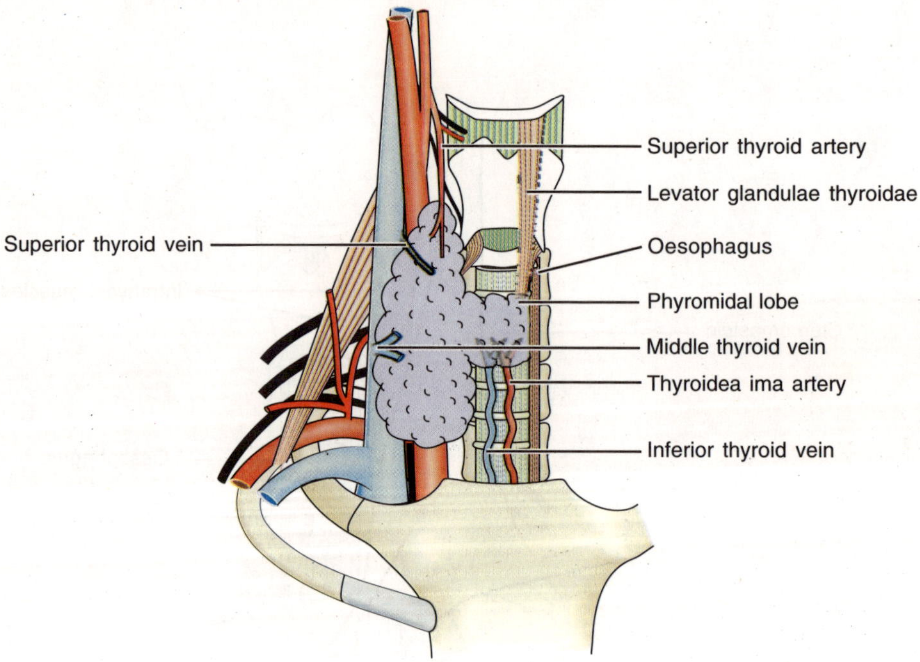

Fig. 18.6 The thyroid gland—Vascular supply

18.7 The parathyroid glands—Posterior aspect

Two pairs of small yellowish brown ductless glands are embedded in the posterior surface of the capsule of thyroid gland, one pair in each lobe. They lie within the pretracheal fascia near the anastomosing artery that joins superior and inferior thyroid arteries.

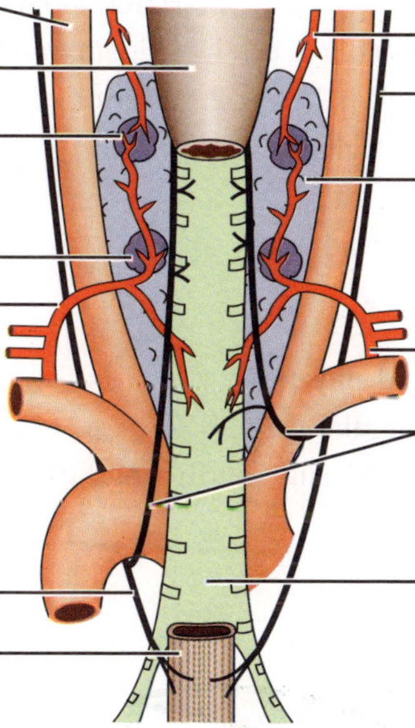

Fig. 18.7 The parathyroid glands—Posterior aspect

18.8 A schematic transverse section through the neck at C7 level. To show the planes of muscles and their relations to each other

Revise the relations of the thyroid gland.

Note the two cervical viscera, trachea and oesophagus, in interrelationship with each other. Both begin immediately below the cricoid cartilage, anterior to the sixth cervical vertebra, and descend into the thorax.

The flat posterior wall of trachea lies against the oesophagus. Lateral to it are the thyroid lobes, the common carotid arteries and the branchio-cephalic trunk on the right side inferiorly. A recurrent laryngeal nerve ascends on each side in the groove between oesophagus and trachea in the neck.

The oesophagus lies between the trachea and the prevertebral fascia overlying the anterior longitudinal ligament and the longus cervics muscle. Its right relations are thyroid lobe and cervical pleura; on left side it is separated from cervical pleura by subclavian artery and thoracic duct.

Relations of a lateral lobe of thyroid gland

- Superficial – Sternohyoid
  – Sternothyroid
  – Superior belly of omohyoid

- Medial
  - Two cartilages
    1. Thyroid
    2. Cricoid
  - Two tubes
    1. Trachea
    2. Oesophagus
  - Two nerves
    1. Recurrent laryngeal
    2. External laryngeal
  - Two muscles
    1. Cricothyroid
    2. Inferior constrictor of pharynx
- Posterior
  - Parathyroid glands
  - Carotid sheath
  - Inferior thyroid artery

Relations of isthmus

- Superficial
  - Cirfrahyoid muscles
  - Anterior jugular vein
- Posterior
  - Second, third and fourth rings of trachea

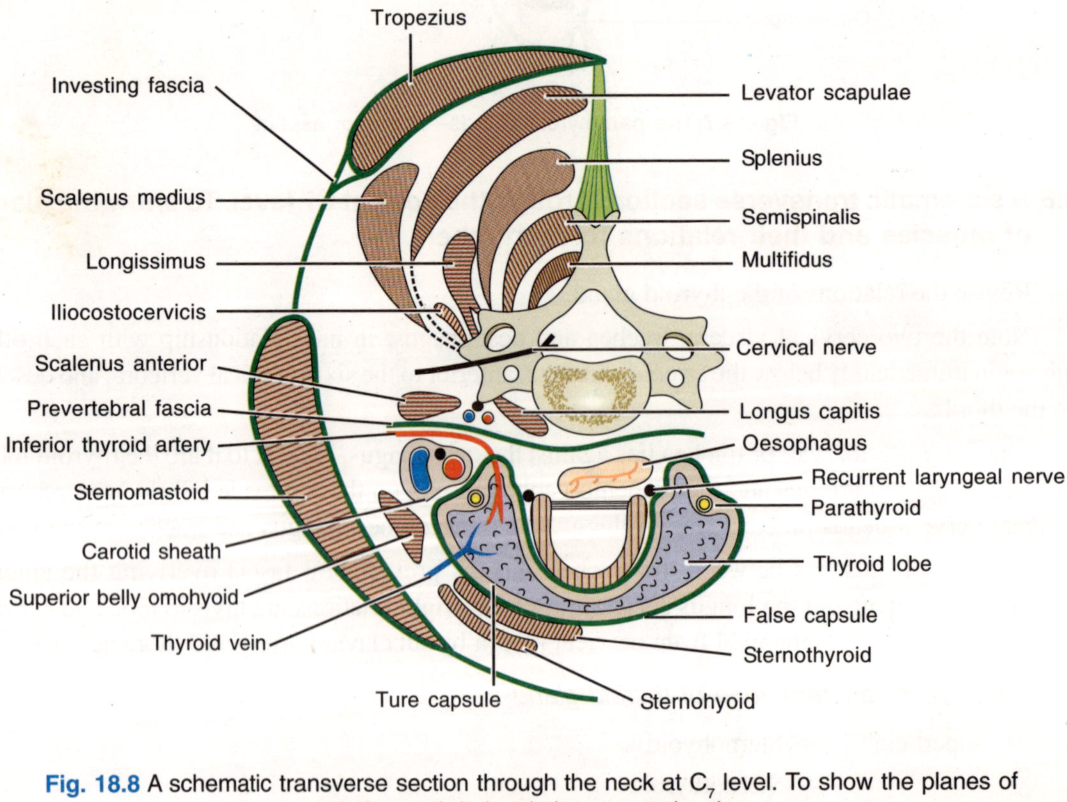

Fig. 18.8 A schematic transverse section through the neck at C_7 level. To show the planes of muscles and their relations to each other

Vessels and Nerves in Upper Part of the Neck

Chapter 19

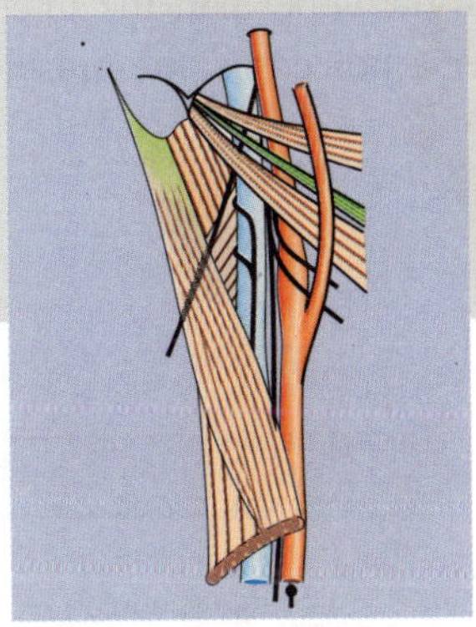

BUILDING UP THE STRUCTURES IN UPPER PART OF THE NECK

19.1 The base of skull near jugular foramen

The carotid canal lies anterior to the jugular foramen and the hypoglossal canal postero-medial to it. The position of these foramina gives a clear picture of the relative positions of the structures at the base of skull.

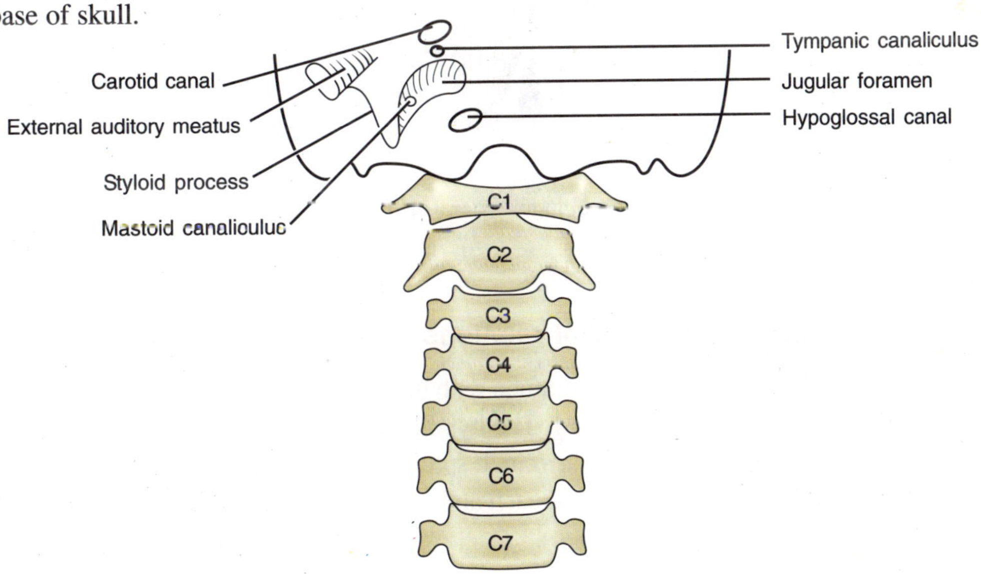

Fig. 19.1 The base of skull near jugular foramen

The ridge of bone between the jugular foramen and carotid canal is perforated by multiple small foramina. One of these is known as canaliculus for tympanic branch, of glossopharyngeal; the others carry carotico tympanic branches from the internal carotid artery and sympathetic filaments from the carotid plexus. In the lateral wall of the jugular foramen is the mastoid canaliculus for the auricular branch of vagus.

19.2 The internal jugular vein—Posterior relations

In the upper part the internal jugular vein lies first on the rectus capitis lateralis next on the transverse processes, the muscles attached to them, the cervical plexus and its branches.

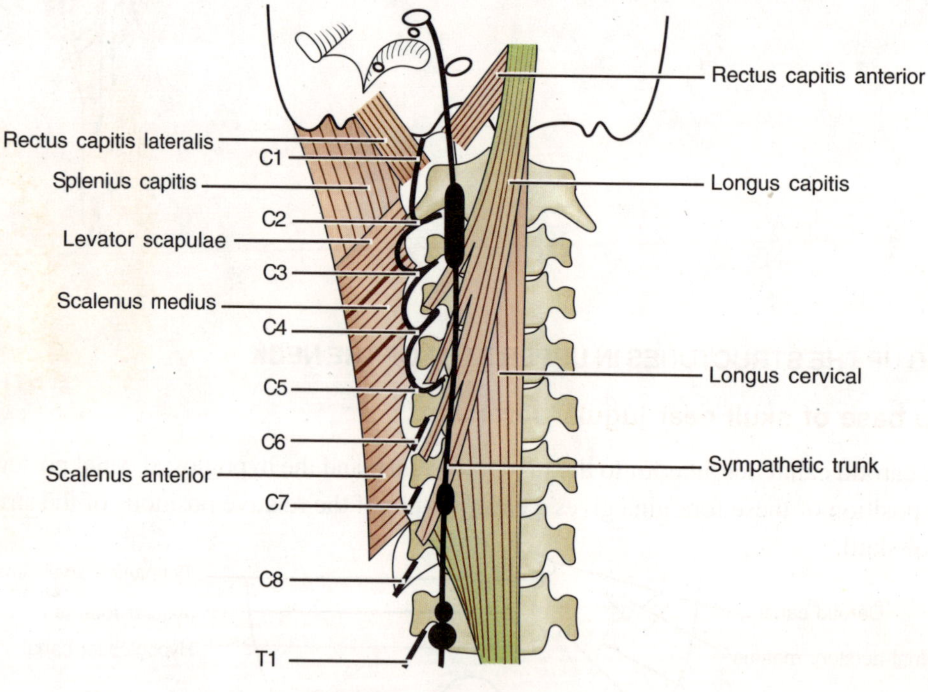

Fig. 19.2 The internal jugular vein—Posterior relations

19.3 The internal jugular vein—Medial relations

It descends vertically from the jugular foramen with the glossopharyngeal, vagus and accessory nerves related anteromedially to its upper end. The hypoglossal nerve leaves the skull through the hypoglossal canal medial to the internal jugular vein. It spirals infero-laterally, behind the other nerves which lie posterior to internal carotid artery, to reach and adhere briefly with the lateral aspect of the vagus. Descending with it in the neuro-vascular bundle, the last four cranial nerves pass through the upper part of the carotid sheath.

The accessory nerve usually crosses the superior bulb of internal jugular vein superficially. The slender inferior root of the ansa cervicalis arises from the ventral rami of the second and third cervical nerves behind the internal jugular vein to come forwards, usually on the lateral surface of the vein.

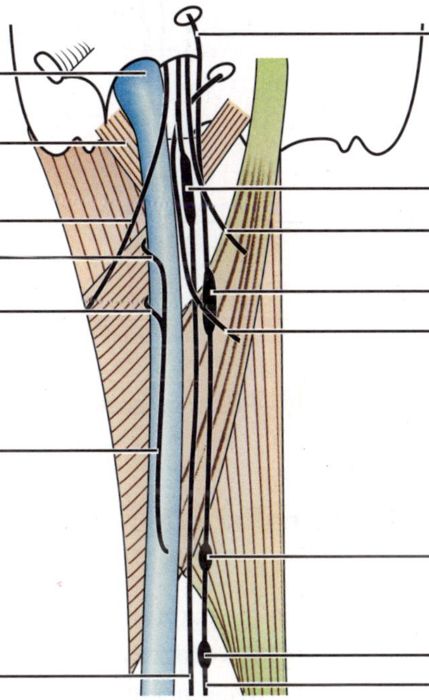

Fig. 19.3 The internal jugular vein—Medial relations

19.4 The internal carotid artery—Posterior, posterolateral and lateral relations

Posterior are the longus capitis and the sympathetic trunk.

Posterolateral are the glossopharyngeal, vagus, accessory and hypoglossal nerves.

Lateral is the internal jugular vein except near the skull where it becomes posterior to the internal carotid artery due to the relative position of the openings of carotid canal and jugular foramen at the base of skull.

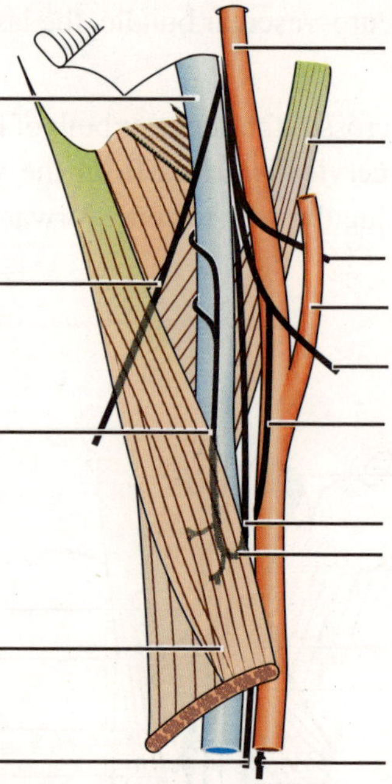

Fig. 19.4 The internal carotid artery—Posterior, posterolateral and lateral relations

19.5 The internal carotid and external arteries—Structures intervening between them

The external carotid artery lies buried in the parotid gland. Apart from (i) the deep lobe of the parotid gland, the other structures intervening between the arteries are (ii) the styloid process, (iii) the stylo-pharyngeus muscle, (iv) the glossopharyngeal nerve, (v) the pharyngeal branch of vagus, (vi) the styloglossus muscle and (vii) the stylohyoid ligament.

These structures are also superficial relations of internal carotid artery. Three nerves are superficial to this artery, two are mentioned here, they cross under posterior belly of digastric. The third viz., the hypoglossal is shown if Figure 19.7 *(Refer page 146)* and crosses the internal carotid artery in the carotid triangle.

19.6 The internal and external carotid arteries—Medial relations

The internal carotid artery lies medially on superior laryngeal nerve, middle and superior constrictors of pharynx and levator palati muscle.

The medial relations of external carotid artery are external and internal laryngeal branches of superior laryngeal nerve, pharyngeal branch of vagus and middle constrictor of pharynx. The stylopharyngeus muscle, glossopharyngeal nerve and styloid process are related at the higher level.

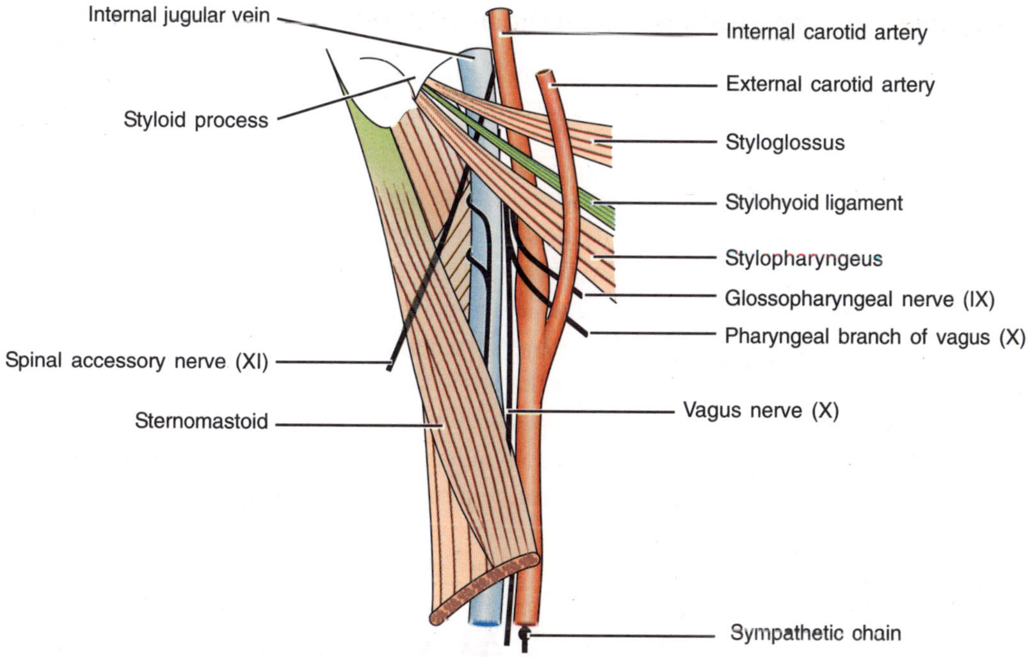

Fig. 19.5 The internal and external carotid arteries—Structures interveining between them

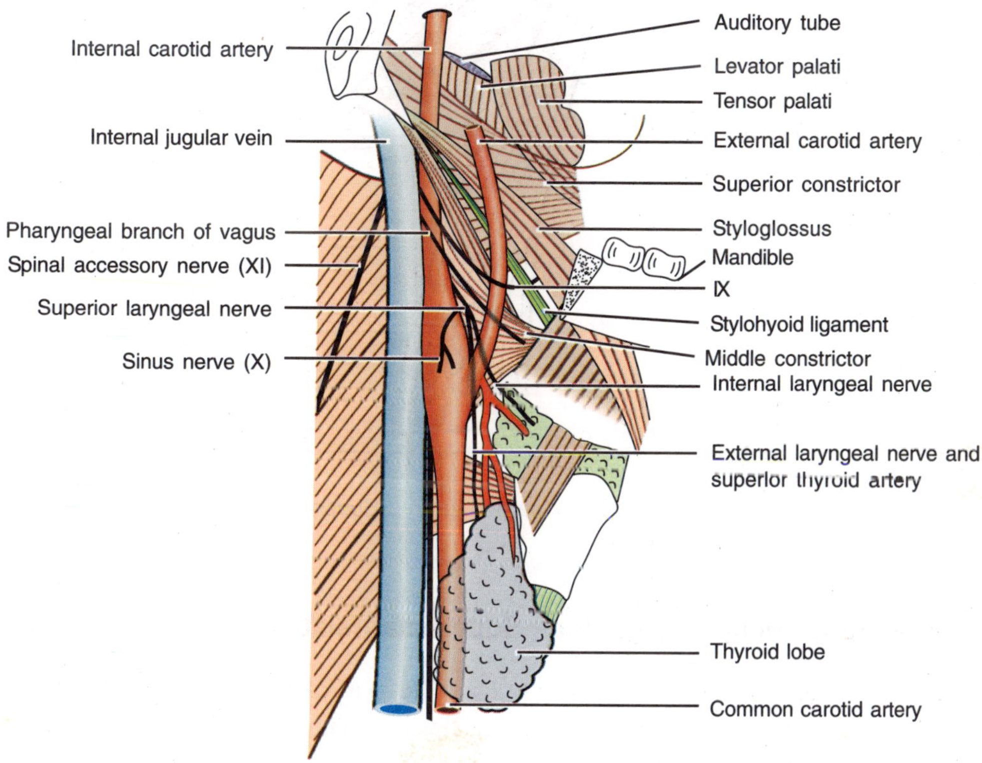

Fig. 19.6 The internal and external carotid arteries—Medial relations

19.7 The external carotid artery—Superficial relations

The superficial relations are (i) the post belly of digastric, (ii) the stylohyoid muscle and (iii) the stylomandibular ligament. The posterior belly of digastric is the key muscle in the upper part of the neck.

It is important to visualise the deep relations of the posterior belly of the digastric here. Note that it crosses the internal jugular vein, both carotid arteries, the origin of the facial artery and the loop of the lingual artery. Under cover of the lower border of the muscle, the occipital artery runs towards the scalp and the posterior auricular runs along the upper border. The ascending pharyngeal arises from the deep aspect of the external carotid. Accessory nerve lies between the internal jugular vein and the posterior belly. The hypoglossal is in the angle between the internal jugular vein and the internal carotid artery. The glossopharyngeal passes downwards and forwards between the internal jugular vein and the internal carotid artery. Stylohyoid and stylopharyngeus muscle lie close to the upper border of the muscle. The muscle is therefore a ready guide to many structures.

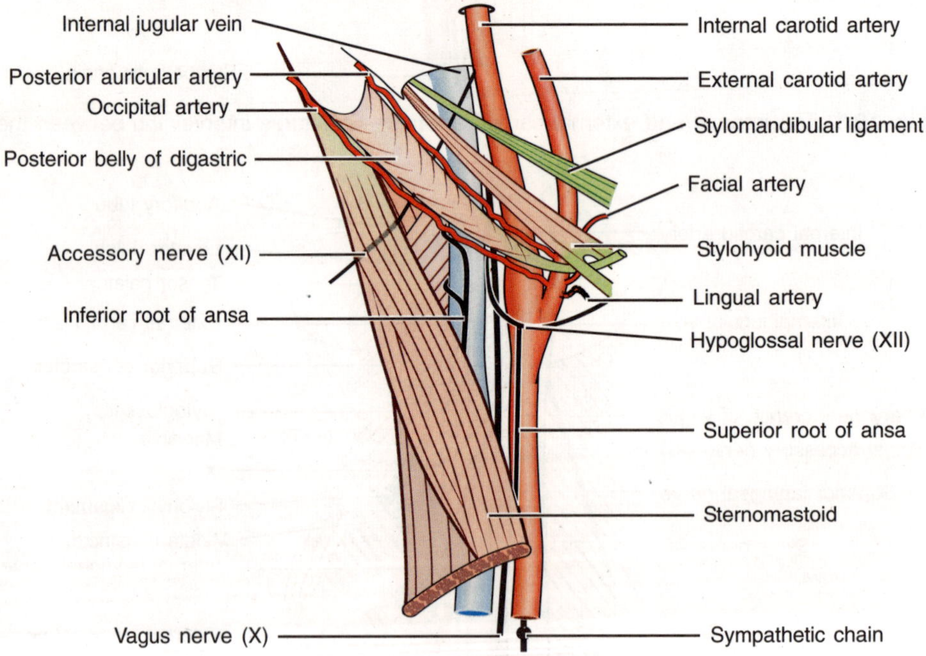

Fig. 19.7 The external carotid artery—Superficial relations

19.8 The posterior belly of digastric—Superficial relations

The posterior belly of digastric is deep to the lower part of the parotid gland and the angle of mandible. It is crossed superficially by common facial vein and is overlapped by submandibular gland and runs obliquely across the neurovascular bundle of the neck.

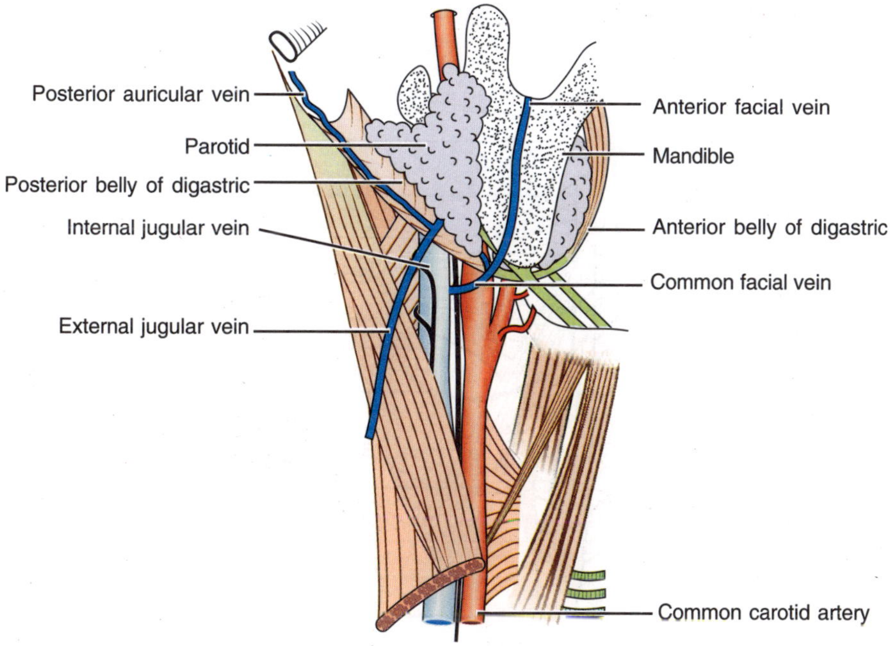

Fig. 19.8 The posterior belly of digastric—Superficial relations

THE LAST FOUR CRANIAL NERVES AND CERVICAL SYMPATHETIC CHAIN

19.9 The glossopharyngeal nerve

It passes through the anterior part of jugular foramen in its own dural sheath, and has a superior and inferior ganglion. The nerve descends between internal jugular vein and internal carotid artery, curves round the stylopharyngeus, between the internal and external carotid arteries, lies in the gap between the superior and middle constrictors of pharynx and then passes into the tongue deep to the hyoglossus.

The branches are (i) the tympanic nerve, from the superior ganglion, which enters the tympanic canaliculus and forms the tympanic plexus on the promontory on the medial wall of middle ear, (ii) the nerve to stylopharyngeus (motor), (iii) the pharyngeal branches for pharyngeal plexus on middle constrictor, (iv) carotid sinus nerve (v) sensory branches to posterior on third of tongue, palatine tonsil, sofe palate and epiglottis.

19.10 The vagus nerve

It leaves the skull, with the accessory nerve in the same sheath of duramater, through the middle compartment of jugular foramen. It has superior and inferior ganglia and descends vertically

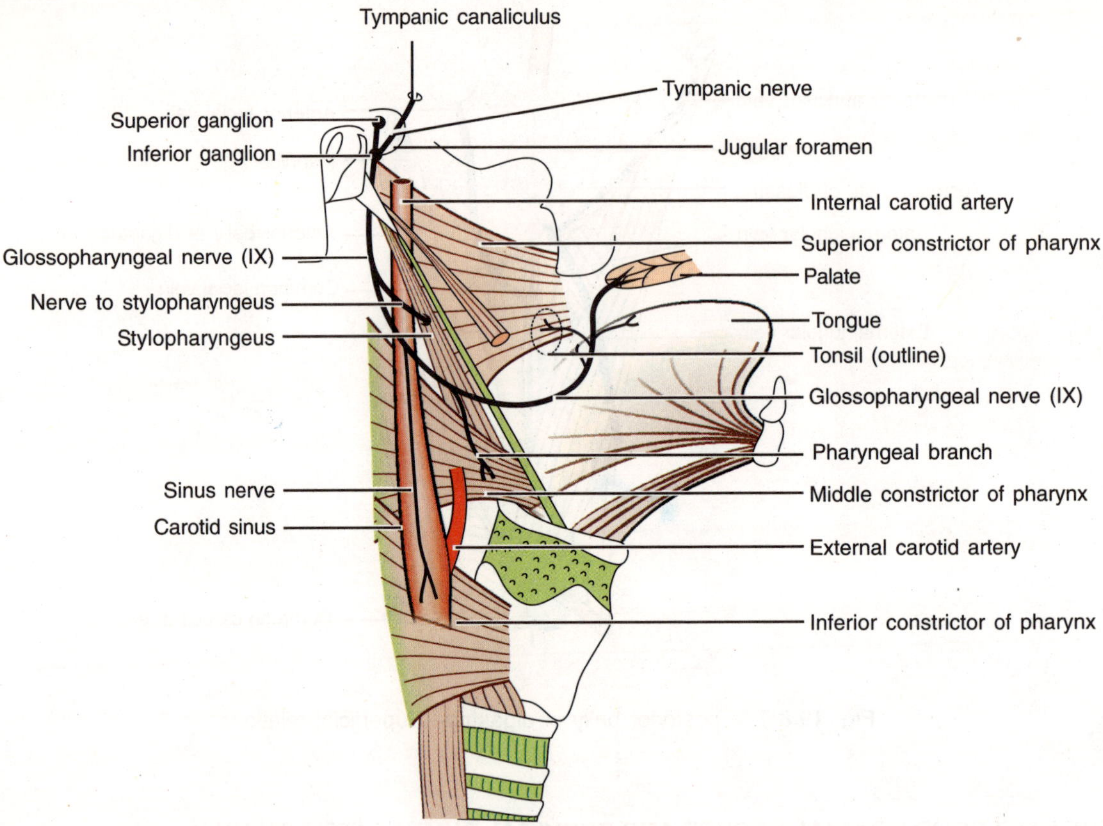

Fig. 19.9 The glossopharyngeal nerve

in the carotid sheath. At the root of the neck it crosses the anterior surface of the subclavian artery. The cranial part of accessory nerve joins it below the inferior ganglion. The branches are as follows:

From superior ganglion:

The meningeal branch for duramater of posterior cranial fossa; the auricular branch (Alderman's nerve or Arnold's nerve) which enters the mastoid canaliculus and supplies the postero-inferior quadrant of the outer surface of tympanic membrane and a small adjacent area of skin of the external acoustic meatus, and a little of the corresponding skin behind the auricle.

From inferior ganglion:

The pharyngeal branch to pharyngeal plexus on the middle constrictor; the superior laryngeal nerve which divides into internal (sensory) and external (motor) laryngeal nerves, twigs to carotid sinus and carotid body.

From vagal trunk:

Superior and inferior cervical cardiac branches, two on each side, the recurrent laryngeal nerve which hooks around the ligament arteriosum on left side and around the subclavian artery on the right side.

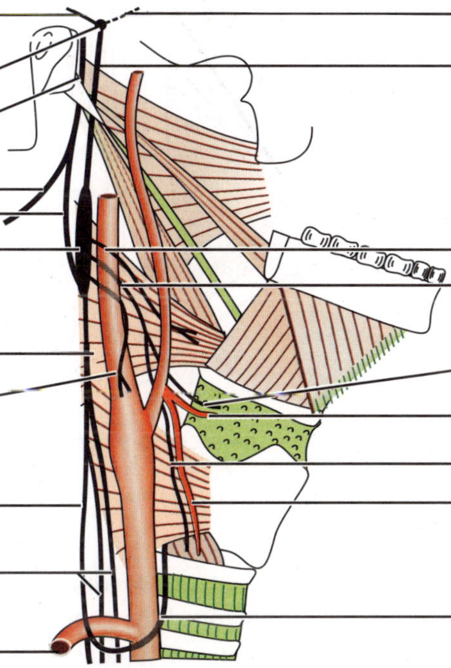

Fig. 19.10 The vagus nerve

19.11 The accessory nerve

The accessory nerve occupies the middle compartment in jugular foramen. The cranial part joins vagus to be distributed to the striped muscles of the pharynx, palate and larynx through the pharyngeal branch of vagus.

The spinal part descends between the internal jugular vein and internal carotid artery, then turns and passes anterior or posterior to internal jugular, to cross the transverse process of the atlas. It passes under the posterior belly of the digastric and the occipital artery and enters the anterior border of the sternomastoid muscle. It emerges from the posterior border of this muscle to cross the posterior triangle and ends in the substance of trapezius at the lowest point of its origin (i.e., Th 12 spine).

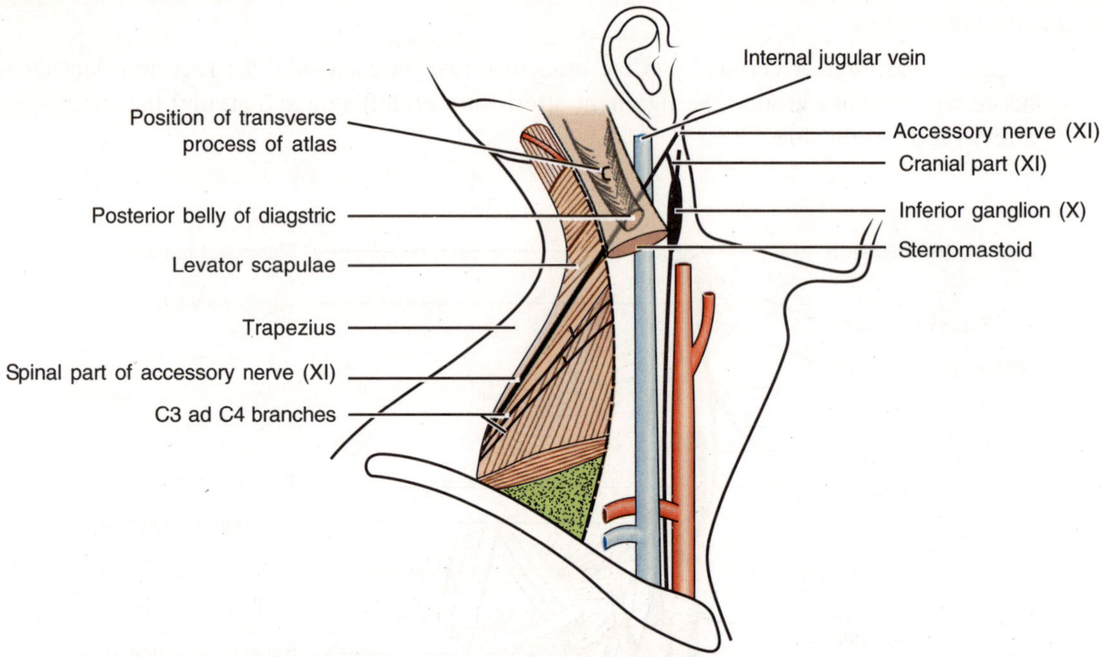

Fig. 19.11 The accessory nerve

19.12 The hypoglossal nerve

The hypoglossal nerve emerges from the anterior condilar canal and is joined by a substantial branch from the ventral ramus of C1. It spirals round the ganglion nodosum (inferior) of vagus to emerge between the internal carotid artery and internal jugular vein, deep to the styloid muscles and posterior belly of digastric. It then crosses the internal and external carotid arteries and loop of lingual artery to pass to the tongue.

The true hypoglossal fibres supply all the intrinsic and extrinsic muscles of the tongue except palatoglossus. The C1 fibres are given off as (i) the meningeal branch, (ii) the superior root of ansa cervicalis, (iii) the nerve to thyrohyoid and (iv) the nerve to geniohyoid.

19.13 The cervical sympathetic trunk

The trunk runs almost vertically in the prevertebral fascia anterior to the longus cervicis and longus capitis muscles on the roots of transverse processes and posterior to the carotid sheath.

Note the superior cervical ganglion opposite the second and third cervical vertebrae and the middle cervical ganglion at the level of the sixth cervical vertebrae. The inferior cervical ganglion is anterior to the eighth cervical ventral ramus when separate; when it is fused with the first thoracic ganglion (cervico-thoracic ganglion), it lies across the neck of the first rib behind the common carotid and vertebral arteries.

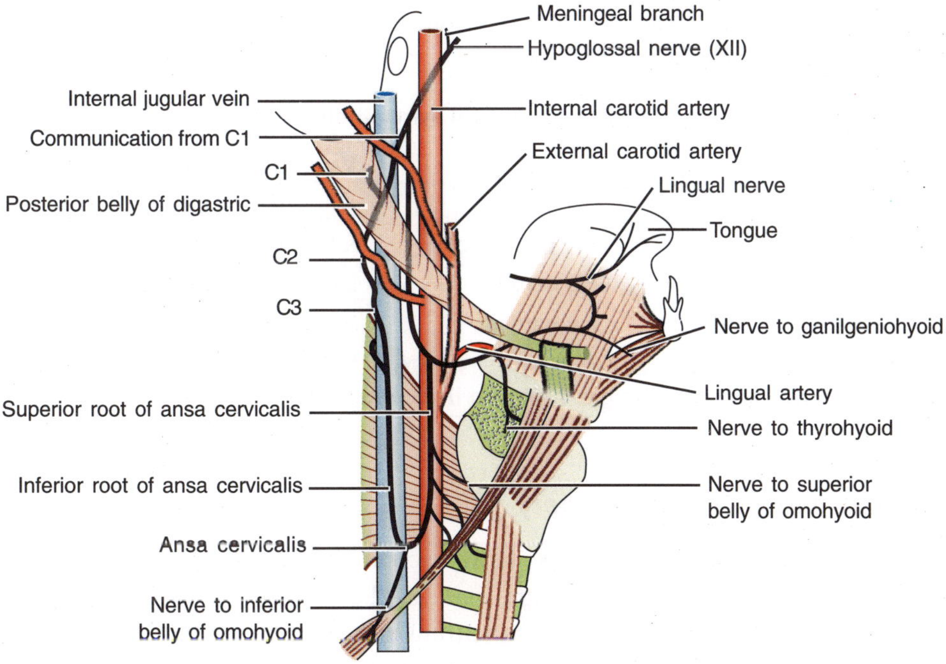

Fig. 19.12 The hypoglossal nerve

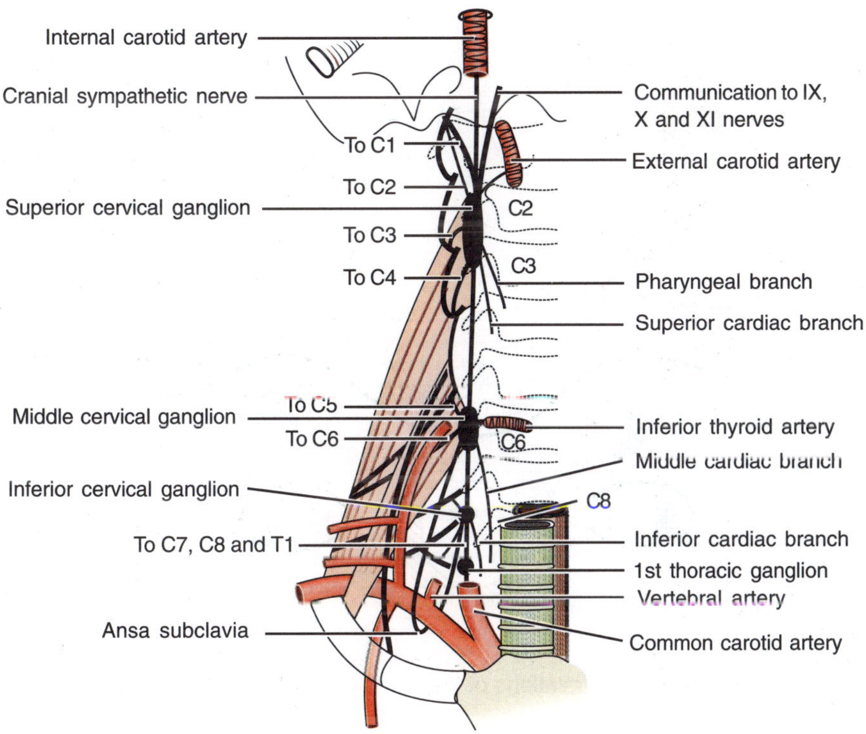

Fig. 19.13 The cervical sympathetic trunk

Each of the three ganglia gives (i) grey rami thatcommunicates to the cervical nerves, (ii) a cardiac nerve and (iii) a plexus to an artery.

Table: Branches of cervical sympathetic ganglia.

Branches	Somatic	Visceral	Vascular
Superior	C1, 2, 3 and C4	One cardiac and One pharyngeal	Internal and external carotid arteries
Middle	C5 and C6	One cardiac	Inferior thyroid artery
Inferior	C7, 8 and T1	One cardiac	Vertebral artery and subclavian arteries

The superior cervical ganglion also gives twigs to IX, X and XII nerves.

19.14 The first part of vertebral artery

The first part of the vertebral artery is posterior to common carotid and inferior thyroid arteries and its own vein. It lies anterior to the ventral rami of the C7 and C8 which have the seventh transverse process between them. The sympathetic trunk lies along its medial side and the cervico-thoracic ganglion is partly behind the artery. It is crossed by the thoracic duct on the left side.

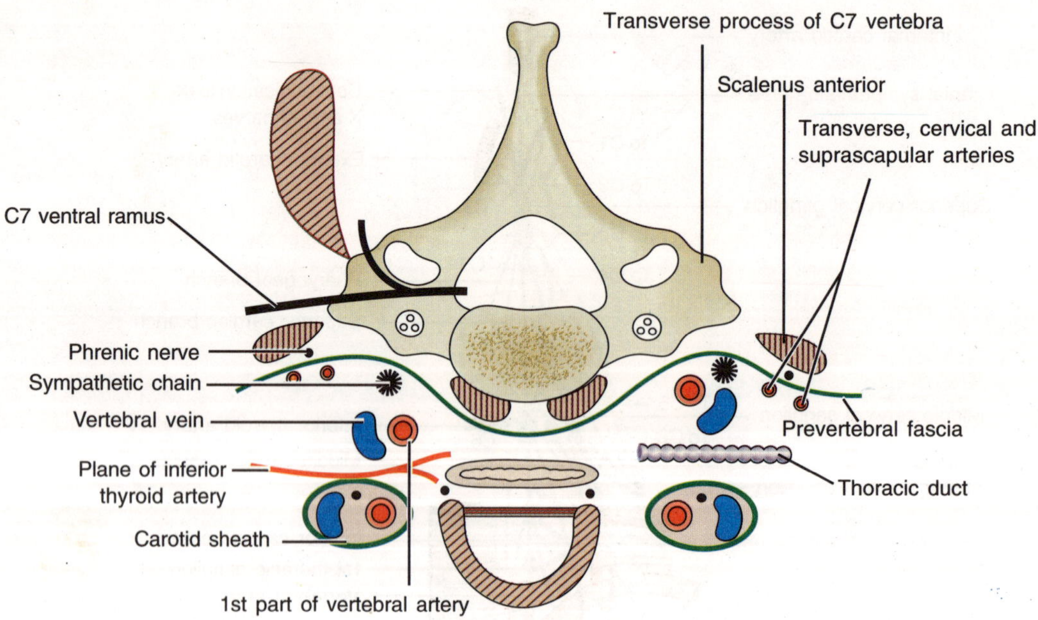

Fig. 19.14 The relations of first part of vertebral artery

19.15 The second part of vertebral artery

The second part lies in the foramina transversaria of C6 to C1 in front of the ventral rami of cervical nerves. It is accompanied by the vertebral venous plexus and a plexus of sympathetic nerve fibres derived from the cervico-thoracic ganglion.

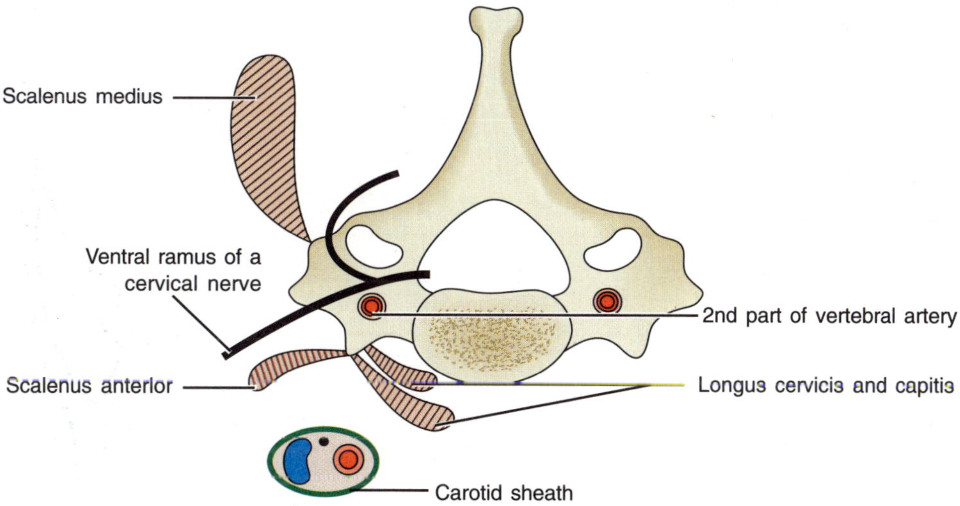

Fig. 19.15 The relations of the second part of vertebral artery

19.16 The third part of vertebral artery

The third part lies on the posterior arch of atlas in the suboccipital triangle. The first cervical nerve and the lateral mass of atlas are on its medial side and rectus capitis lateralis is on its lateral side when it turns backwards after emerging from the foramen transversarium of atlas. As it turns medially behind the upper articular process of atlas, the trunk of the first cervical nerve lies below it, on the posterior arch of atlas, and the dorsal ramus enters the triangle from beneath its lower border.

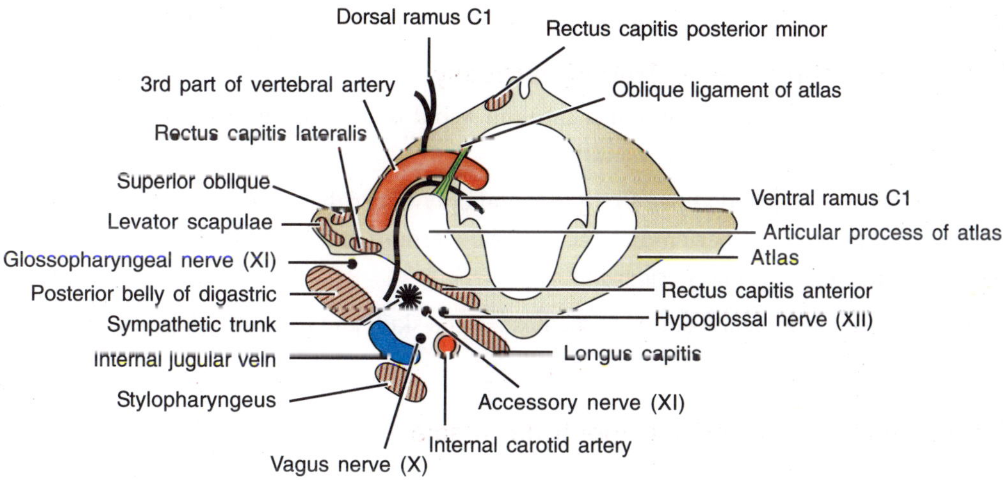

Fig. 19.16 The relations of the third part of vertebral artery

The Cervical Fascia

Chapter 20

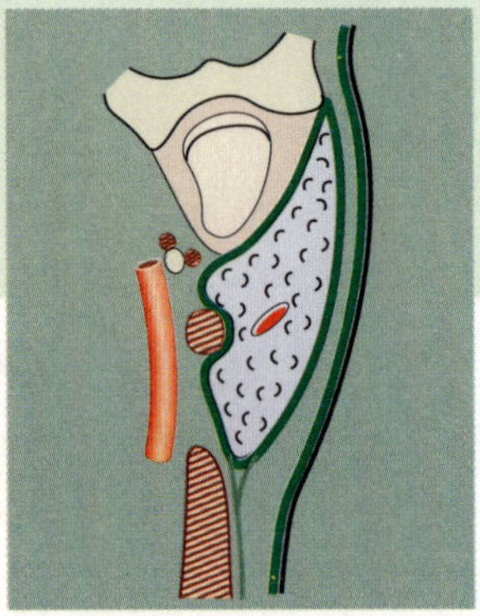

20.1 (a) The deep fascia of neck

It has three layers viz., an investing, a prevertebral and a pretracheal layer which surround the neck like a collar, hence the name "Fascia Colli". The investing layer surrounds all the important structures in the neck; the prevertebral layer surrounds the vertebral column and the muscles closely connected with it and the pretracheal layer helps to form a visceral compartment around the chief viscera viz., trachea, oesophagus and thyroid. In the anterolateral part of the neck where these layers are closely associated, they from the carotid sheath around the great vessels of the neck.

(b) The investing layer—Traced vertically

It is attached below to the clavicle and above to the hyoid bone, after which it continues from the hyoid bone to the lower border of the mandible.

The pretracheal layer is attached above to thyroid and cricoid cartilages and below it blends with the connective tissue between the pericardial sac and the sternum and with the adventitia of the great vessels as they leave or enter the pericardial sac.

The prevertebral fascia is attached above to the base of the skull and inferiorly it is attached to the T4 vertebra.

20.2 The investing layer and clavipectorial fascia

The two layers of the investing layer that adhere to the middle third of the clavicle (between sternomastoid and the trapezius) represent above the clavicle, the two layers of clavipectoral fascia

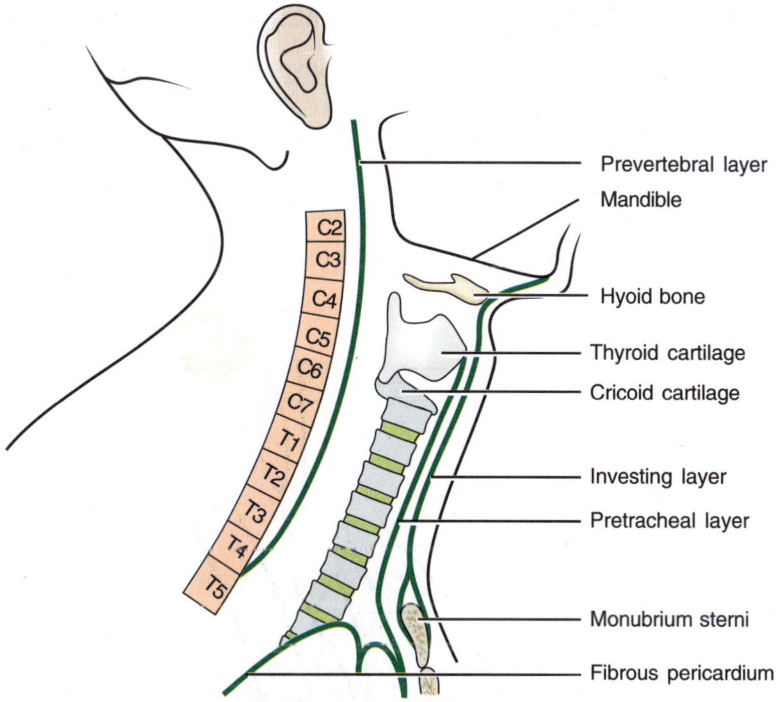

Fig. 20.1 The deep fascia of neck

that enclose the subclavius muscle. The deeper layer of the investing layer splits around the inferior belly of the omohyoid forming a fascial sling which binds the muscle down to the clavicle.

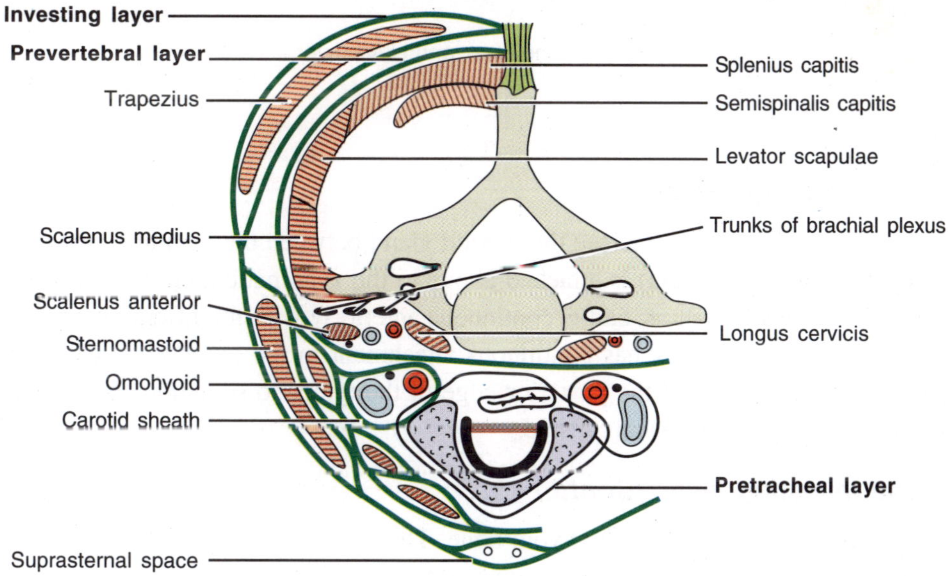

Fig. 20.2 The investing layer—Traced vertically

20.3 The investing layer—Traced horizontally from behind forwards

From its attachment to ligamentum nuchae it splits to enclose the trapezius, then forms the roof of the posterior triangle, and again splits to enclose the sternomastoid and forms the deep fascia in front of the neck. It gives fascial capsule to submandibular and parotid glands. In the posterior triangle, it gives a deep lamella which encloses the inferior belly of omohyoid. It also gives off delicate laminae that pass between and behind the muscle in front of the trachea. In front of the neck, above the manubrium, it splits to encolse the suprasternal space of Burns.

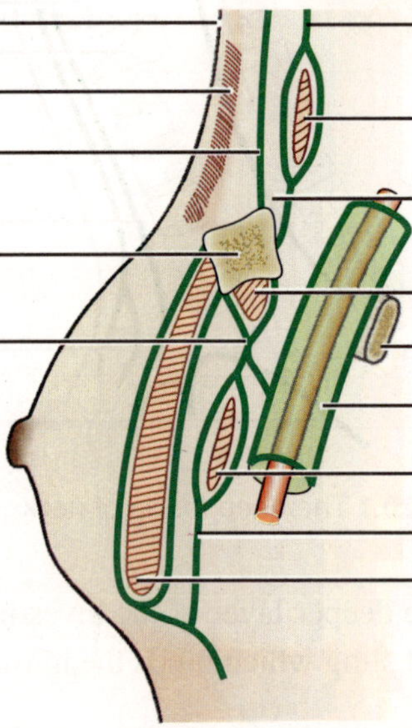

Fig. 20.3 The investing layer and clavipectorial fascia

20.4 (a) The investing layer

The investing layer splits to enclose the parotid gland between the mandible and the ear. The superficial layer (the parotid fascia) is attached above to the zygomatic arch and the cartilaginous part of the external acoustic meatus, and is continuous anteriorly with the fascia over masseter (the masseteric fascia). The deep layer has continuous attachment to the lower edge of the tympanic temporal, the styloid process, and the posterior edge of the tympano-squamous fissure behind the attachment of the temporomandibular capsule.

(b) The investing layer *(Contd.)*

The layer splits into two above the hyoid bone. The superficial layer is attached to the lower margin of the mandible and the deep layer is attached to the mylohyoid line, thus forming a capsule for the submandibular salivary gland. Posterior to the gland the enclosing fasciae fuse to form a flattened band, the stylomandibular lig. The ligament occupies a coronal plane of the ramus of the mandible laterally. It is in contact with posterior pole of the submandibular gland anteriorly and the parotid gland posteriorly.

The investing layer is remarkable for the frequency with which it splits into two. It splits to enclose two muscles (trapezius and sternomastoid), two salivary glands (parotid and submandibular) and two spaces (supraclavicular and suprasternal).

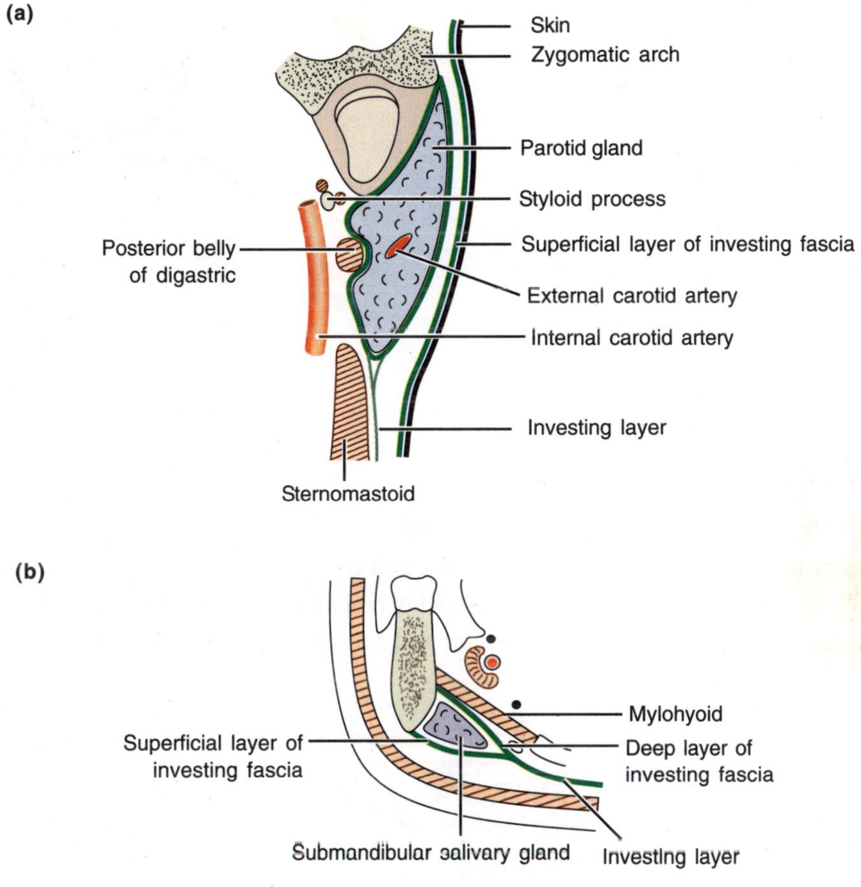

Fig. 20.4 The investing layer

The Lymphatic Drainage

Chapter 21

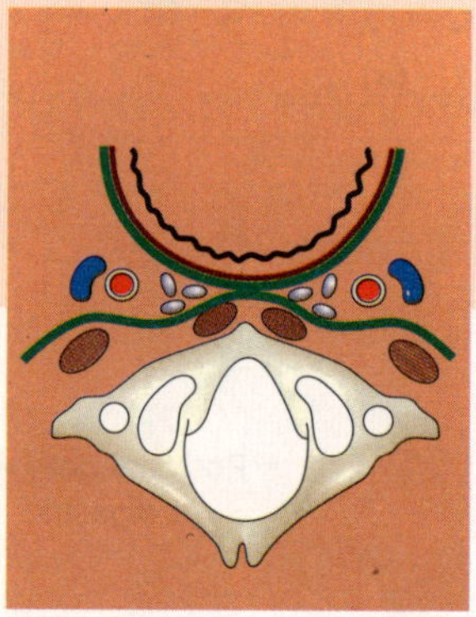

21.1 Superficial cervical lymph nodes

These are situated along the superficial veins according to the general plan. The superficial nodes are arranged in the form of a circle at the junction of the head and neck. This is called the 'Pericervical Collar' or 'Cervical Collar' and consists of occipital, retro-auricular (mastoid), superficial parotid (pre-auricular), deep parotid, submandibular and submental nodes.

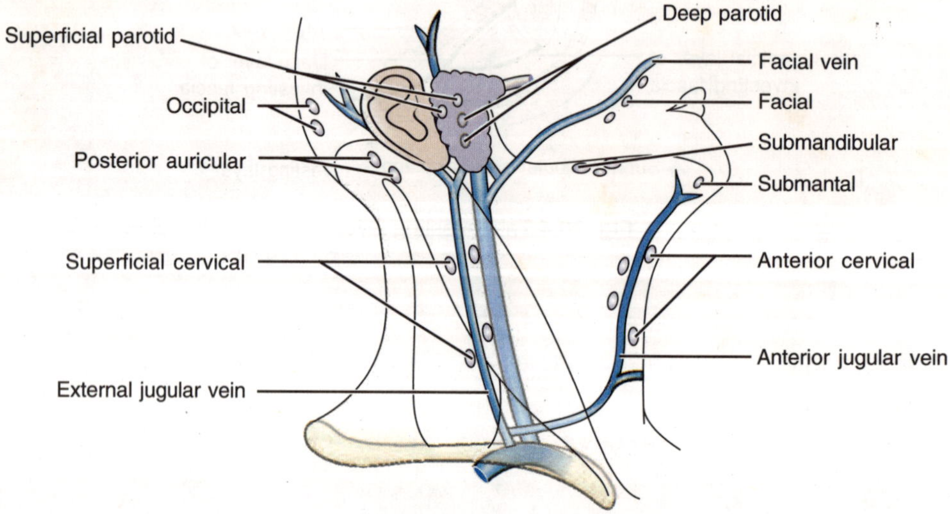

Fig. 21.1 Superfical cervical lymph nodes

In addition to these well-defined situations, there are a few extensions at certain sites:

- Facial nodes along facial vein are upward extension of submandibular nodes.
- Anterior cervical lymph nodes along the course of anterior jugular vein are extensions of submental lymph nodes.
- Superficial cervical nodes along external jugular vein are off-shoots of the superficial parotid nodes.

21.2 Deep cervical lymph nodes

These lymph nodes lie deep to the sternomastoid muscle along the length of the carotid sheath. They are divided into superior and inferior groups and are, respectively, above and below the level of belly of omohyoid. There is an extension of this group comprising the retropharyngeal set in the retropharyngeal space between the pharyngeal wall and the pretracheal fascia.

In the superior group a constant node lies at the point where the posterior belly of digastric crosses the internal jugular vein (jugulo-digastric node). It receives the lymphatics from the palatine tonsil and posterior part of the tongue.

The jugulo-omohyoid node lies where omohyoid crosses the internal jugular vein. It drains anterior and deep regions of the tongue.

The inferior (or supraclavicular) cervical nodes communicate with the axillary nodes and lymph vessels from breast. Some project beyond the posterior border of sternomastoid. The left supraclavicular nodes are known as Virchow's glands and are common sites of metastases of gastric, testicular and oesophageal carcinoma.

The laryngeal and tracheal nodes are scattered over the anterior and lateral aspects of the larynx, trachea and oesophagus by projecting beyond the anterior border of sternomastoid.

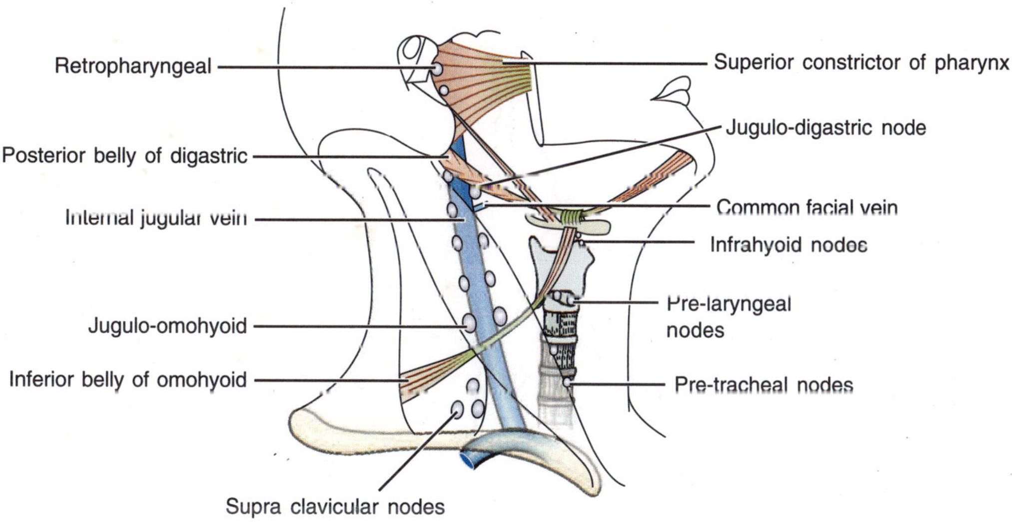

Fig. 21.2 Deep cervical lymph nodes

21.3 The relations of retropharyngeal lymph nodes

The prevertebral fascia is bound to the buccopharyngeal fascia in the midline. These lymph nodes lie in front of the prevertebral fascia.

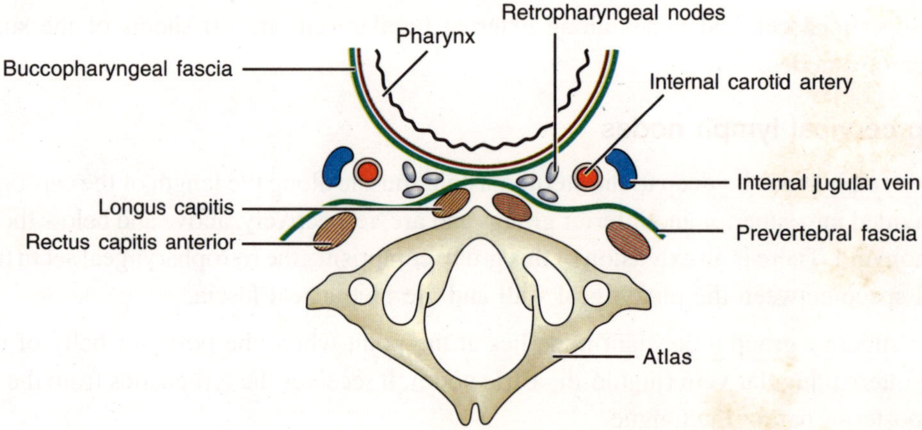

Fig. 21.3 The relations of retropharyngeal lymph nodes

21.4 Waldeyer's lymphatic rings

At the entrance to the pharynx there is a considerable amount of lymphoid tissue which is grouped in a circular fashion, formed superiorly by pharyngeal tonsil, inferiorly by lingual tonsil and laterally by palatine tonsils and tubal tonsils.

This internal ring of Waldeyer drains into pericervical chain and deep cervical nodes which constitute the external ring of Waldeyer.

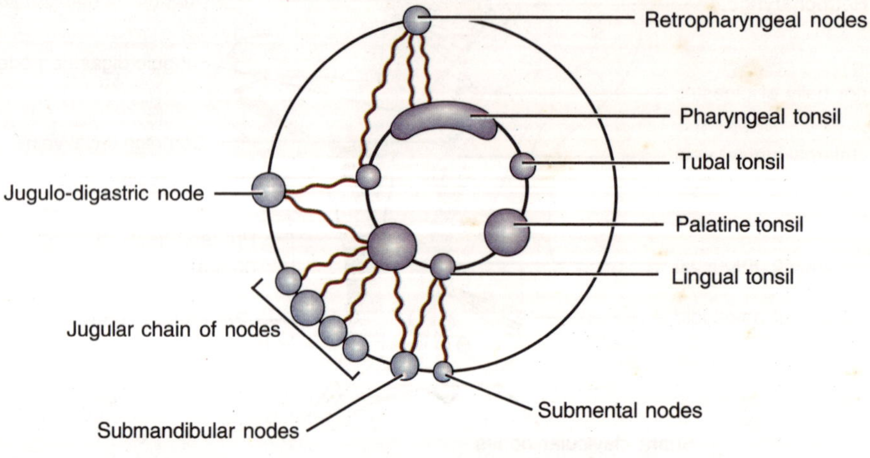

Fig. 21.4 Waldeyer's lymphatic rings

The Joints of the Neck

Chapter 22

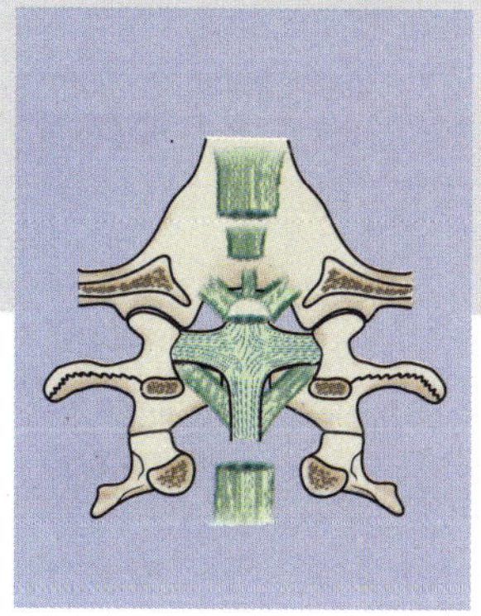

The altanto-axial joints are three in number. On either side is a synovial joint between the lateral masses of the two vertebrae. In the midline is the pivot joint between the back of the anterior arch of atlas and the odontoid process of axis. All are synovial joints.

The accessory ligaments of these joints are the membrane tectoria, the cruciform ligament, the apical and alar ligaments (of the odontoid) and the accessory atlanto-axial ligaments.

22.1 The membrane tectoria

It extends from the back of the body of the axis to the inner surface of the basiocciput, a short distance away from the margin of the foramen magnum. It is the cranial continuation of the posterior longitudinal ligament.

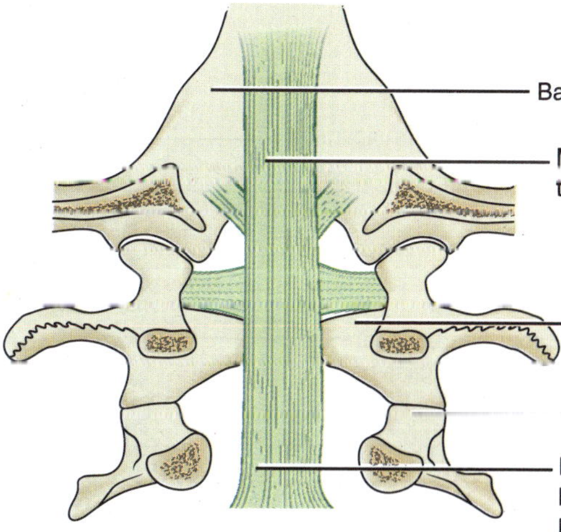

Fig. 22.1 The membrana tectoria

22.2 The cruciform ligament

The membrane tectoria has been cut above and below to expose the cruciform ligament, which consists of the following:

(i) A strong transverse band running across the back of the odontoid process from one lateral mass of atlas to the other

(ii) A weak vertical band extending from the body of the axis to the occipital bone where it is attached under the membrane tectoria.

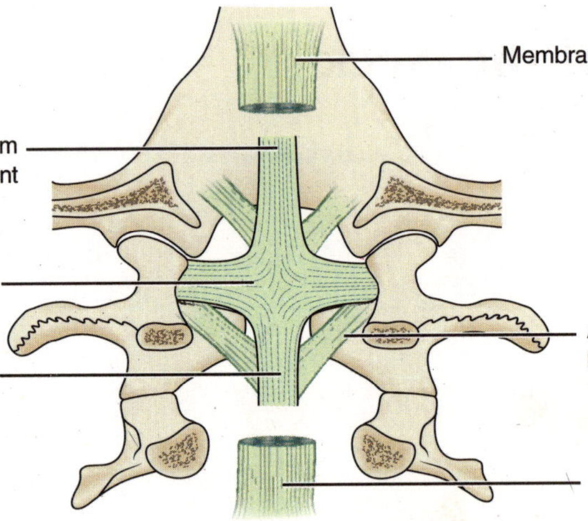

Fig. 22.2 The cruciform ligament

22.3 The apical and alar ligaments

The superior limb of cruciform ligament has been cut to expose from behind:

(i) The apical ligament extends from the apex of the odontoid process to the anterior margin of foramen magnum. It is the fibrous remnant of notochord.

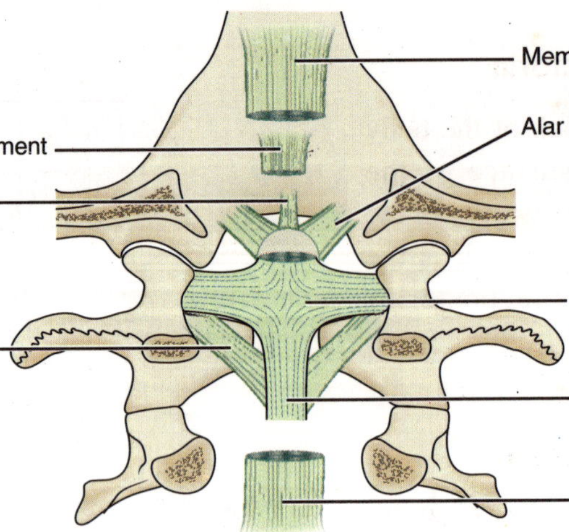

Fig. 22.3 The apical and alar ligaments

(ii) The alar ligaments lie on either side of the apical ligament and extend from the dens to the medial margins of the occipital condyle.

The accessory atlanto-axial ligaments pass from the back of the body of the axis to the corresponding lateral mass of the atlas.

22.4 Median section through atlanto-occipital and atlanto-axial regions

The apical ligament is attached to the tip of the dens and the anterior edge of the foramen magnum. The membrane tectoria passes upwards from the axis, behind the cruciform ligament and dens and through the foramen magnum, to be attached to the upper surface of the basiocciput. The anterior arch of atlas is connected to the anterior margin of the foramen magnum by the anterior atlanto-occipital membrane, strengthened in the middle by fibres continuous with the anterior longitudinal ligament.

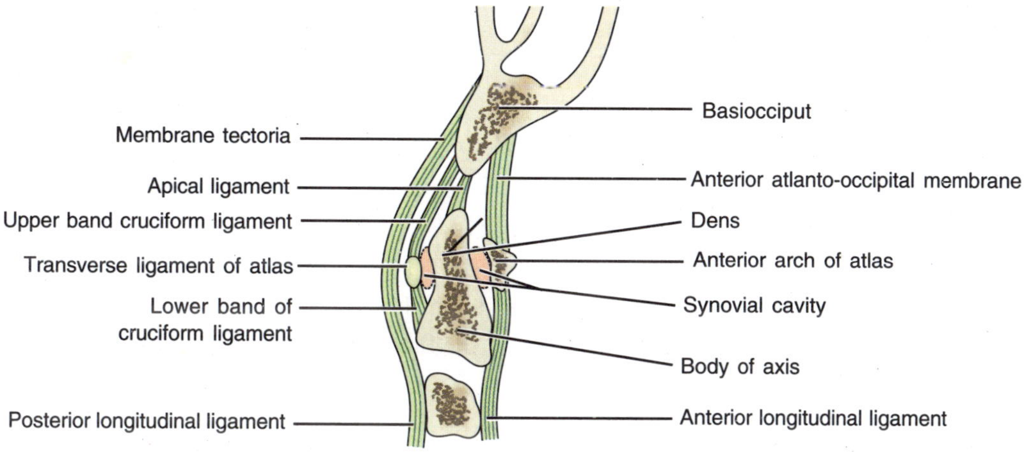

Fig. 22.4 Median section through atlanto-occipital and atlanto-axial regions

The Mouth

Chapter 23

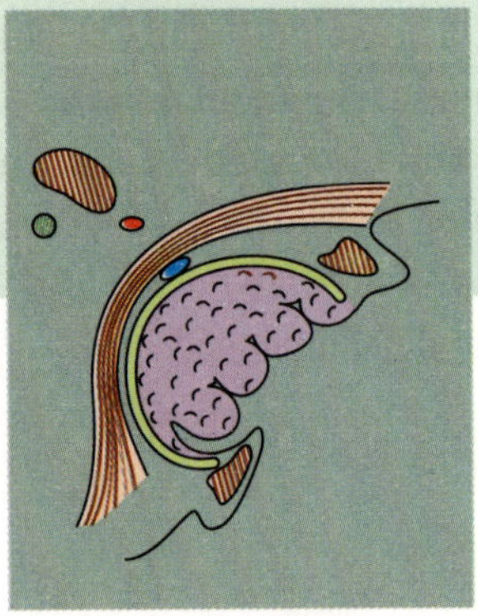

23.1 Open mouth cavity proper

The mouth cavity is bounded by gums and teeth, has a roof and floor and communicates posteriorly with the pharynx through the isthmus of the fauces. In the roof are hard and soft palates

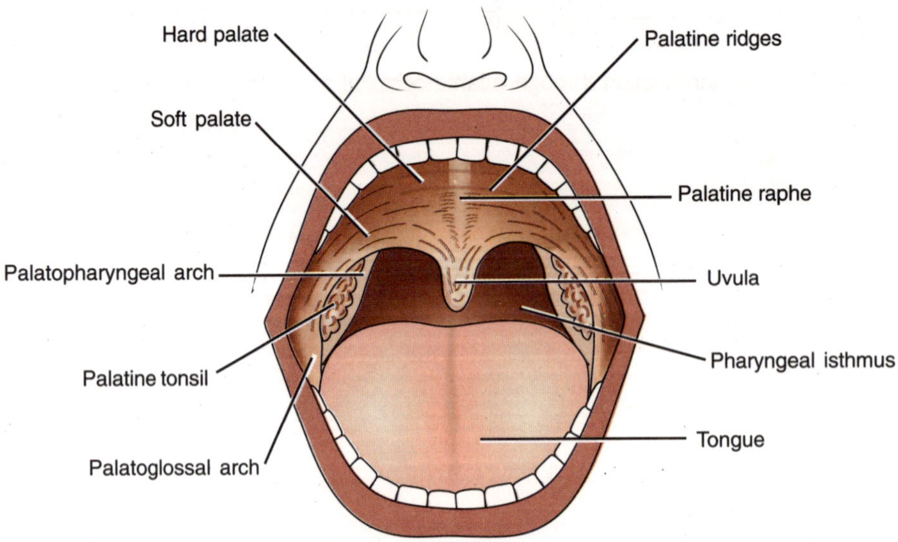

Fig. 23.1 Open mouth cavity proper

with the uvula hanging down from the posterior end of the soft palate. There are two folds of mucous membrane extending down from the soft palate. The anterior fold is called the palatoglossal arch and this forms the posterior limit of the oral cavity. The posterior fold is the palatopharyngeal arch and it lies in oral part of the pharynx.

23.2 Open mouth with tongue raised

The mucous membrane has been removed from the right side.

Floor of the mouth is formed by the mucous membrane which connects the tongue to the mandible. Note the frenulum connecting the inferior surface of the tongue to the floor of the mouth. On both sides of the frenulum the sublingual gland bulges upwards to form the sublingual fold which ends anteriorly in the sublingual papilla.

Study the structures exposed on the undersurface of the tongue on the right side after the removal of mucous membrane.

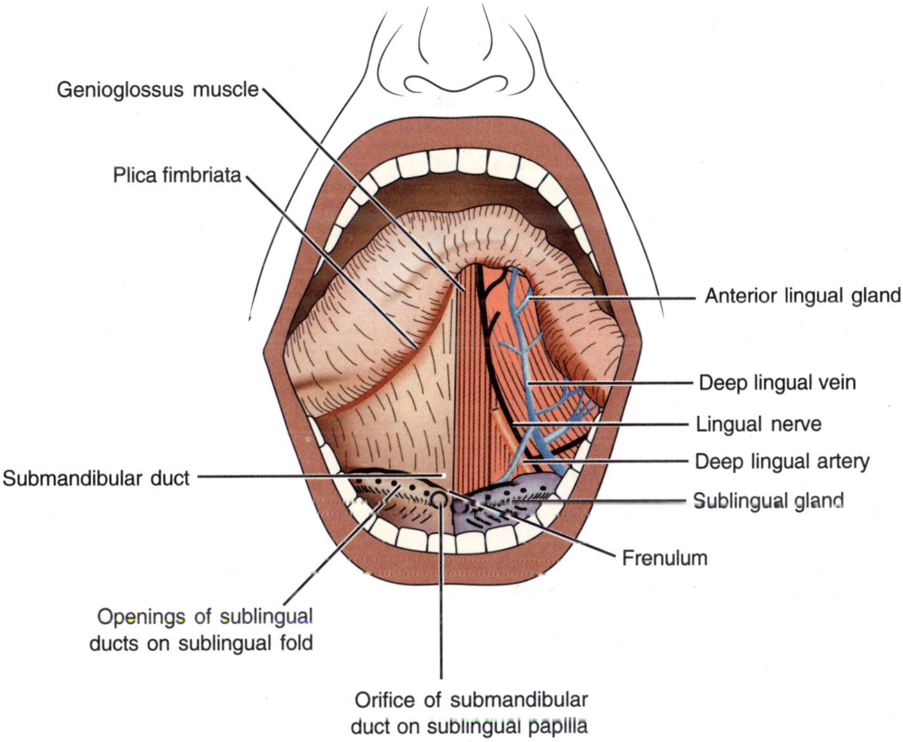

Fig. 23.2 Open mouth with tongue raised and structures on the left side of mouth exposed

23.3 Palatine tonsil in the fauces

Fauces is the part of the oro-pharynx which contains the two palatine tonsils between the palatoglossal and palatopharyngeal arches.

The triangular fold is a fold of mucous membrane passing from the lower part of the tonsil to the palatoglossal arch.

The semilunar fold is an occasional fold crossing the upper part of the tonsillar fossa.

The intratonsillar cleft is the remains of the second pharyngeal pouch which penetrates the tonsil and may pass into the soft palate. It is a convenient site for bacteria to set up inflammation.

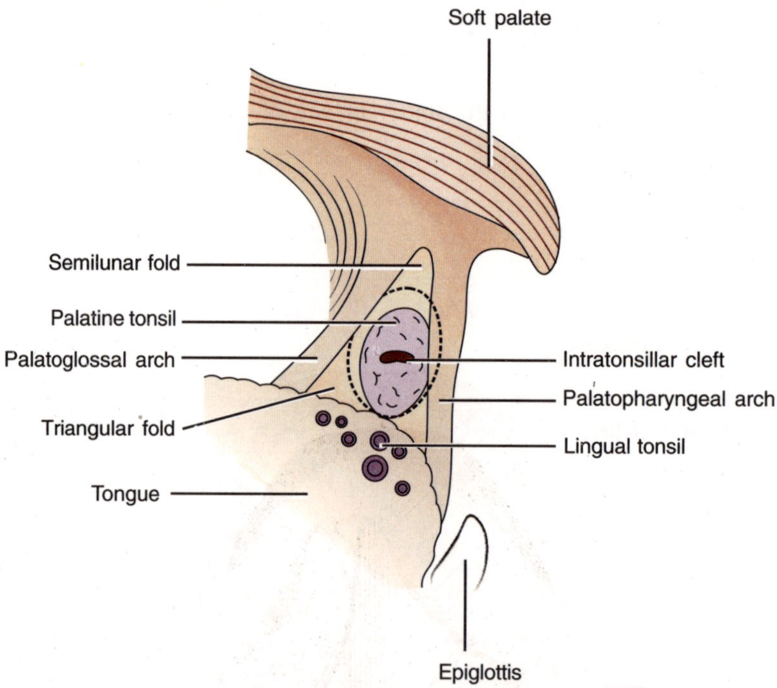

Fig. 23.3 Palatine tonsil in the fauces

23.4 Horizontal section through tonsil

The capsule of the tonsil is a thin but strong fibrous structure, continuous with the pharyngeal aponeurosis. It covers the deep surface of the tonsil and extends into it to form septa that conduct nerves and vessels. The capsule is therefore removed with the tonsil in a tonsillectomy.

On the medial surface are the openings of 12–20 crypts of tonsil.

The lateral surface is separated from the superior constrictor by lax connective tissue. The superior constrictor separates the tonsil from the ascending palatine and tonsillar arteries, the glossopharyngeal nerve and the stylohyoid ligament.

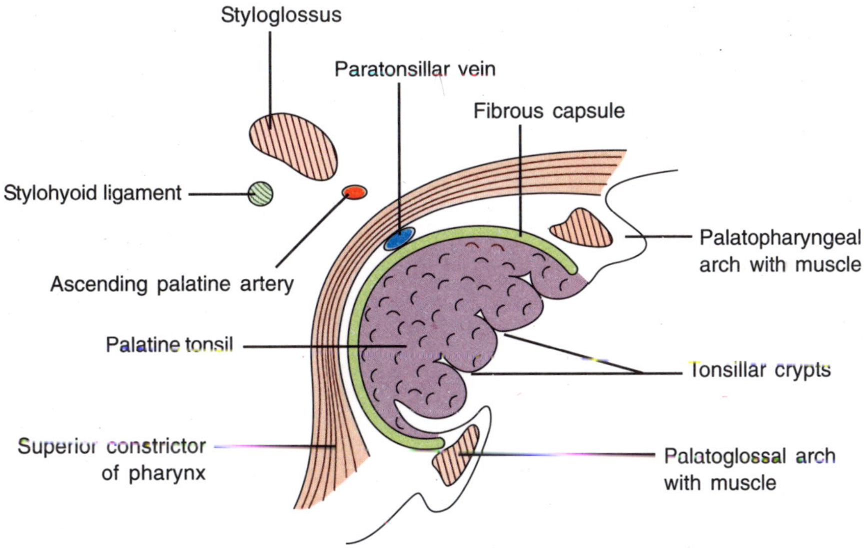

Fig. 23.4 Horizontal section through tonsil

The Pharynx

Chapter 24

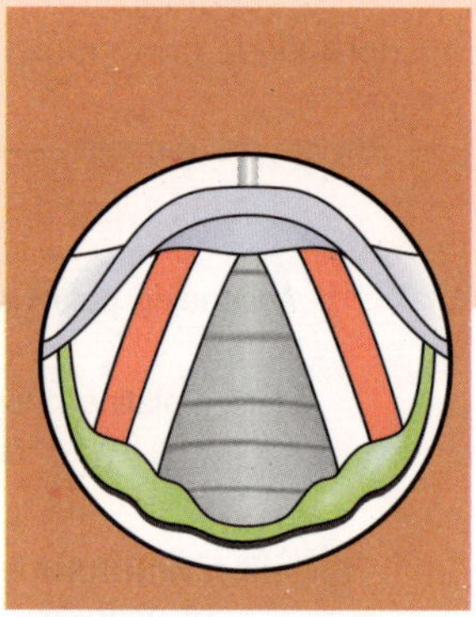

24.1 Scheme of pharynx

The pharynx acts as a common channel for both air and food pathways. It is divided into nasal (nasopharynx), oral (oropharynx) and laryngeal (laryngopharynx) parts. Pharynx extends from the base of the skull to the lower border of cricoid cartilage (C6).

The nasopharynx communicates with the oropharynx through the pharyngeal isthmus. The choanae form the junction between the nasopharynx and the nasal cavity proper.

24.2 The nasopharynx

The anterior wall is formed by the sloping upper or posterior surface of the soft palate. The posterior wall presents in its upper part an irregular swelling, the pharyngeal tonsil containing lymphoid tissue. The lateral wall shows the pharyngeal ostium of the auditory tube with torus tubarius above and salpingopharyngeal fold going downwards. The pharyngeal recess is the vertical slit behind the fold.

24.3 The structures seen by posterior rhinoscopy

Inspection of back part of the nasal cavity is performed by inserting a postnasal mirror through the mouth and pharynx. Note the living anatomy seen.

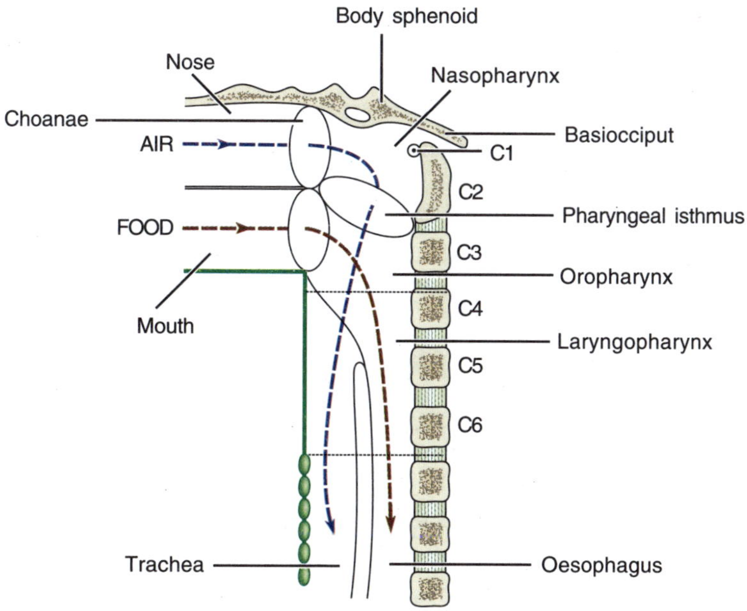

Fig. 24.1 Scheme of pharynx

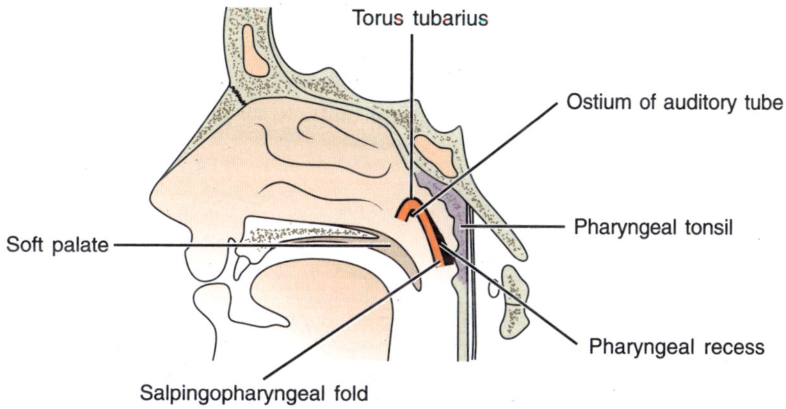

Fig. 24.2 The nasopharynx

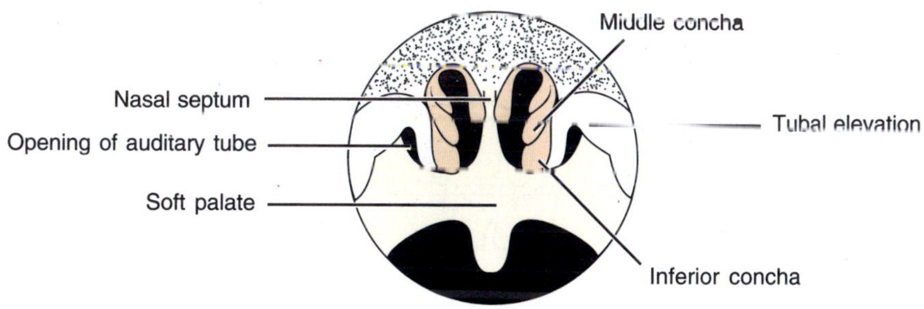

Fig. 24.3 The structures seen by posterior rhinoscopy

24.4 The Oropharynx

The anterior wall is formed by the pharyngeal part of the dorsum of the tongue, behind which is the upper end of the epiglottis. The lateral wall is the tonsillar fossa occupied by the palatine tonsil and bounded anteriorly by the palatolgossal arch and posteriorly by the palatopharyngeal arch.

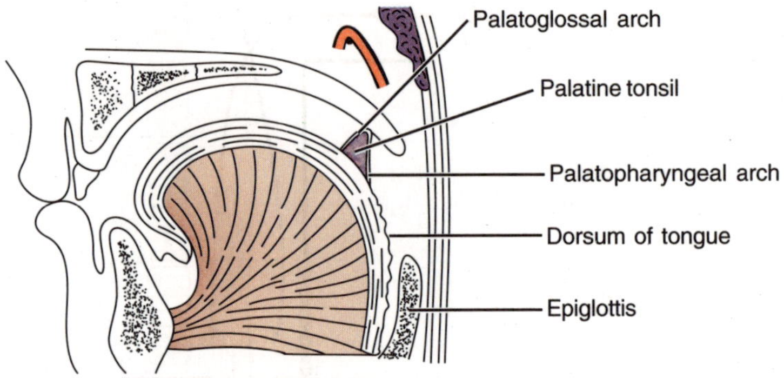

Fig. 24.4 The Oropharynx

24.5 The laryngopharynx

The anterior wall is formed by the laryngeal aditus and the soft tissues covering the back of the arytenoids and the cricoid lamina. The lateral walls present the small pyriform recess.

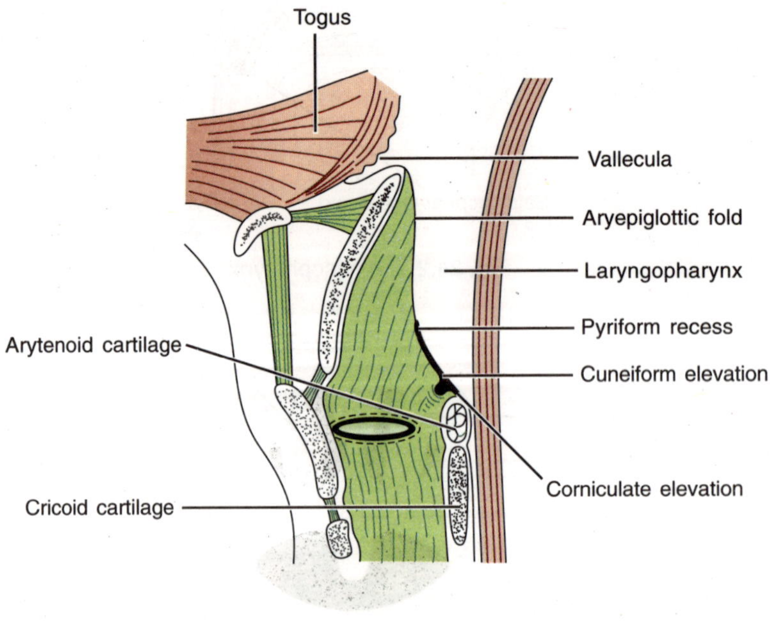

Fig. 24.5 The laryngopharynx

24.6 The structures seen on indirect laryngoscopy

An angled laryngeal mirror is placed against the anterior aspect of uvula. Light reflected into the subjects mouth illuminates the laryngeal mirror, on which an image of the larynx can be seen. The cartilaginous rings of the upper part of the trachea can be seen through the open glottis.

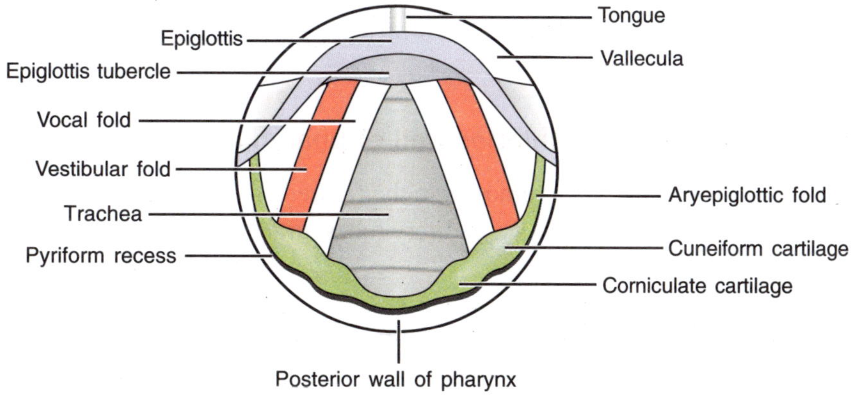

Fig. 24.6 The structures seen on indirect laryngoscopy

24.7 The muscles of the pharynx—posterior aspect

The raphe on the posterior wall of the pharynx is attached to the pharyngeal tubercle on the basiocciput. There is an interval between the upper border of superior constrictor and the base of skull. The pharyngobasilar fascia is attached to the base of skull and is thickened above the upper edge of superior constrictor at the pharyngeal recess.

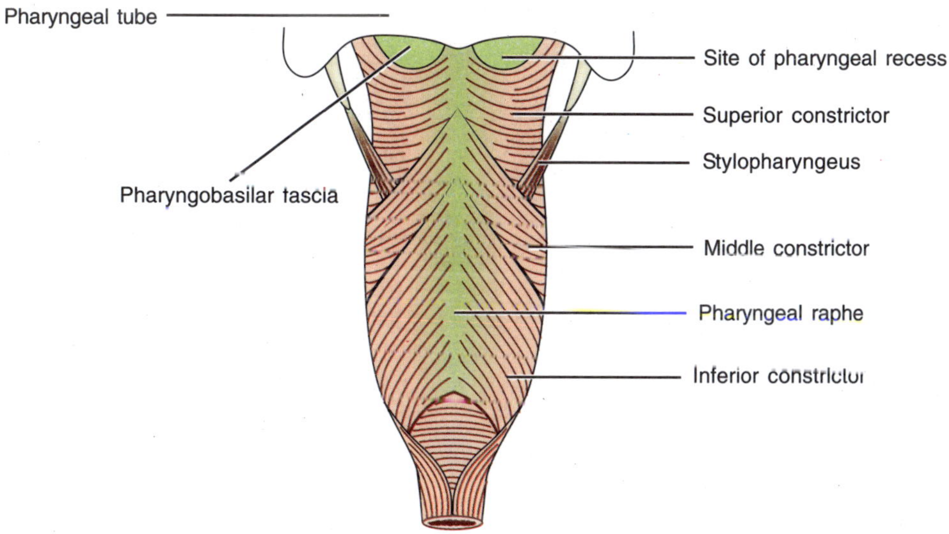

Fig. 24.7 The muscles of the pharynx—posterior aspect

In the posterior part, the muscles are so arranged that they overlap each other from below upwards. The junction of pharynx with oesophagus is the least dilatable part of the alimentary canal.

The inferior constrictor muscle contains two parts: (i) upper oblique fibres (thyropharyngeus) and (ii) lower horizontal fibres (cricopharyngeus). In between these fibres on the posterior aspect of pharyngeal wall there is a potential area of weakness which is known as 'Killians Dehiscence' through which the pharyngeal may herniate and form a deiverticulum known as Pulson's deiverticulum.

24.8 The posterior aspect of anterior wall of pharynx

Part of posterior wall has been removed in the figure. Note the various cavities with which the pharynx communicates viz., nasal cavity, auditary tubes, oral cavity, larynx and oesophagus.

Nerve Supply

All the muscles of the pharynx are supplied by the pharyngeal plexus except stylopharyngeus, which is supplied by the glossopharyngeal nerve.

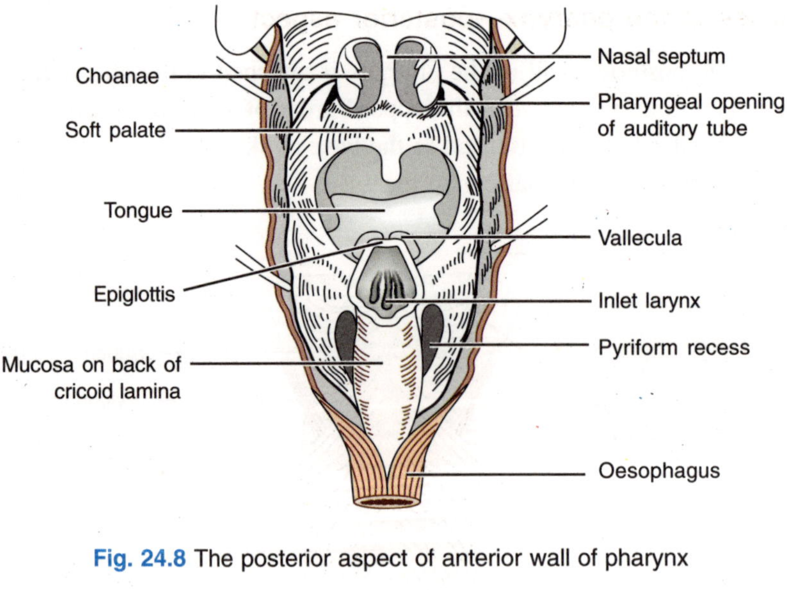

Fig. 24.8 The posterior aspect of anterior wall of pharynx

The Soft Palate

Chapter 25

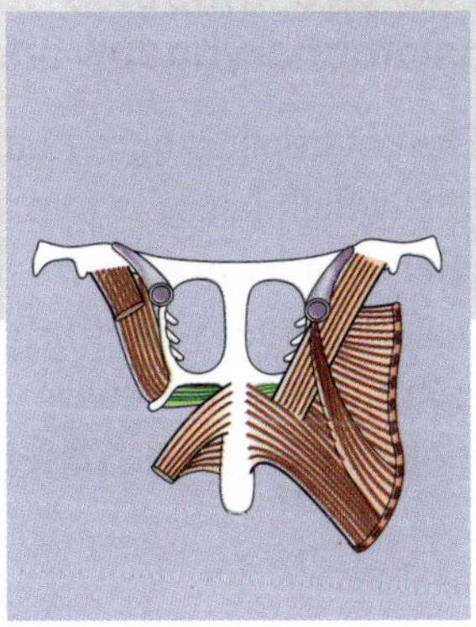

25.1 The two muscles entering the soft palate from above viz., Tensor palati and levator palati

The tensor veli palatini, which is outside the pharynx is attached to the base of the skull (the scaphoid fossa of the pterygoid process of the sphenoid bone, the lateral surface of the auditory tune

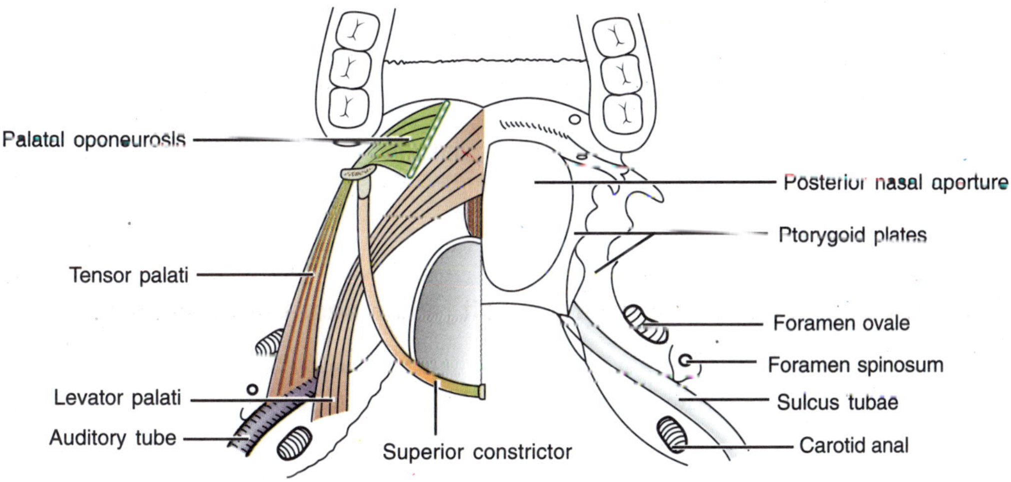

Fig. 25.1 The two muscles entering the soft palate from above viz., Tensor palati and levator palati

and the spine of sphenoid) and passes downwards. Its tendon hooks around the pterygoid hamulus to pass medially to become internal to pharynx and enters the soft palate as palatal aponeurosis.

The levator palati, which is inside the pharynx, is attached to the medial surface of the auditory tube and the adjacent part of the petrous temporal antero-medial to the carotid canal. The muscle passes downwards and enters the soft palate in which it lies between the two layers of palatopharyngeus muscle.

25.2 The two muscles leaving the soft palate and passing downwards viz., palatopharyngeus and palatoglossus

The palatopharyngeus attached to the aponeurosis and posterior edge of the hard palate has two layers which laterally join and pass downwards in the palatopharyngeal arch behind the palatine tonsil. Between its two layers lie levator veli palatini and the musculus uvulae. The stronger of the two layers lies antero-inferiorly between the levator palati and the tendon of tensor palati (right side of diagram). The thin postero-superior layer lies under the mucous membrane of the nasopharyngeal surface of the soft palate (left side of the diagram).

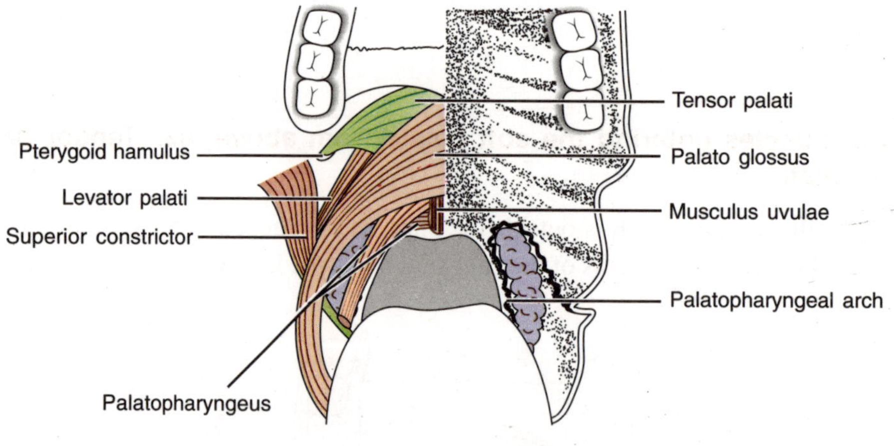

Fig. 25.2 Two muscles (palatopharyngeus and palatoglossus) leave the soft palate to pass downwards

25.3 One muscle hangs down from the soft palate near the midline into the uvula

Musculus uvulae are slips of muscles running antero-posteriorly into the uvula. It arises from the posterior edge of the hard palate near the midline and is inserted into the muucous membrane of uvula.

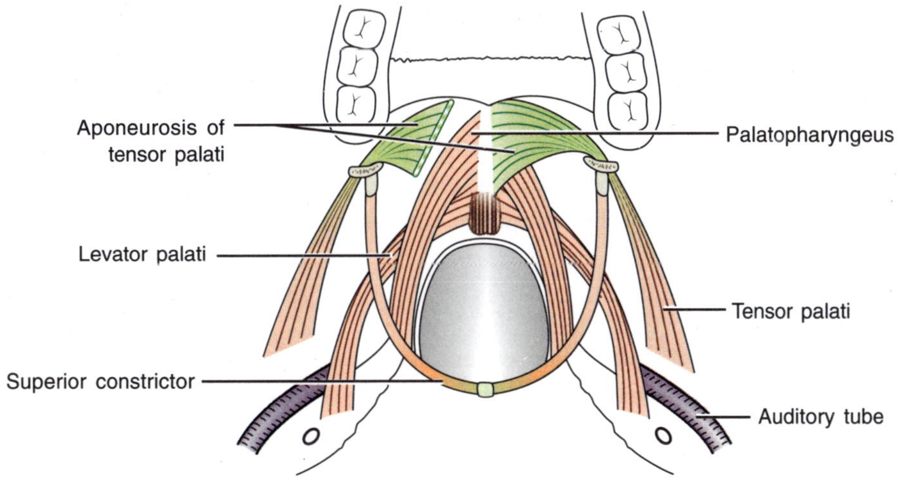

Fig. 25.3 One muscle (musculus uvula) hangs down from the soft palate into the uvula

25.4 (a) The palatal musculature as seen from the superior or pharyngeal surface of soft palate

The salpingopharyngeus comes from the lower part of the cartilage at the pharyngeal opening of the auditory tube. It passes downwards inside the constrictor muscle and blends with the palatopharyngeus.

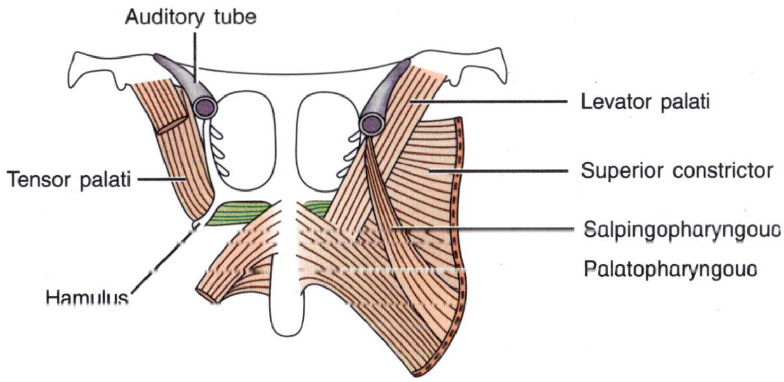

Fig. 25.4a The palatal musculature seen from the superior or pharyngeal surface of the soft palate

(b) Scheme of the muscular composition of the soft palate

The soft palate consists of a dense fibrous framework called the palatine aponeurosis, formed by the expanded tendons of the paired tensor palati muscles. To this aponeurosis the other four pairs fo palatine muscles are attached. The inferior surface is covered with stratified squamous epithelium. Columnar pseudo-startified ciliated epithelium (respiratory epithelium) covers most of the superior surface. Much of the substance of the soft palate consists of mucous glands, and diffused amongst them is lymphoid tissue.

Nerve Supply

- All the muscles of soft palate except tensor palati are supplied by motor fibres in pharyngeal plexus, which come from the cranial part of the accessory nerve.
- Tensor palati is supplied by a branch of the mandibular nerve which passes through the otic ganglion without relaying in it.

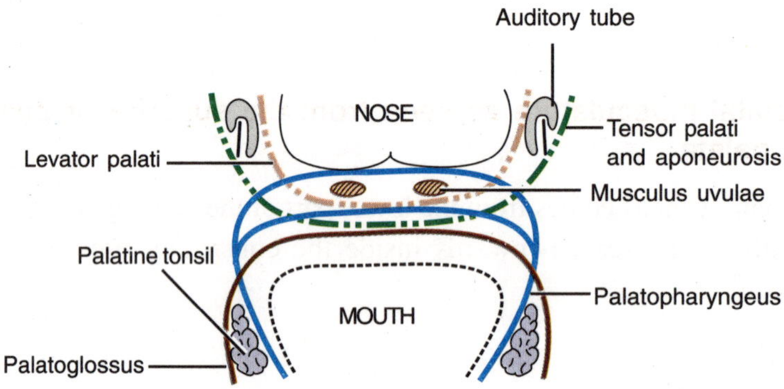

Fig. 25.4b Scheme of the muscular composition of the soft palate

The Nose

Chapter **26**

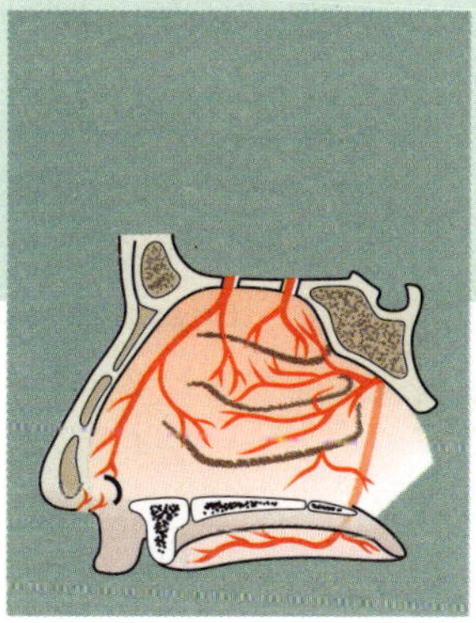

26.1 The nasal cavities in coronal section

The nasal cavities appear pear shaped being much broader at the floor, which is the palate. Each cavity has a floor, a roof, a medial wall or septum and a lateral wall.

Note the adjacent air sinuses.

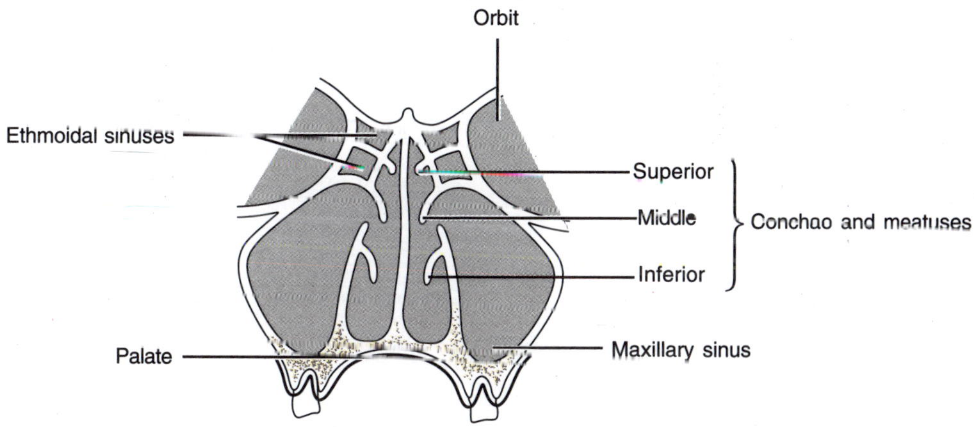

Fig. 26.1 The nasal cavities in coronal section

26.2 The bony and cartilaginous skeleton of external nose: Profile

The upper part is bony, formed by the nasal bones and frontal processes of maxillae. The lower part consists of hyaline cartilages in several pieces to permit movement of the alae. They do not extend to the free margins of the nostrils which are formed by fibro-fatty tissue.

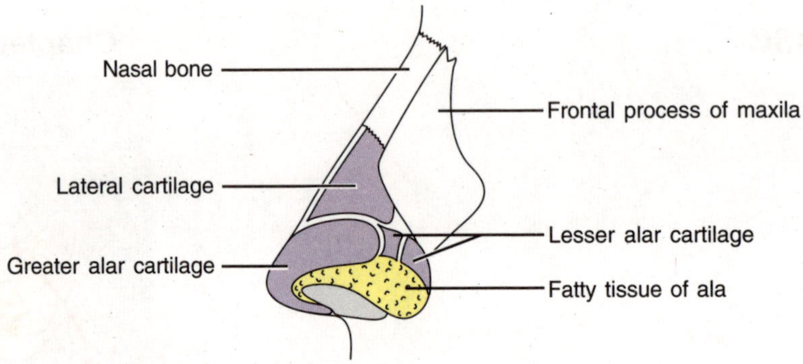

Fig. 26.2 The bony and cartilaginous skeleton of external nose

26.3 Skeleton of nasal septum

The nasal septum is partly bony and partly cartilaginous. The bony part is posterior and is formed by the perpendicular plate of ethmoid bone superiorly and the vomer inferiorly. The septal cartilage lies in the anterior angle, formed by the above two bones and extends forwards to become attached to the external nasal cartilage superiorly and anteriorly but not inferiorly.

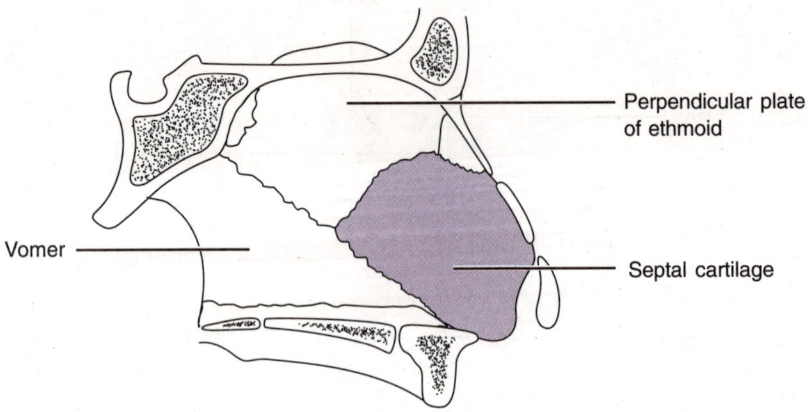

Fig. 26.3 Skeleton of nasal septum

26.4 The nerves in the nasal septum

The olfactory area comprising the upper third of the septum has branches of olfactory nerve spread over it.

The lower or respiratory area is supplied by nasopalatine which passes downwards and forwards to reach the floor of the nose, and then through the incisive canal and median incisive foramen to end in the mucous membrane of the anterior part of the hard palate. The posterior superior medial nasal nerves supply the postero-superior part of the septum. The medial nasal branches of the anterior ethmoidal nerve supply the anterior part of the septum.

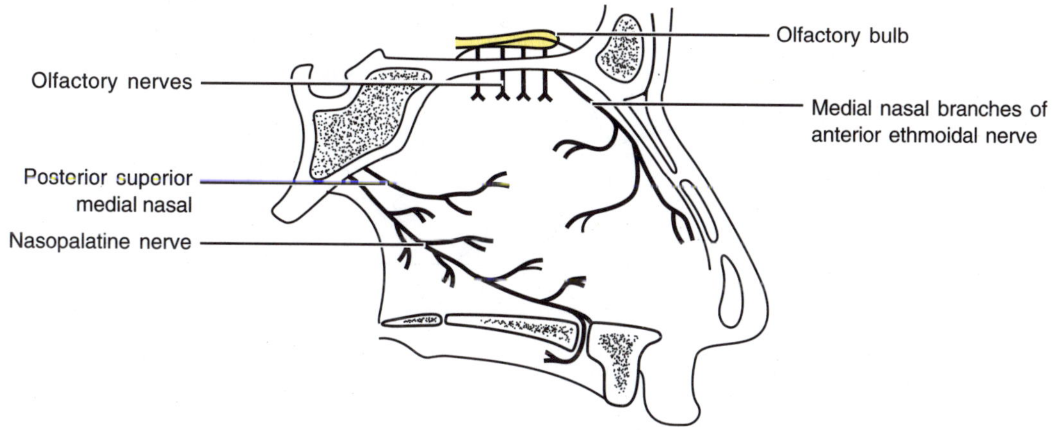

Fig. 26.4 The nerves in the nasal septum

26.5 The medial or nasal surface of right maxilla

It presents the large, irregular opening of the maxillary sinus. The other features and areas of articulation are labelled.

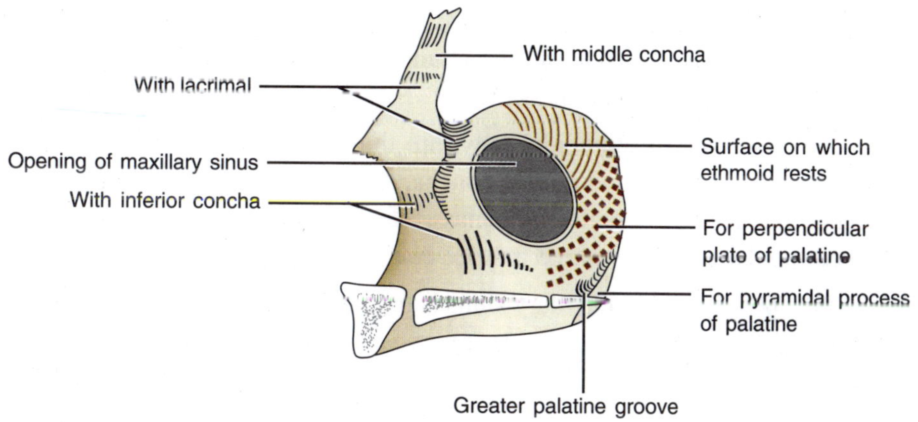

Fig. 26.5 The medial or nasal surface of right maxilla

26.6 The bones articulating with the nasal surface of maxilla

The posterior third or more of the nasal surface of maxilla has the perpendicular plate of the palatine applied to it, which also closes in the aperture of the sinus. In front of the sinus the naso-lacrimal groove is covered, in its upper part, by the lacrimal bone which also encroaches to a slight extent on the upper and front part of the orifice of the sinus. The lower part of the opening is filled by the down-turned maxillary process of the inferior nasal concha.

The lacrimal process of inferior nasal concha extends up to meet the lacrimal bone, covering the lower part of the naso-lacrimal groove. The ethmoidal process projects upwards in the opening.

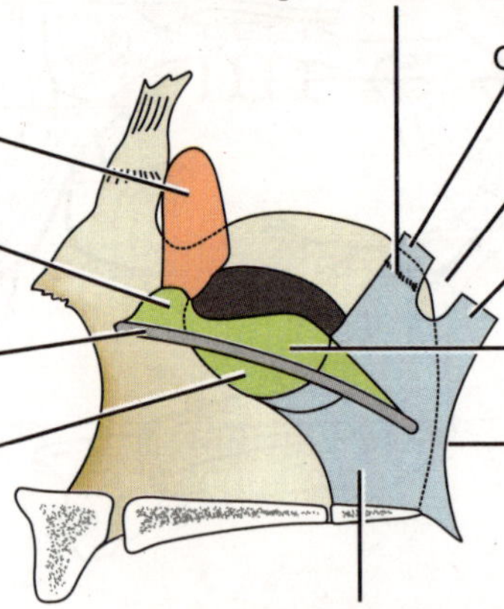

Fig. 26.6 The bones articulating with the nasal surface of maxilla

26.7 The bones articulating with the nasal surface of maxilla *(Contd.)*

The upper sloping part of the nasal surface of maxilla has the ethmoidal labyrinth resting on it. It covers the upper part of the opening of the sinus. The upper end of the perpendicular plate of palatine passes up between the maxilla and the ethmoid separating them and appearing between them in the extreme back part of the orbital floor.

From the medial surface of ethmoidal labyrinth thin sheets of bone curve downwards and laterally and are known as superior and middle concha. An uncinate process passes downwards and backwards from the front and lower parts of the mass, lateral to the middle concha, to articulate with the lacrimal and ethmoidal processes of the inferior concha.

The size of the opening of the maxillary sinus is reduced by all the bones articulating with the nasal surface of maxilla. It is further reduced to a very small size by mucous membrane.

The body of sphenoid converts the spheno-palatine notch into the spheno-palatine foramen.

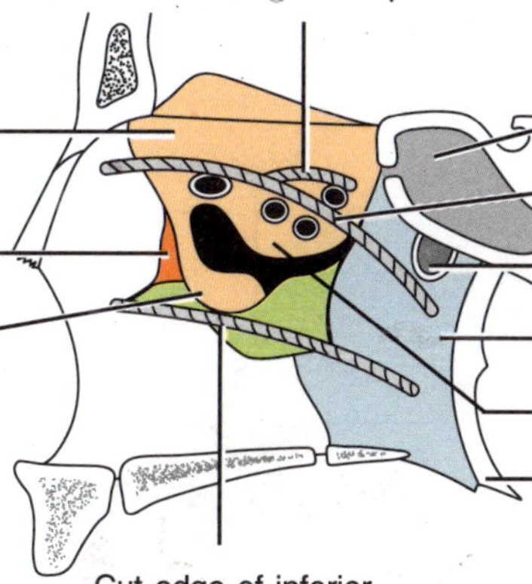

Fig. 26.7 The bones articulating with the nasal surface of maxilla

26.8 The completed bony lateral wall of nasal cavity

Note the flat medial surface of the ethmoidal labyrinth from which the superior and middle conchae project. Inferior nasal concha is a separate bone.

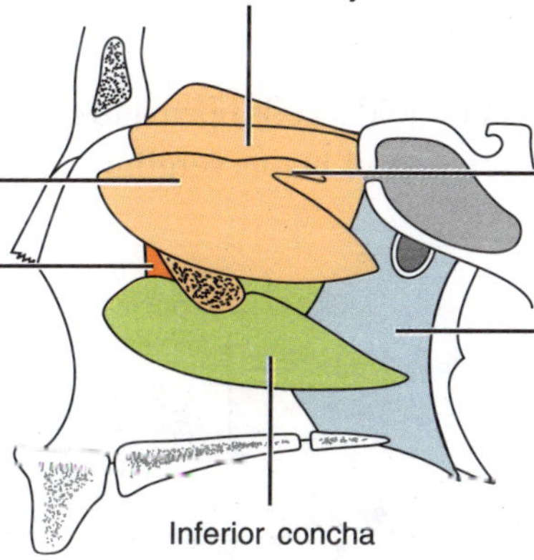

Fig. 26.8 The completed bony lateral wall of nasal cavity

26.9 The lateral wall of right nasal cavity with mucous membrane in position

Note the three conchae. Beneath each concha is the corresponding meatus. The superior concha is shorter and straighter than the others. It is placed across the posterior-superior corner of the wall, and subdivides the area above the middle concha into the spheno-ethmoidal recess above and behind, and the superior meatus below and in front. The sphenoidal air sinus opens into the spheno-ethmoidal recess.

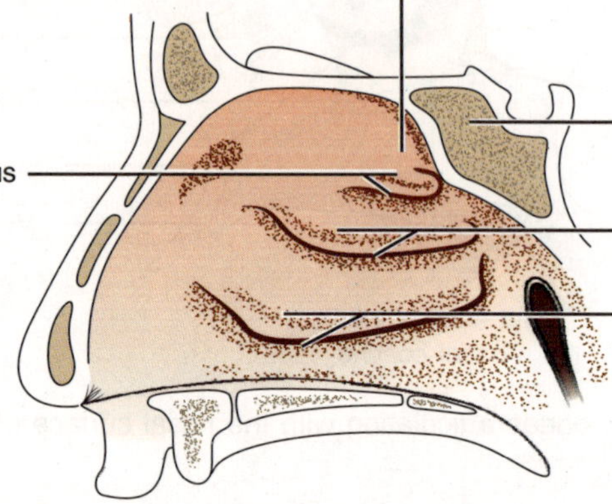

Fig. 26.9 The lateral wall of right nasal cavity with mucous membrane in position

26.10 The opening in the meatuses

The three conchae are shown cut to expose the meatuses and their openings. The bulla in middle meatus is bound in front and below by a curved hiatus, hiatus semilunaris, which leads upwards into a passage in the ethmoid, the infundibulum.

The frontal sinus and the anterior ethmoidal cells open into infundibulum, i.e., the middle meatus. The maxillary sinus opens into the back part of hiatus semilunaris.

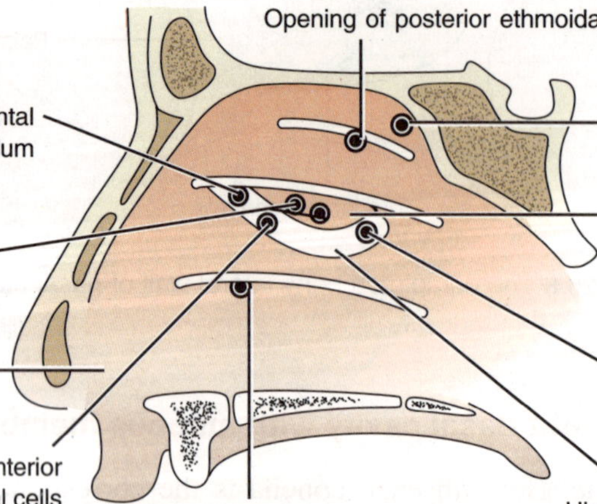

Fig. 26.10 The openings in the meatuses

26.11 Innervation of the lateral wall of nasal cavity

Olfactory nerves are largely confined over the superior concha.

The posterior superior lateral nasal nerves are direct branches from the pterygopalatine ganglion. The posterior inferior nasal nerves are distributed to the posterior parts of the middle and inferior meatuses and the inferior concha. The anterior part of the nasal cavity is innervated largely through the anterior ethmoidal nerve.

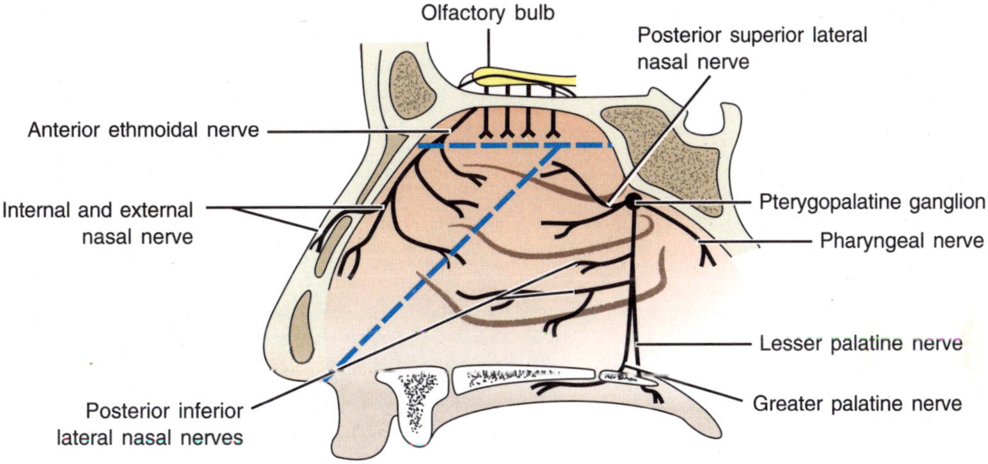

Fig. 26.11 Innervation of the lateral wall of nasal cavity

26.12 The arteries of the nose

The arteries run in general with the larger nerves.

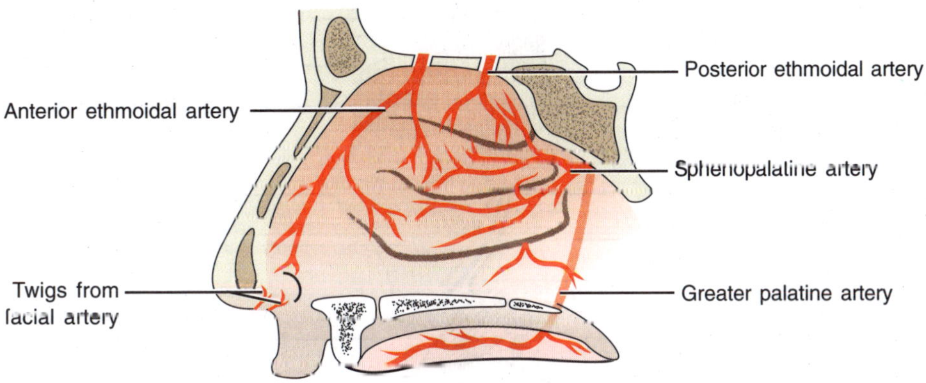

Fig. 26.12 The arteries of the nose

The Larynx

Chapter 27

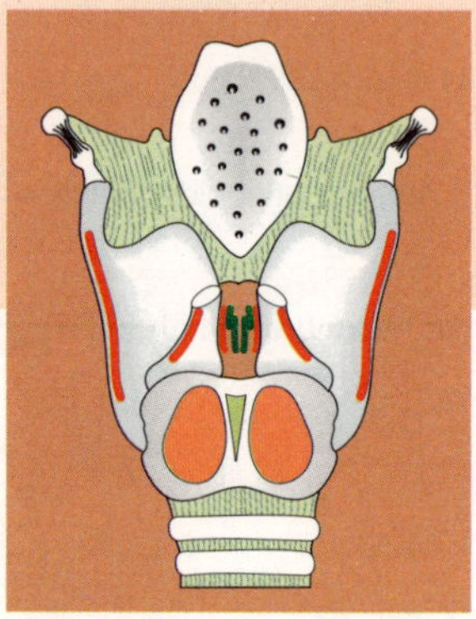

27.1 The lateral view of larynx—Cartilages, ligaments and muscular attachments

The outer surface of thyroid cartilage is marked by an oblique line which gives origin to thyrohyoid and inferior constrictor of pharynx and insertion to sternothyroid muscle. Note that the inferior

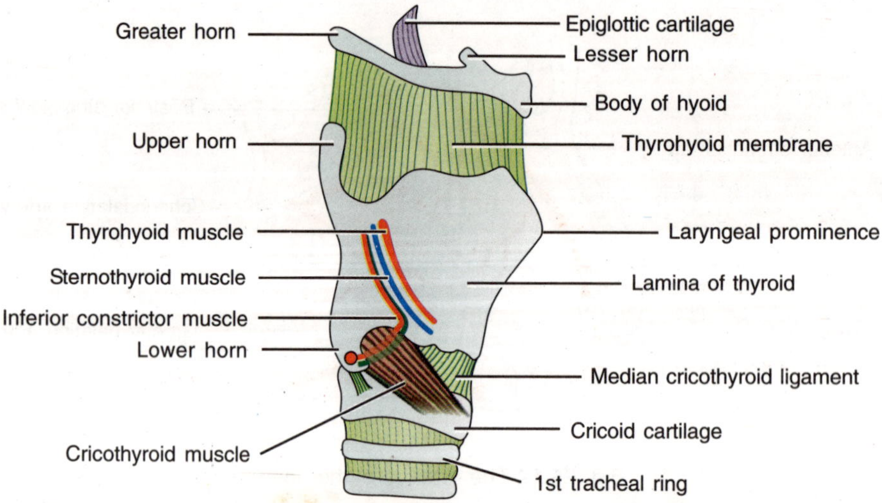

Fig. 27.1 The lateral view of larynx—Cartilages, ligaments and muscular attachments

constrictor also arises from the side of the cricoid cartilage, from a fine tendinous band thrown across the cricothyroid and from the inferior cornu of thyroid cartilages.

27.2 The internal framework of larynx on median section

The triangular cricothyroid membrane is attached below to the whole length of the upper border of the arch of the cricoid, in front it blends with the median cricothyroid ligament; and after curving medial to the lower border of the thyroid cartilage, it ends above in a free upper border, the vocal ligament, which forms the framework of the vocal fold or true cord. The three ligaments viz., median cricothyroid ligament, cricothyroid membrane and vocal ligament, constitute the conus elasticus.

The quadrangular membrane curves backwards from the lateral broder of the epiglottic cartilage to the lateral broder of the arytenoid cartilages. Its free upper border is thickened to form the aryepiglottic ligament; the free lower border is markedly thickened to form the vestibular ligament which is the basis of the vestibular fold or false vocal cord.

The internal framework of larynx formed by arytenoid and epiglottic cartilages, the two fibro-elastic membranes and median cricothyroid ligament is covered with a sheet of muscles on the outside and is lined by mucous membrane on the inside.

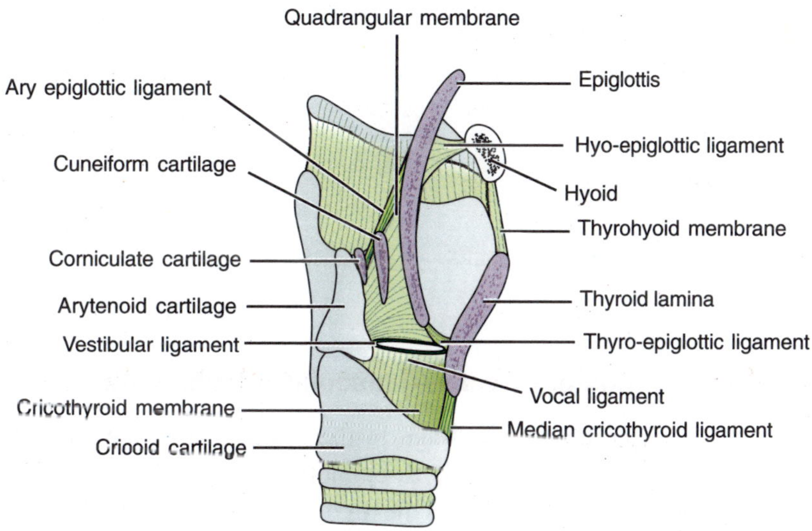

Fig. 27.2 The internal framework of larynx on median section

27.3 The intrinsic muscles of larynx in lateral view after removal of thyroid cartilage

Laterally they form a sheet in five parts. The lateral cricoarytenoid is lateral to the cricothyroid membrane, the thyroarytenoid to the vocal and vestibular ligaments, the thyro-epiglotticus and aryepiglotticus to the quadrangular membrane. The vocalis is the most medial bundle of fibres of thyro-arytenoid.

27.4 The interior of larynx in hemisection

The cavity of larynx is divided into three parts: (i) the vestibule, extending from the aditus or entrance to the vestibular folds, (ii) the ventricle lying between the vestibular and vocal folds, (iii) the infraglottic cavity lying below the vocal folds and extending downwards to the lower border of the cricoid cartilage.

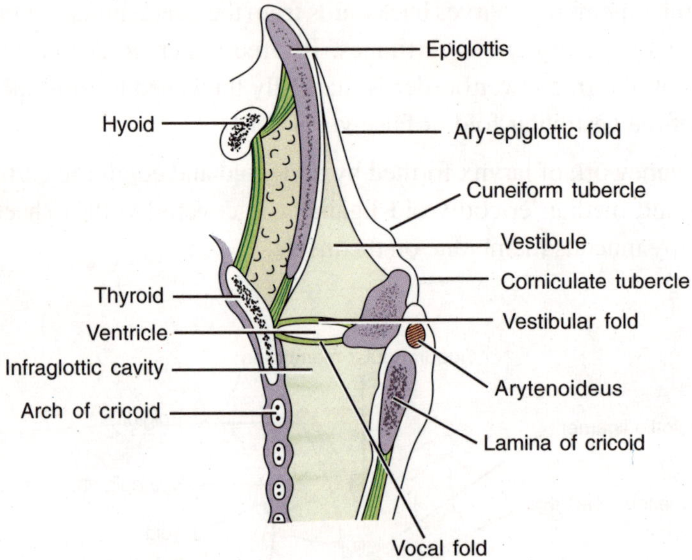

Fig. 27.4 The interior of larynx in hemisection

27.5 Cartilages of larynx, posterior view—Muscular attachments

The internal surface of the thyroid cartilage in the upper part of the angle formed by the junction of the laminae gives attachment to the thyro-epiglottic ligament; below this and on each side of midline, the vestubular and vocal ligaments and the thyro-arytenoid, thyro-epiglotticus and vocalis muscles gain attachment.

The transverse arytenoid arises from the muscular process and lateral border of the arytenoid cartilage, and is inserted into the corresponding parts of the cartilage on the opposite side. The oblique arytenoid passes from the back of the muscular process of one arytenoid cartilage to the apex of the opposite cartilage.

The posterior crico-arytenoid arises from the infero-medial region of the broad depression on the corresponding half of the posterior surface of the lamina of the cricoid cartilage.

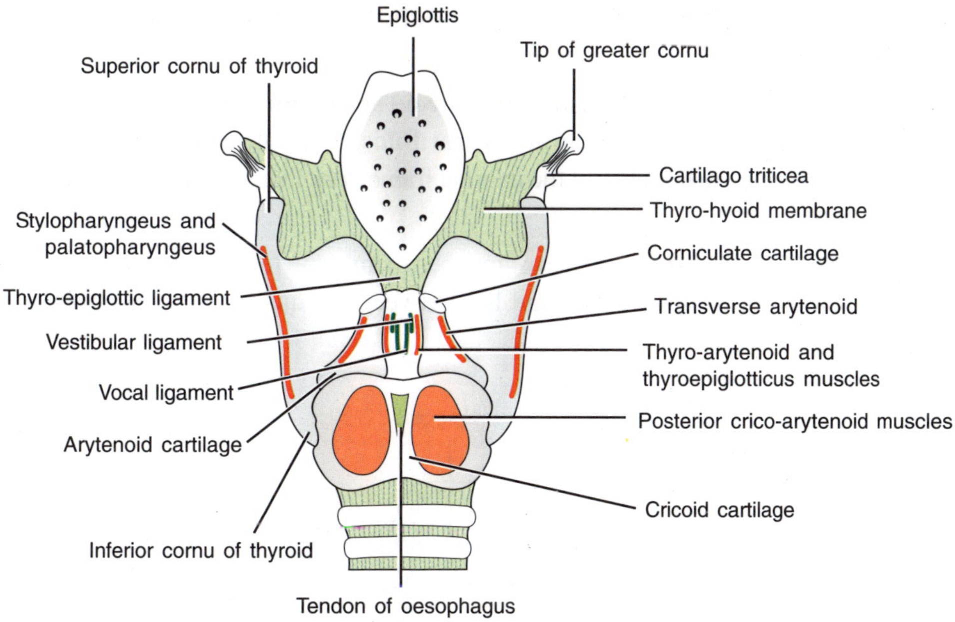

Fig. 27.5 Cartilages of larynx, posterior view—Muscular attachments

27.6 The muscles of the larynx—Posterior aspect

Posteriorly the sheet of muscles has two parts viz., the arytenoideus its oblique fibres partly continue as the aryepiglotticus, and the posterior crico-arytenoid which is most important as it is the only muscle which widens rima glottidis (safety muscle).

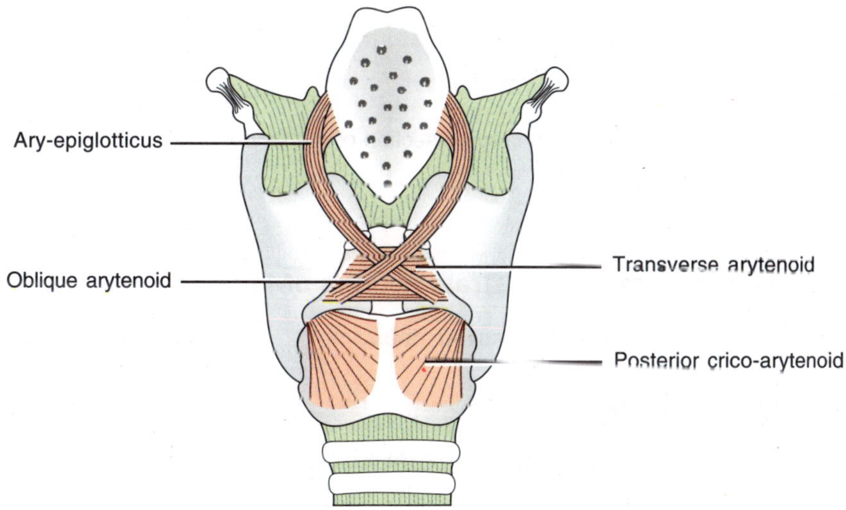

Fig. 27.6 The muscles of the larynx—Posterior aspect

27.7 The posterior aspect of a coronal section of the larynx and the upper end of trachea

Note the external framework made up of cricoid and thyroid cartilages, the internal framework here is represented by the vestibular and vocal folds. The intrinsic muscles of larynx (except cricothyroid) are applied to the sides of the internal framework like a sphincter, imperfectly subdivided into several parts.

The laryngeal saccule is acul de sac of mucous membrane from the anterior end of the ventricle. It extends upwards for about 1.25 cm and lies between the quadranular membrane and the thyro-arytenoid and thyro-epiglotticus.

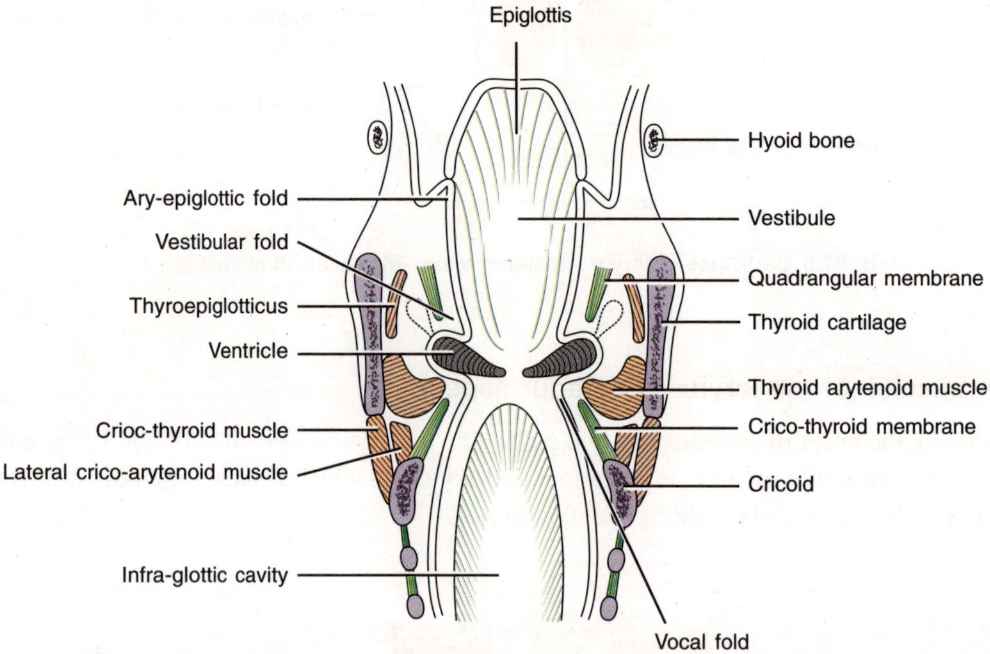

Fig. 27.7 The posterior aspect of a coronal section of the larynx and the upper end of trachea

27.8 (a) Schematic diagram to illustrate actions of laryngeal muscle

Arrows indicate the line of pull of various muscles.

(b) Abduction of vocal folds

The arrows indicates the line of pull of posterior crico-arytenoid, the only abductors. The abducted vocal folds and the abducted, retracted and laterally rotated arytenoid cartilages are shown in dotted lines.

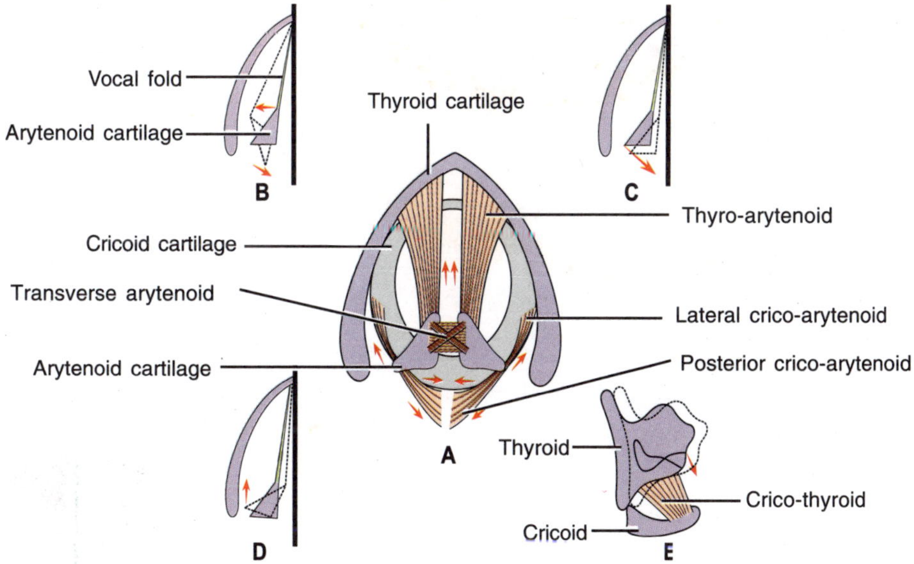

Fig. 27.8 Schematic diagram to illustrate actions of laryngeal muscle

(c) Closure of the rima glottidis

The arrow indicates the line of pull of the transverse arytenoid muscle. Both the vocal folds and the arytenoid cartilages are abducted, but there is no rotation of the latter.

(d) Abduction of vocal folds

The arrow indicates the line of pull of the lateral crico-arytenoid muscles. The abducted vocal folds and the medially rotated arytenoid cartilages are shown in dotted outlines.

(e) Tension of the vocal folds

It is produced by the action of the crico-thyroid muscle by flexion of the thyroid cartilage upon the cricoid cartilage.

Relaxation of the vocal folds is produced by the action of thyro-arytenoid muscles, which draw the arytenoid cartilages ventrally.

Nerve Supply

- All the intrinsic muscles of the larynx are supplied by the recurrent laryngeal nerve except crico-thyroid which is supplied by the external laryngeal nerve.

The Tongue

Chapter 28

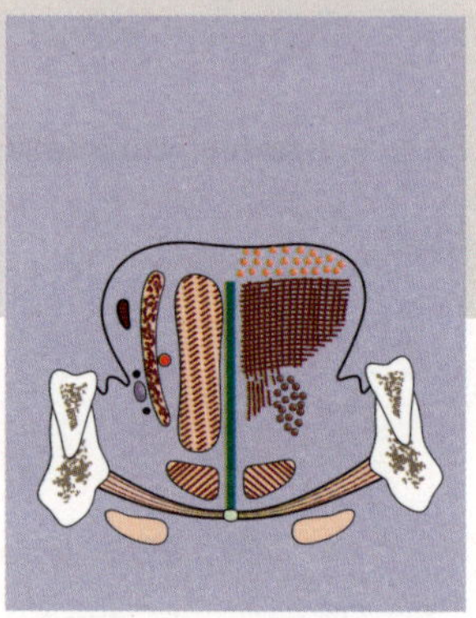

28.1 The dorsum of the tongue and the palatine tonsil

The left side of the figure shows the distribution of the papillae and the right side areas of sensory nerve supply of tongue.

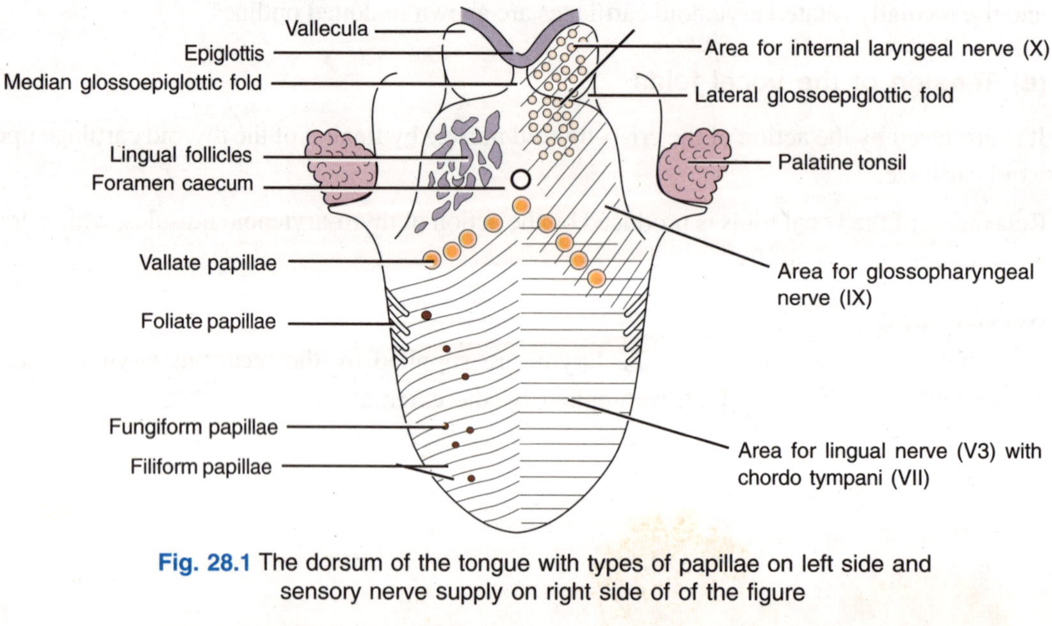

Fig. 28.1 The dorsum of the tongue with types of papillae on left side and sensory nerve supply on right side of of the figure

28.2 Lymphatic drainage of tongue

The lymphatics drain in the following way:

(a) The lymphatics from the tip pierce the mylohyoid to end in the submental nodes of both sides. Some cross the hyoid bone superficially to reach the jugulo-omohyoid node.

(b) Vessels from the margin of the tongue cross both surfaces of the hyoglossus and end in the jugulo-digastric and jugulo-omohyoid nodes. Others pass both superficial and deep to the sublingual salivary gland, pierce the mylohyoid and reach the submandibular, jugulodigastric and jugulo-omohyoid nodes.

(c) Vessels from the central part of the tongue descend between the genioglossi and terminate in the submandibular, jugulo-digastric and jugulo-omohyoid nodes; some cross the median plane.

(d) Vessesls from the base of the tongue pierce the superior constrictor muscle of the pharynx to end in the jugulo-digastric node of both sides.

It is important to note that in 50% of cases, the lymphatic vessels draining the anterior two-third of the tongue and the floor of the mouth traverse the periosteum of the mandible on their way to submental and submandibular lymph nodes.

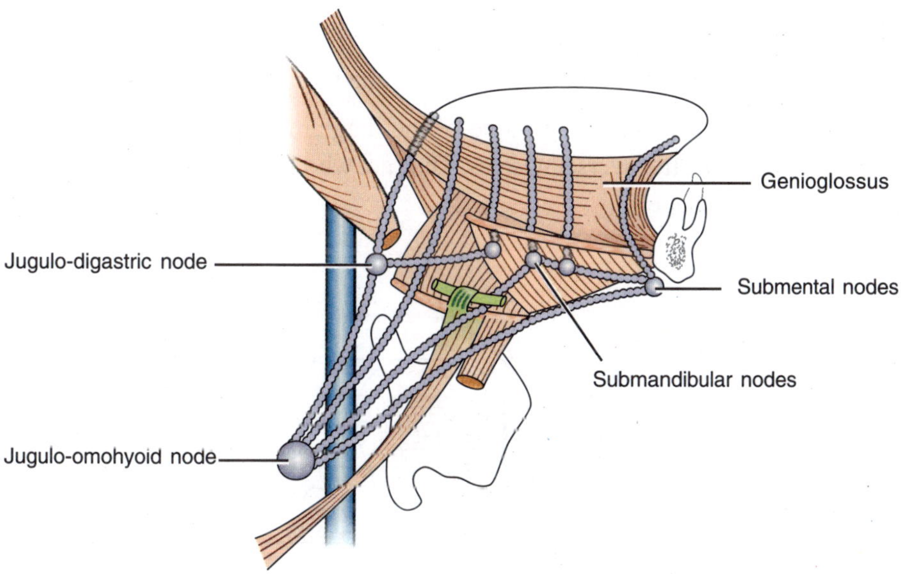

Fig. 28.2 Lymphatic drainage of tongue

28.3 The extrinsic muscles of the tongue

The extrinsic group comprising of genioglossus, hyoglossus, styloglossus and palatoglossus is shown. These muscles take origin from parts outside the tongue, and can therefore move the tongue as well as alter its shape.

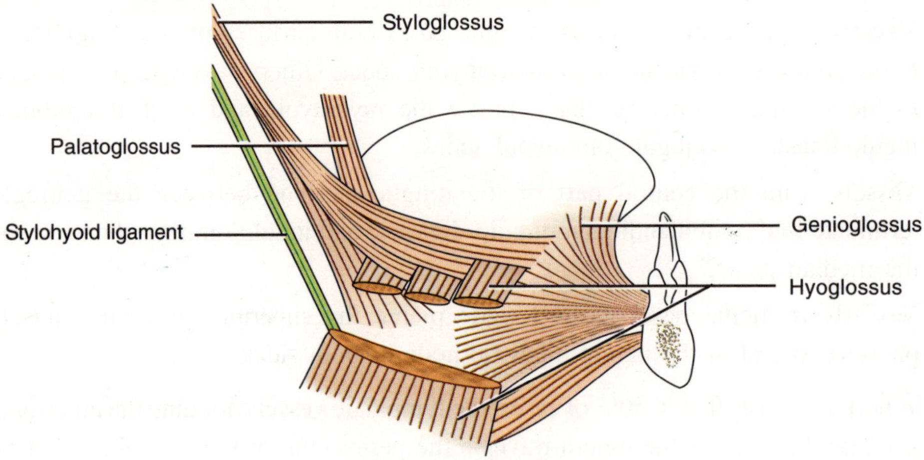

Fig. 28.3 The extrinsic muscles of the tongue

28.4 Schematic transverse section of tongue

The intrinsic muscles are shown on the right side of the figure.

The intrinsic muscles shown on the lift side of the diagram consist of superior longitudinal inferior longitudinal, vertical and transverse muscles. They are wholly inside the tongue and, therefore, can produce only changes in shape.

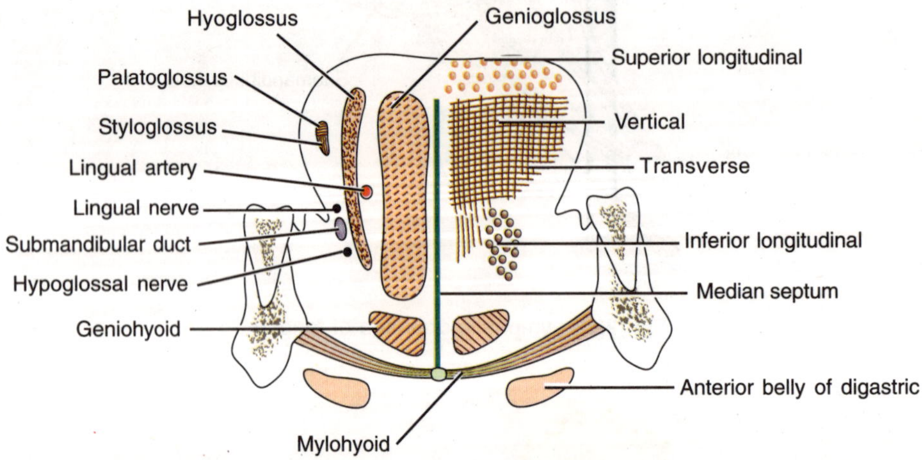

Fig. 28.4 Schematic transverse section of tongue to show intrinsic muscles

The longitudinal muscles are arranged in two relatively narrow bands, the superior on the dorsum of the tongue, immediately beneath the mucous membrane, and the inferior towards the lower surface. The transverse and vertical muscles are actually somewhat oblique.

The septum is a median fibrous partition which is strongest posteriorly where it is attached to the hyoid bone. It does not reach the mucous membrane of the dorsum, but is separated from it by the superior longitudinal muscle.

The extrinsic muscles are shown on the left side of the figure.)

Nerve Supply

- All the extrinsic and intrinsic muscles of the tongue are supplied by hypoglossal nerve, except palatoglosses, which is innervated by the pharyngeal plexus.

The Teeth

Chapter 29

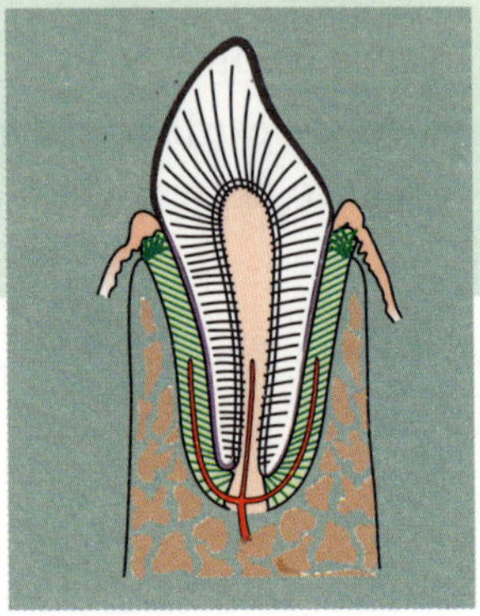

29.1 Dental terminology

Special terms are used to describe the surfaces of teeth. The surface adjacent to the lip or cheek is known as labial or buccal surface. The surface adjacent to the tongue is the lingual (lower jaw teeth) or palatal surface (upper jaw teeth). The premolars and molars have medial and distal surfaces. The median point between the central incisors is the datum point for these terms. Because the dental arch is curved, it will be noted that the mesial surfaces of these postcanine teeth face anteriorly and distal surfaces posteriorly.

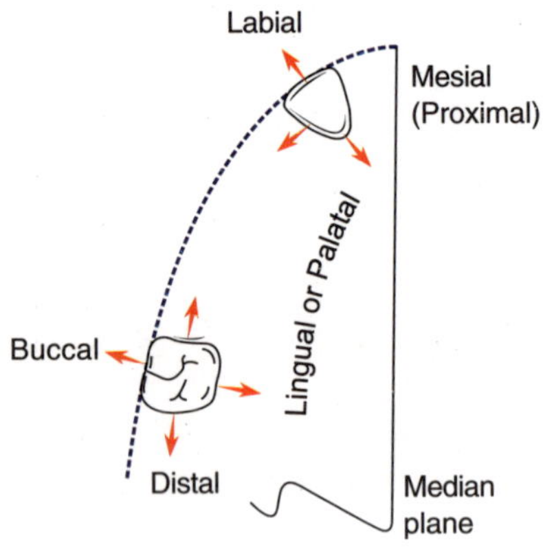

Fig. 29.1 Dental terminology

29.2 The deciduous or \primary teeth (Milk teeth)

The primary teeth are twenty in number, ten in each jaw, that is five in each quadrant; two incisors, one canine and two molars (I.2; C.I; M.2). They appear between half and two and half years. The first teeth to erupt are the lower central incisors at about 6 months. The lower teeth frequently precede the upper in eruption.

The approximate number of deciduous teeth at a particular age is equal to the age of the child in months minus six. The diagram shows average time of eruption in months.

They start shedding round about 6–7 years of age.

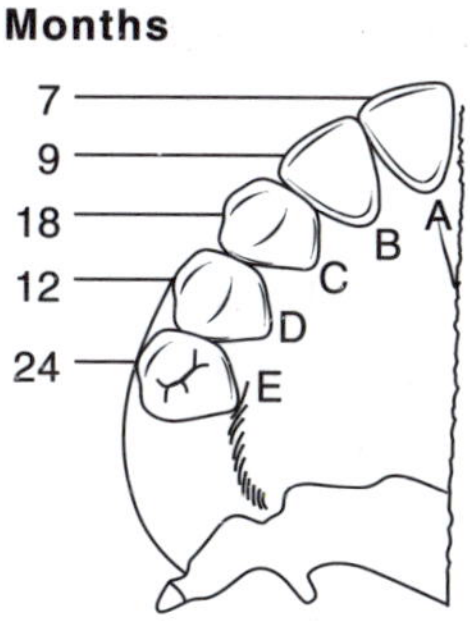

Numbering of teeth in each quadrant

E	D	C	B	A	A	B	C	D	E
E	D	C	B	A	A	B	C	D	E

Symbol for right first upper molar

D|

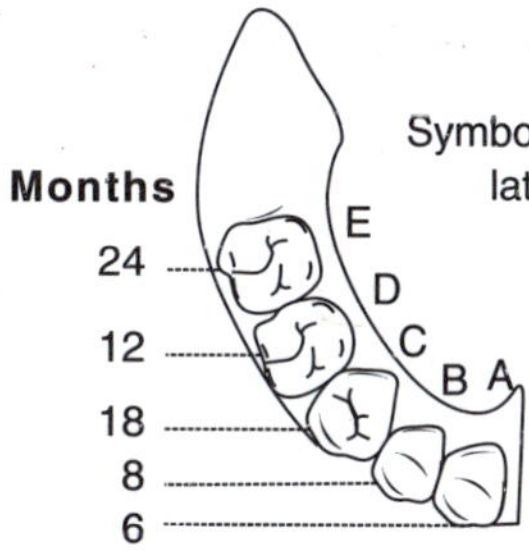

Symbol for right lower lateral incisor

B|

Fig. 29.2 The deciduous or primary teeth (Milk teeth)

29.3 The permanent teeth

They begin to appear about the 6th year and replace the deciduos teeth by about the 12th year. They are 32 in number that is eight in each quadrant; two incisors, one canine, two premolars and three molars (I.2; C.I; P.2; M.3). The time of eruption is given in years. The first to erupt is the first molar. Approximately four teeth are replaced every year.

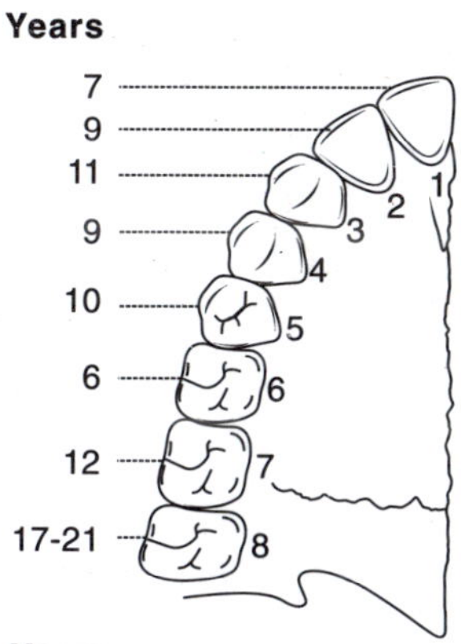

Numbering of teeth in each quadrant

8	7	6	5	4	3	2	1	1	2	3	4	5	6	7	8
8	7	6	5	4	3	2	1	1	2	3	4	5	6	7	8

Symbol for right upper canine

3|

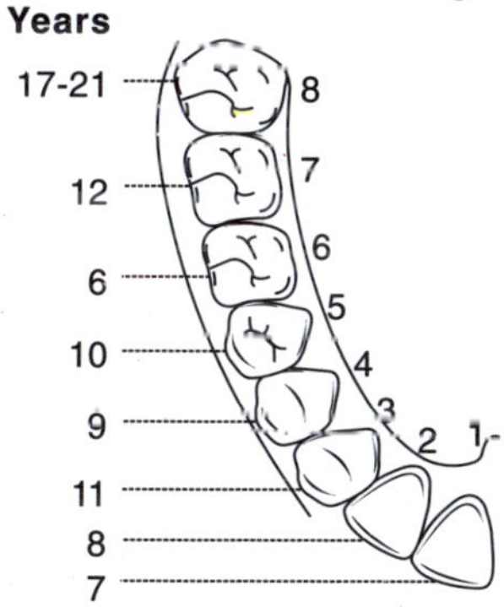

Symbol for right lower first molar

6|

Fig. 29.3 The permanent teeth

29.4 A bucco-lingual longitudinal section of a young lower first premolar tooth and its environs

The bulk of a tooth is composed of dentine. The enamel covering the crown is about 1.5-mm thick, while the cement covering the root is usually very much thinner. The dentine contains a central canal, the pulp cavity. At its coronal end, the cavity is expanded into a pulp chamber, and in the root region it is narrowed into a pulp canal opening at or near the tip of the root into an apical foramen. The cement of the root is separated from the bony socket by soft tissue, the periodontal ligament, which is about 0.2-mm wide.

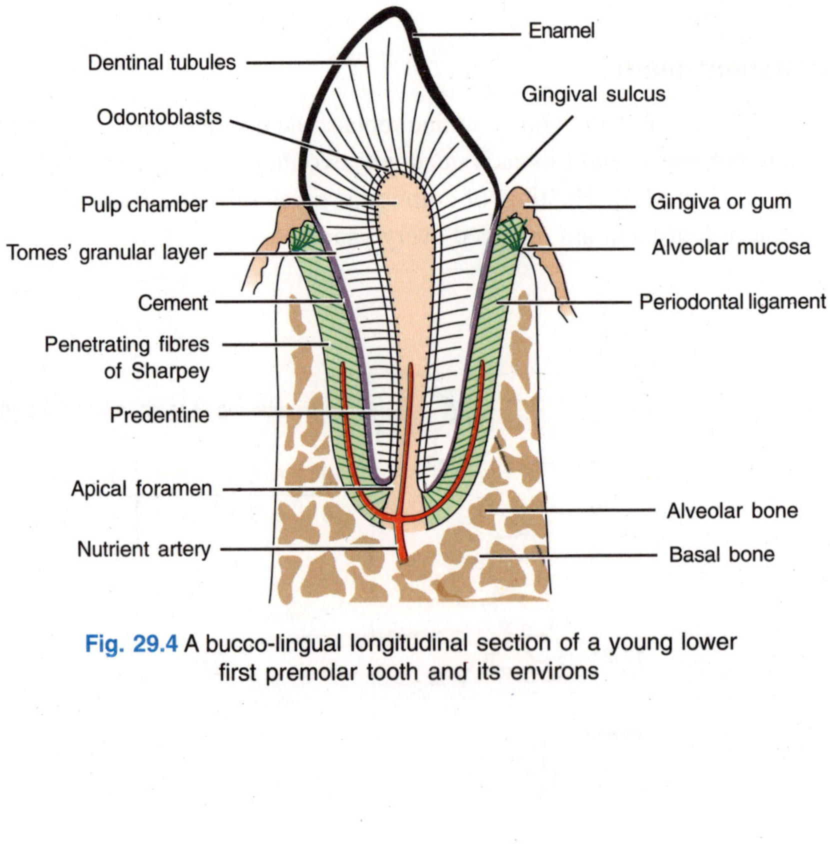

Fig. 29.4 A bucco-lingual longitudinal section of a young lower first premolar tooth and its environs

The Ear

Chapter 30

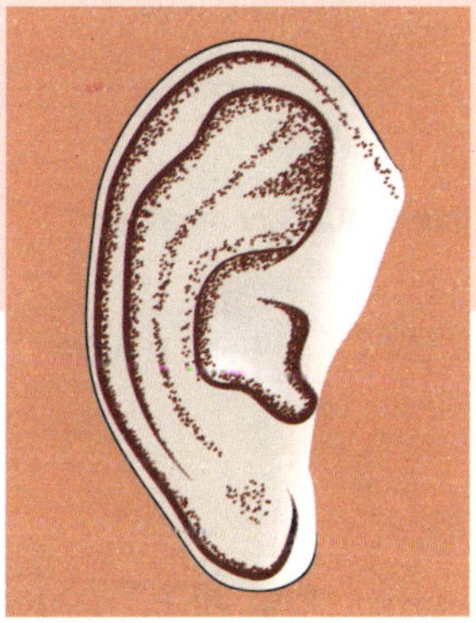

30.1 Topographic overview of the vestibulo-cochlear apparatus located within the right temporal bone

The scheme shows the parts of the right auditory apparatus as if viewed through a semi-transparent temporal bone. The tympanic cavity is bounded laterally by the tympanic membrane; medially by the lateral wall of the internal ear; it communicates posteriorly with the tympanic antrum and through it with the mastoid air cells, and anteriorly with the auditory tube.

30.2 The features of the right auricle

The external ear consists of the auricle or pinna, and the external acoustic meatus. The lateral surface of the auricle, as shown here, is irregularly concave, looks slightly anteriorly, and presents numerous eminences and depressions.

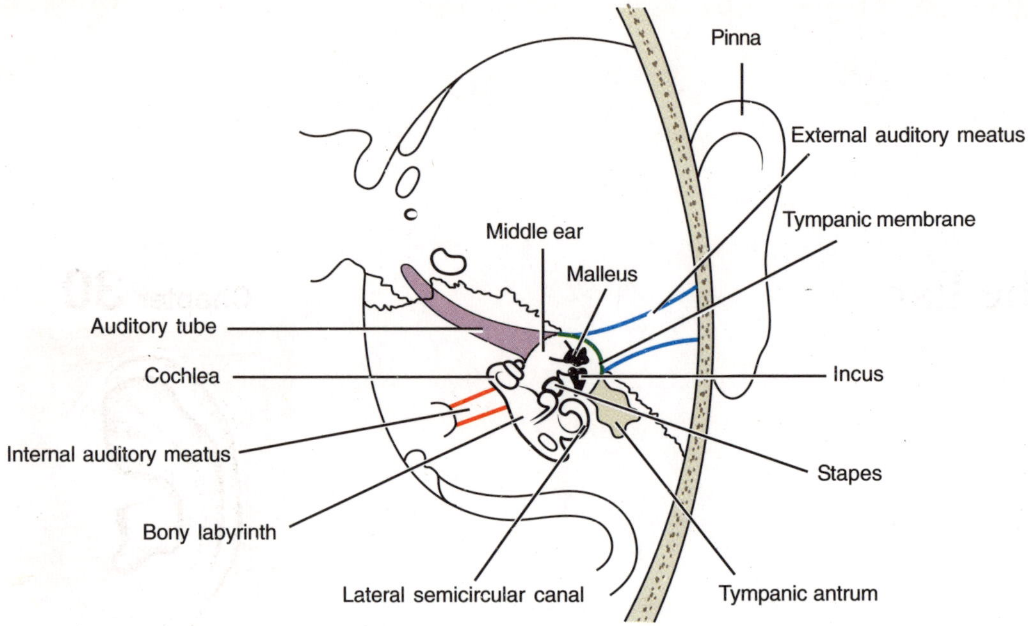

Fig. 30.1 Topographic overview of the vestibulo-cochlear apparatus located within the right temporal bone

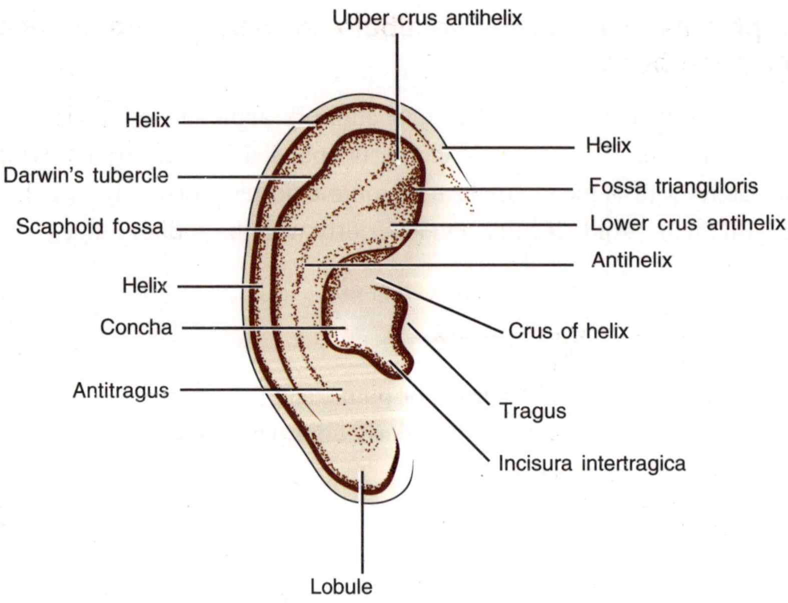

Fig. 30.2 The features of the right auricle

30.3 The ossicles of the right ear—viewed from lateral aspect

The various processes and articulations are depicted in the diagram.

The tympanic cavity contains a chain of three movable ossicles. The malleus is attached to the tympanic membrane and the base of stapes to the circumference of the fenestra vestibuli, while the incus is placed between and articulates with both malleus and stapes.

The lower end of the long process of incus bends medially and terminates in a rounded projection, the lenticular process, the medial surface of which is covered with cartilage, and articulates with the head of the stapes which is directed laterally and has a small cartilage covered depression. The base of stapes is fixed to the margin of the fenestra vestibuli by the annular ligament.

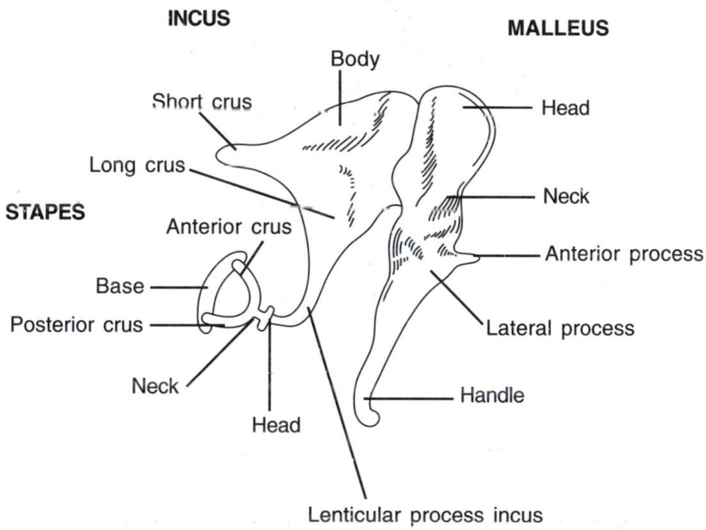

Fig. 30.3 The ossicles of the right ear—Viewed from lateral aspect

30.4 The right tympanic membrane as it appears through an otoscope

The quadrants are indicated in the figure. The quadrants are determined by a line through the handle of malleus and another line at right angles to this. These lines are not perpendicular and horizontal due to slant of the handle.

The cone of light is a reflection of light from the membrane.

The head of malleus is situated within the epitympanic recess. The handle is connected by its lateral margin with the tympanic membrane. The lateral process is attached to the upper part of the tympanic membrane and by means of the anterior and posterior malleolar folds to the extremities of the notch at the upper part of the tympanic sulcus.

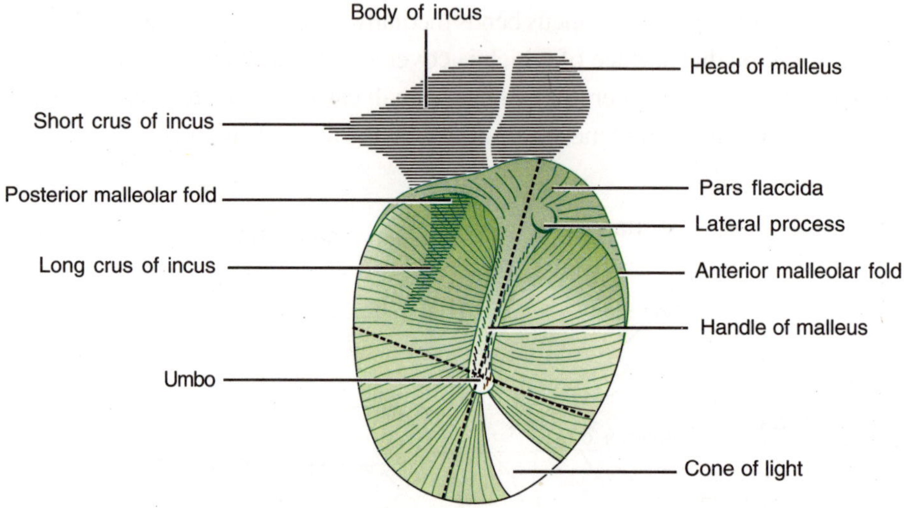

Fig. 30.4 The right tympanic membrane as it appears through an otoscope

30.5 The lateral end (fundus) of the right internal acoustic meatus

It is shown abutting on the medial wall of the vestibule and the base of the modiolus.

The facial nerve passes laterally with the eighth nerve into the internal acoustic meatus, surrounded by a sheath of meninges. Here the nerves intermedius joins the seventh nerve which pierces the meninges at the lateral end of the internal acoustic meatus to enter the facial canal.

The vestibulo-cochlear nerve consists of a superior (vestibular) root and an inferior (cochlear) root. These unite to form the vestibulo-cochlear nerve which passes into the internal acoustic meatus inferior to the facial nerve and nerves intermedius. Near the funds of the meatus, two or more vestibular ganglia appear. Distal to the ganglia, the vestibular part divides into superior and inferior parts, the inferior part lying with the cochlear part. The superior part pierces the superior vestibular area in the fundus of the meatus.

The cochlear nerve enters through the tractus spiralis foraminosus.

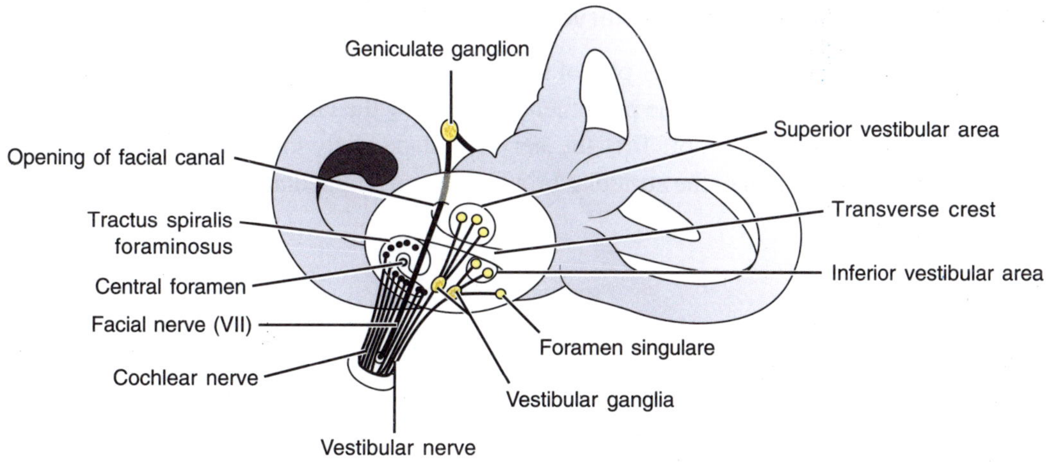

Fig. 30.5 The lateral end (fundus) of the right internal acoustic meatus

30.6 Intrapetrous course of facial nerve

The facial nerve continues laterally in the bony facial canal lying above and between the cochlea and vestibule. At the hiatus for greater petrosal nerve, the facial nerve is enlarged by the sensory ganglion (geniculate) and gives off (i) the greater petrosal nerve, (ii) a branch to the tympanic plexus and (iii) a branch to the sympathetic plexus on the middle meningeal artery. The facial nerve then turns abruptly backwards in the bone of the upper part of middle ear cavity.

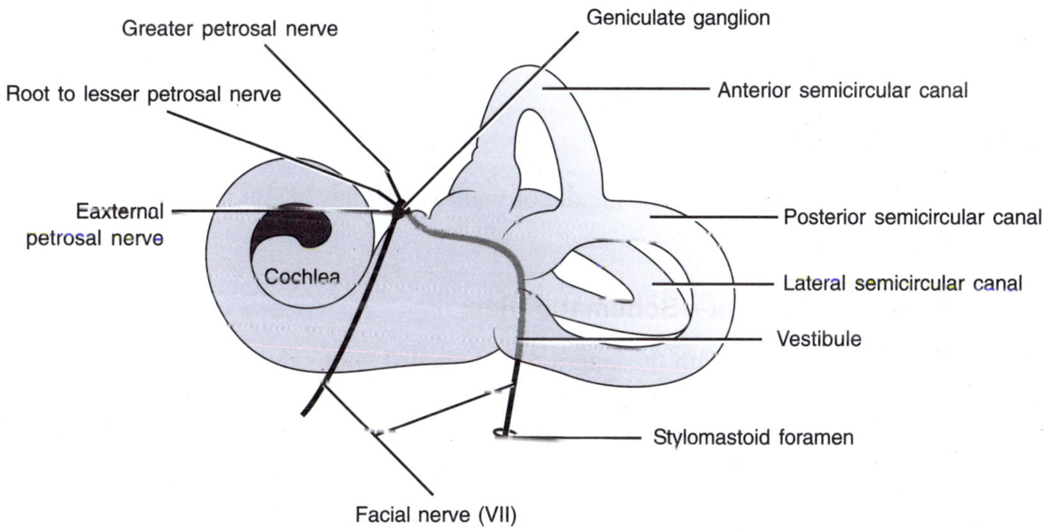

Fig. 30.6 Intrapetrous course of facial nerve

30.7 Intrapetrous course of facial nerve *(Contd.)*

The facial nerve bends in the upper part of the medial wall of the middle ear cavity, superior to fenestra vestibuli and then inferior to the prominence caused by the lateral semicircular canal. It then turns vertically downwards giving off first the nerve to stapendius, then the chorda tympani and finally a communicating branch to the auricular branch of vagus immediately before it emerges from the stylomastoid foramen.

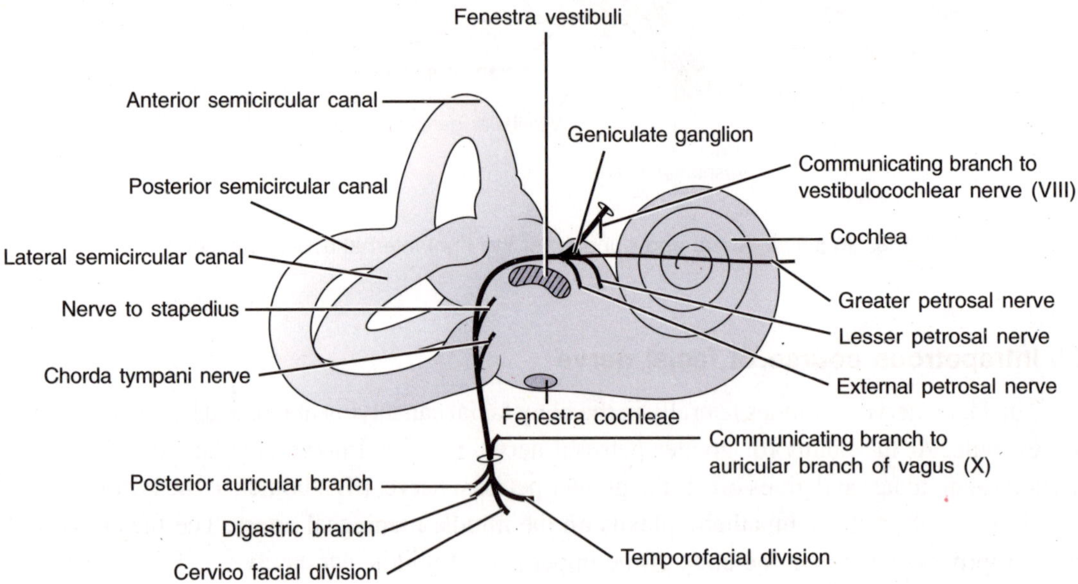

Fig. 30.7 Intrapetrous course of facial nerve

30.8 The chorda tympani

It crosses the medial aspect of the handle of malleus and lies lateral to incus.

30.9 The right middle ear—Schematic view

Interpreted here as a box with the anterior wall opened out to show the internal features.

Lateral or membranous wall has the tympanic membrane. The handle and the lateral process of malleus are embedded in the fibrous layer of the membrane, whereas the head lies above the tympanic membrane. The body and short crus of incus also lie above the tympanic membrane. The long crus lies parallel to and behind the handle of malleus.

Roof or tegmental wall is formed by tegmen tympani of petrous temporal bone and intervenes between the middle ear and the middle cranial fossa.

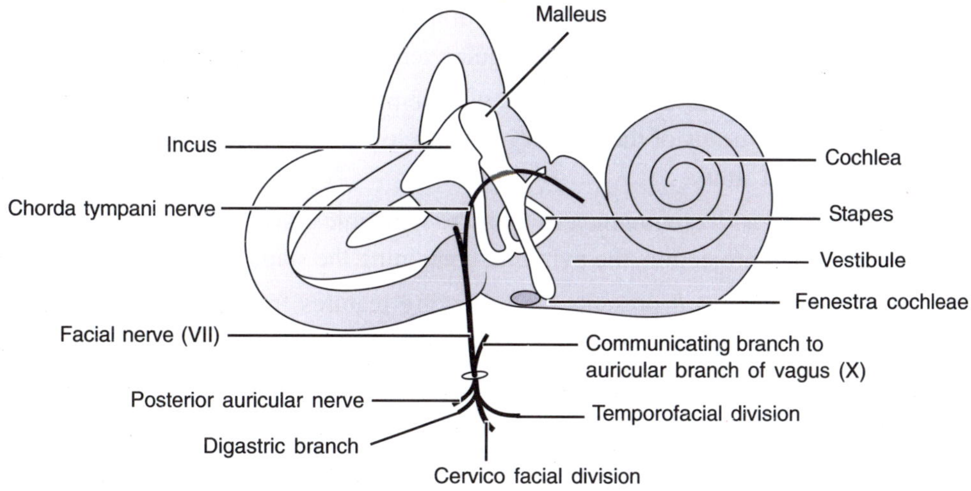

Fig. 30.8 The chorda tympani

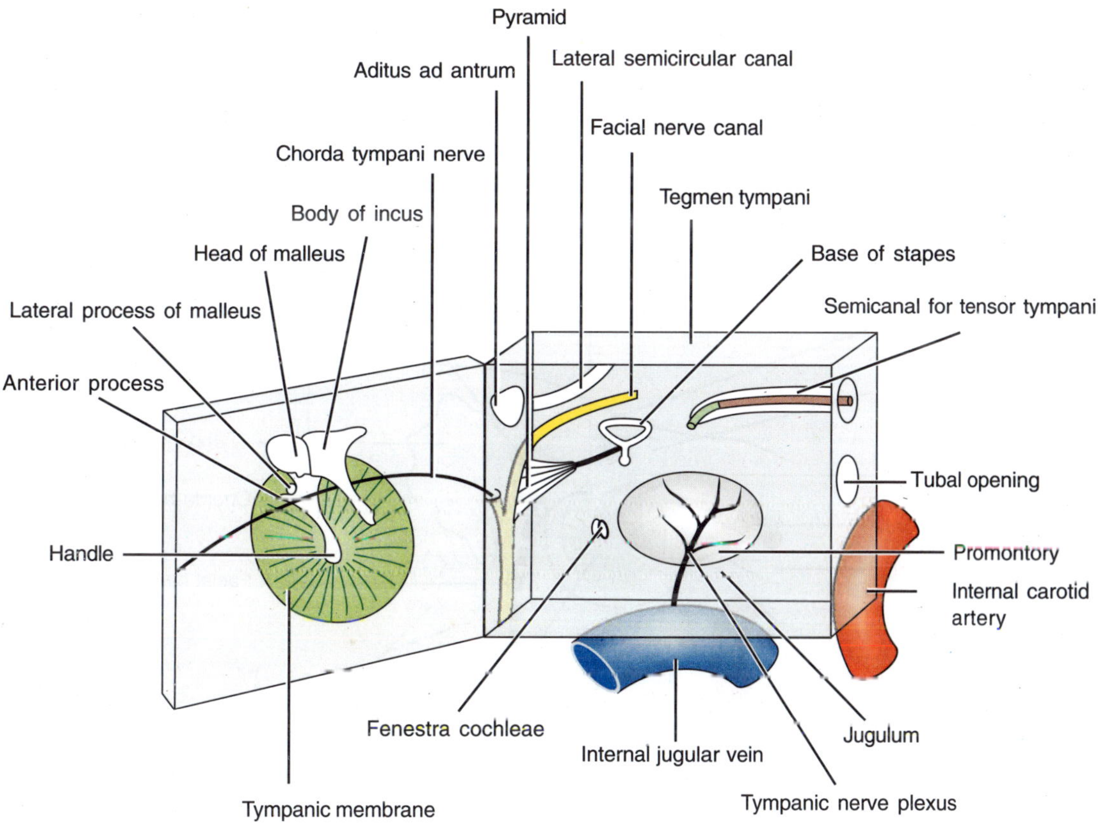

Fig. 30.9 The right middle ear—Schematic view

Floor or jugular wall is formed by jugulum, a thin plate of bone separating it from the jugular fossa which lodges the superior bulb of internal jugular vein.

Anterior or carotid wall has communication with semicanal for tensor tympani muscle above and nasopharynx below by means of the auditory tube. Below the tubal opening is the carotid canal lodging the internal carotid artery.

Posterior or mastoid wall communicates with the tympanic antrum through aditus ad antrum. Below the aditus is a small projection, the pyramid, containing the stapedius muscle.

Medial or labyr inthine wall presents the following features from above downwards:

(i) The prominence of the lateral semicircular canal; (ii) the prominence of the facial nerve canal; (iii) the fenestra vestibuli (oval window); closed by the base of the stapes; (iv) the processus cochleariformis, a bony prominence above the window (v) the promontory, formed by the basal turn of the cochlea and covered by tympanic plexus; and (vi) the fenestra cochleae (round window) covered by the mucous membrane of the middle ear.

30.10 and 30.11 Right tympanic cavity split longitudinally into lateral and medial parts

Note that the lateral wall of the cavity is dominated by the tympanic membrane, malleus, and chorda tympani nerve. The medial wall has a broad bulging, the promontory and the other features already described in Figures 30.10 and 30.11.

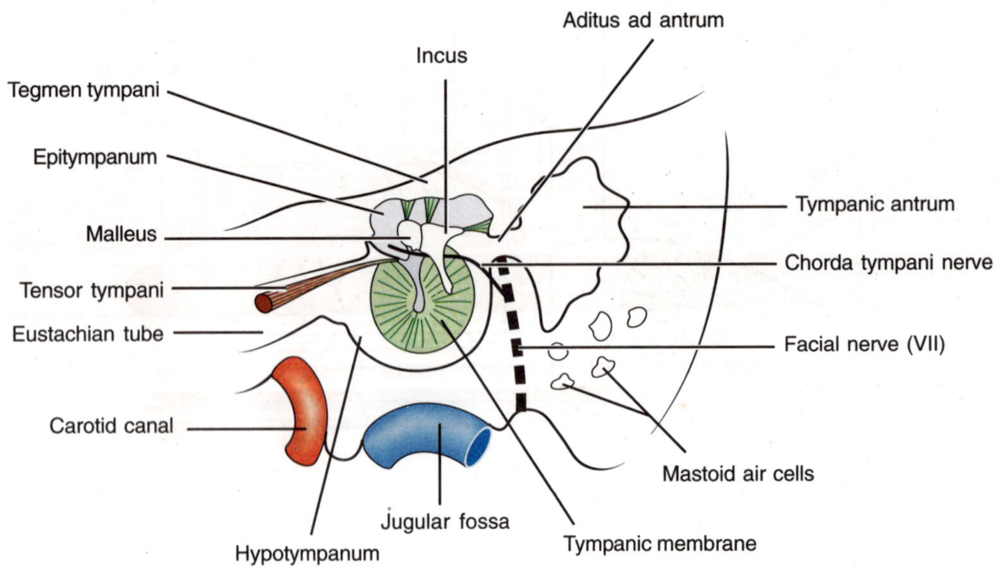

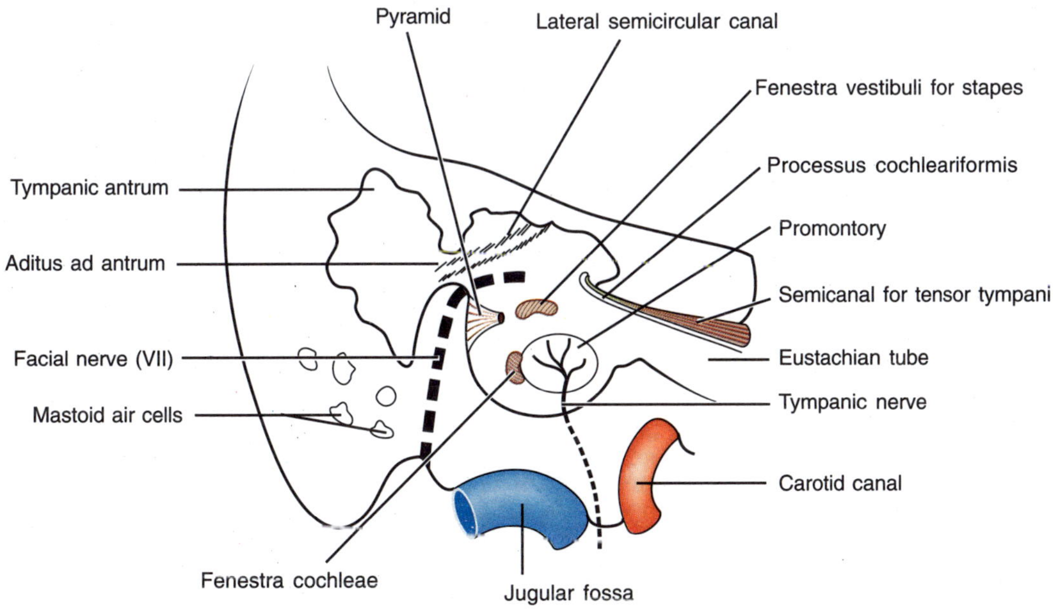

Figs 30.10 and 30.11 Right tympanic cavity split longitudinally into lateral and medial parts

30.12 Coronal section through the right temporal bone seen from infrontic

It shows the internal features of the posterior wall of middle ear cavity.

Note from above downwards the following openings: (i) aditus ad antrum, leading into mastoid antrum, (ii) perforation on the summit of pyramid for the canal of stapedius, (iii) opening through which the chorda tympani nerve enters the tympanum, situated lateral to pyramid.

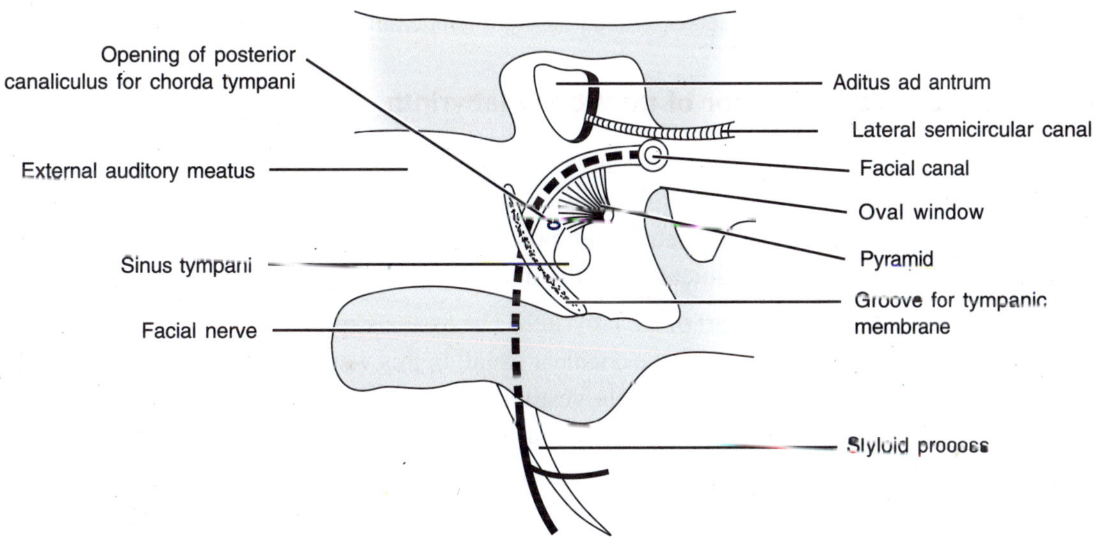

Fig. 30.12 Coronal section through the right temporal bone seen from infrontic

30.13 Coronal section through the right temporal bone seen from behind

It shows the internal features of the anterior wall of middle ear.

Note from above downwards: (i) The opening of the tensor tympani canal, (ii) the orifice of the pharyngo-tympanic tube and (iii) the lamina of bone separating the tympanic cavity from the carotid canal.

The processus cochleariformis is a shelf-like septum between the tube and tensor tympani canal prolonged backwards on the medial wall. The chorda tympani nerve leaves the tympanic cavity through the anterior canaliculus for chorda which is placed at the medial end of the petrotympanic fissure.

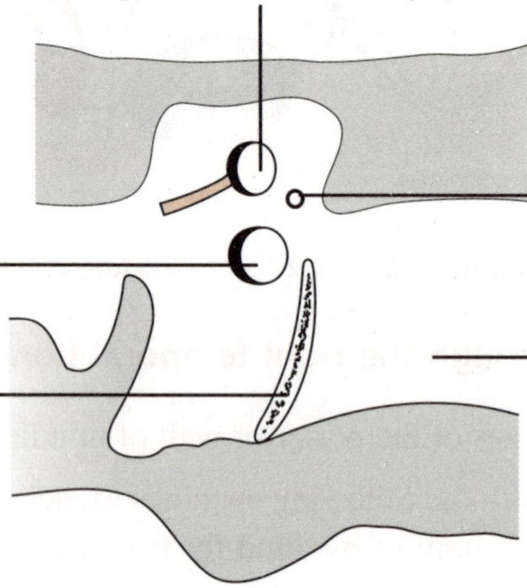

Fig. 30.13 Coronal section through the right temporal bone seen from behind

30.14 Lateral view of interior of right bony labyrinth

The vestibule is the central part of the labyrinth. On its medial wall, a small opening leads into the aqueduct of the vestibule, a tubular extension which leads downwards and backwards and opens on the posterior surface of the petruos temporal. Above and in front of the orifice are groups of minute foramina which communicate with the internal acoustic meatus.

The cochlea is the anterior part of the labyrinth. The osseous spiral lamina is a thin bony shelf which projects from the modiolus into the cochlear canal. In this way the cochlear canal is divided into an apical compartment called the scala vestibili and a basal compartment called the scala vestibuli opens directly into the vestibule. The basal part of scala tympani is shut off from the vestibular cavity and ends at the fenestra cochleae which opens into the tympanic cavity and in the natural state is closed by the secondary tympanic membrane. In the basal wall of the scala tympani, just beyond the fenestra cochleae, is the small orifice of the aqueduct of the cochlea.

The semicircular canals are posterior to the vestibule and open into it.

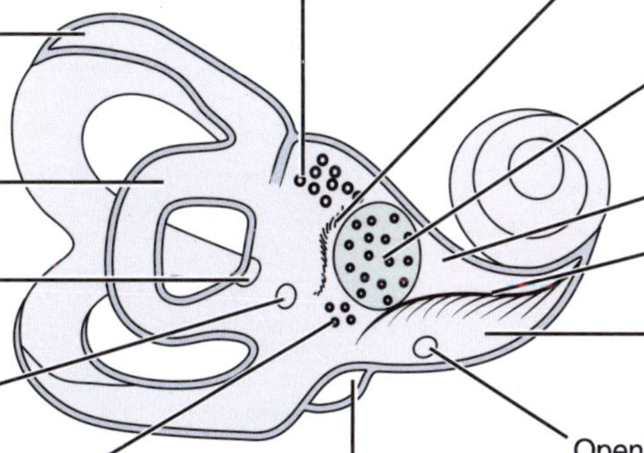

Fig. 30.14 Lateral view of interior of right bony labyrinth

30.15 The distribution of the vestibulo-cochlear nerve to the membranous labyrinth

The superior vestibular part of the vestibular nerve supplies the utricle (utricular nerve), the ampullae of the anterior (superior) and lateral semicircular canal (anterior and lateral ampullary nerves) through the superior vestibular area.

The branches of the inferior vestibular part supply the saccule through the inferior vestibular area and the ampulla of posterior semicircular canal through the foraman singulare (posterior ampullary nerve). The cochlear nerve passes through the tractus spiralis for aminosus as a series of fine bundles which enter the modiolus.

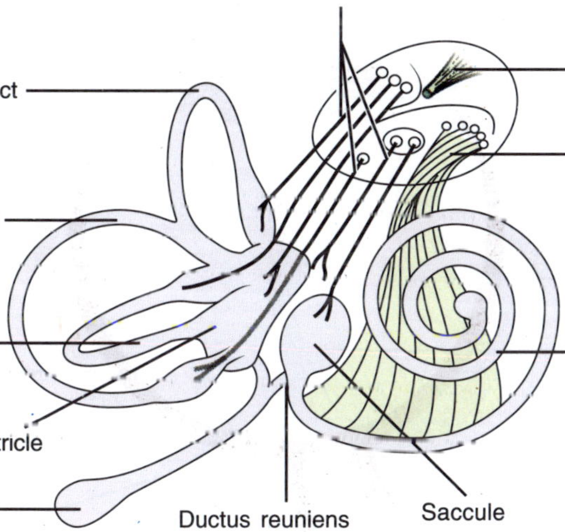

Fig. 30.15 The distribution of the vestibulo-cochlear nerve to the membranous labyrinth

The Eyeball

Chapter 31

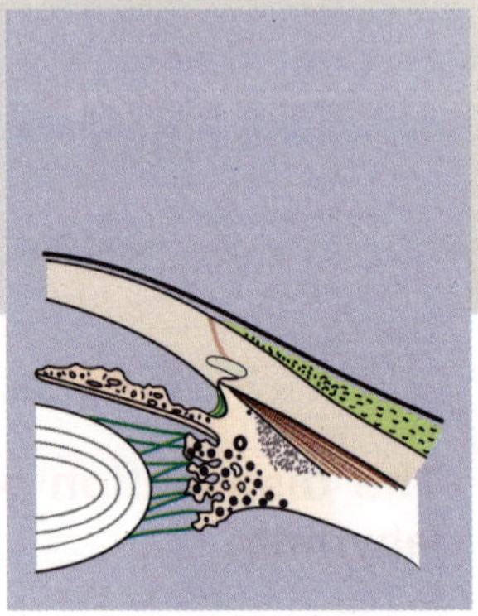

31.1 Horizontal section through the eyeball

Sclera, choroid and retina are the three coats of the eyeball. Cornea is the anterior transparent one-sixth of the sclera. Choroid lines the sclera upto sclero-corneal junction where it is called the

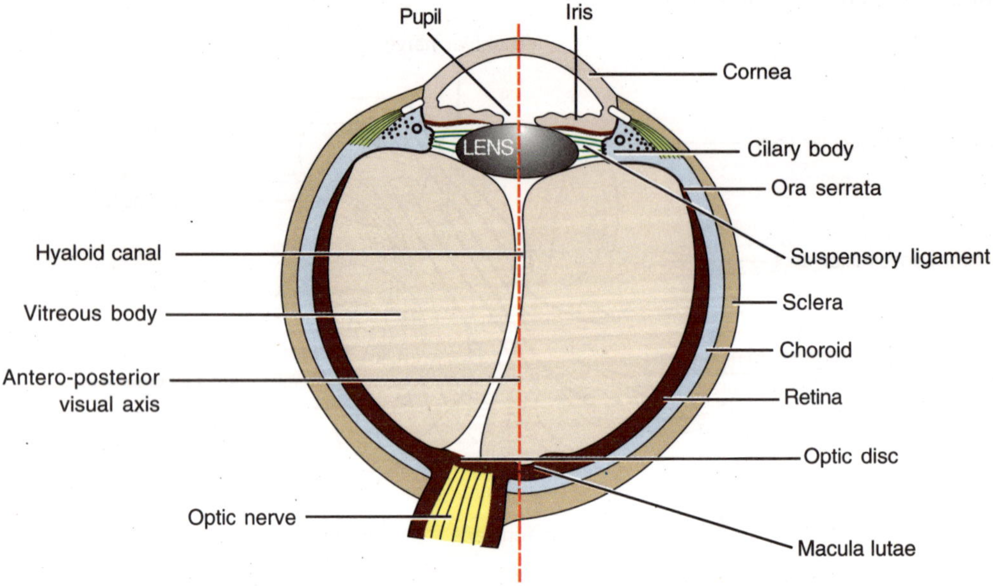

Fig. 31.1 Horizontal Section through the eyeball

ciliary body which becomes the iris more anteriorly. The suspensory ligament of the lens is attached to the posterior surface of the ciliary body. Retina is the innermost coat.

The optic disc (blind spot) is the region where the fibres of the optic nerve converge. About 3 mm lateral to it is a small yellowish area (macula lutea) with a central depressed area (Fovea centralis) where vision is most acute.

31.2 The sclero-corneal junction

Sinus venosus sclerae is a circular space on the inner aspect of the junction. The iris and ciliary body are attached to the scleral spur which is formed by the scleral edge projecting forwards where it is continuous with the cornea. The pectinate ligament connects the iris with the cornea at the irido-corneal angle.

On sagittal section the ciliary body is triangular. The outer part of its anterior side enters into the formation of the angle of anterior chamber. From about its middle part the iris takes origin, and with the remaining part of the anterior surface forms an acute angle which opens in the posterior chamber. The outer side of the triangle corresponds to the ciliary muscle, and lies against the sclera. The outermost fibres (Brucke's muscle) run antero-posteriorly while the inner fibres (Muller's muscle) run circularly. The inner side corresponds to the ciliary processes to which the suspensory ligament is attached.

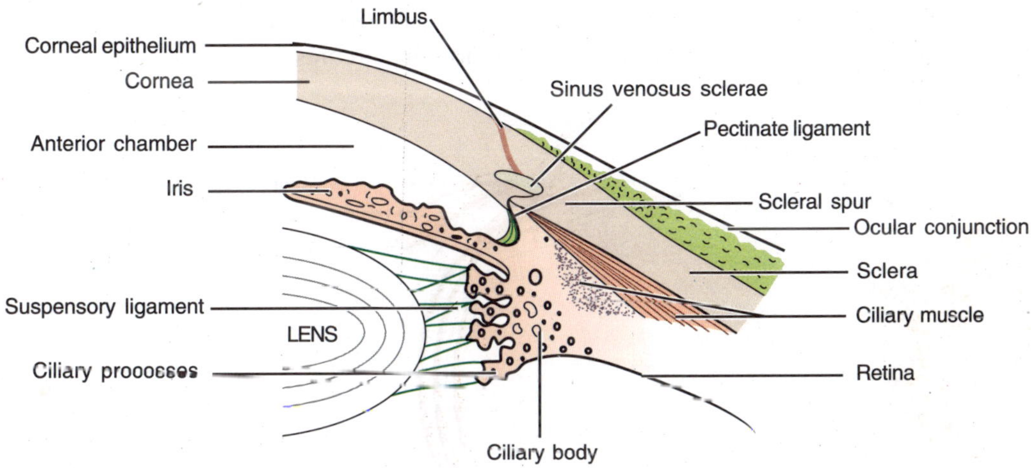

Fig. 31.2 The Sclero-corneal junction

31.3 Anterior half of the eyeball seen from behind

The vitreous body and half of the lens have been removed in the diagram. The ciliary body starts at the ora-serrata. The part beyond ora-serrata is smooth and is known as pars plana or orbicularis ciliaris. Further forwards the inner surface presents radiating ridges of various sizes—the ciliary processes to which are attached the fibres of suspensory ligament.

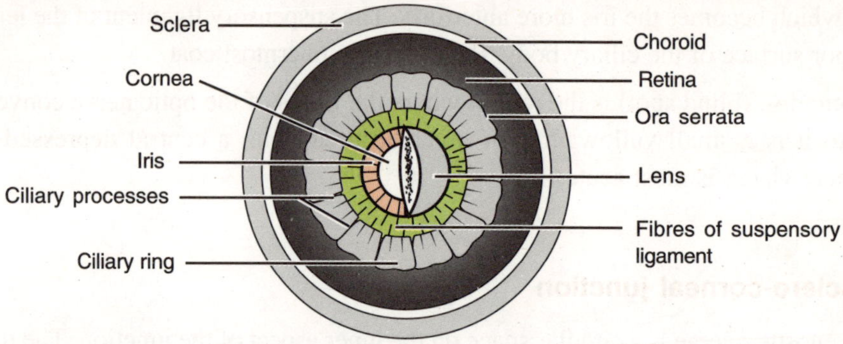

Fig. 31.3 Anterior half of the eyeball seen from behind

31.4 The ciliary arteries

The posterior ciliary arteries divide into 10–20 branches and pierce the sclera and supply the choroid.

The two long posterior ciliary arteries pass through the sclera in a canal. Without giving branches they reach the ciliary muscle, where they divide into two branches which enter the substance of the muscle at its anterior end, anastomose with each other and with the anterior ciliary arteries to from the circulus iridis major.

The anterior ciliary arteries are derived from the arteries to the four recti from whose tendons they emerge. They pass anteriorly from the sclero-corneal junction to enter the ciliary muscle. They anastomose with the long posterior ciliary arteries to form the circulus iridis major.

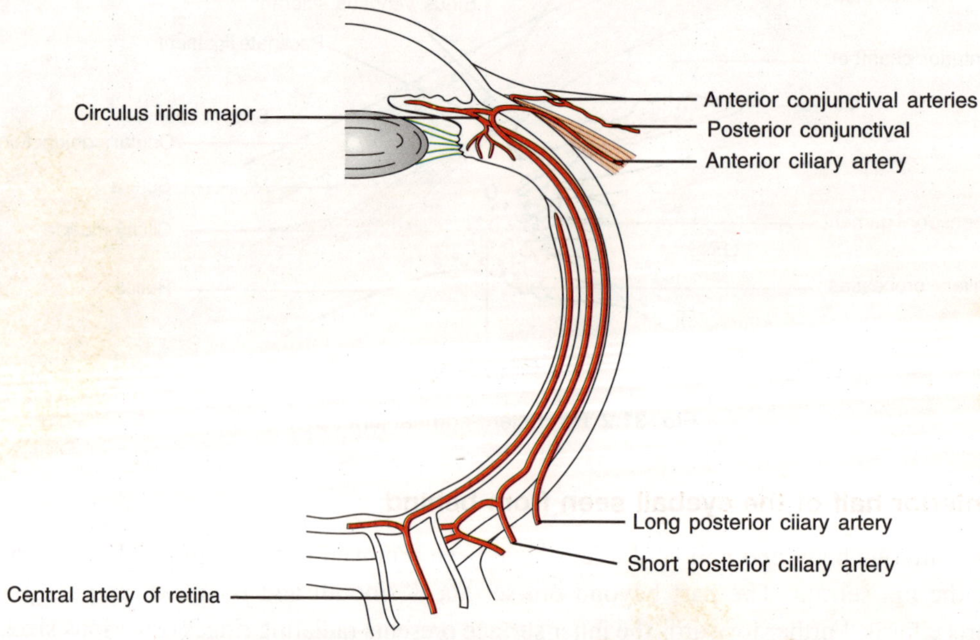

Fig. 31.4 The ciliary arteries

Index

A

B

C

D

M

V

W